THIRD EDITION

Successful Test-Taking

Learning Strategies for Nurses

Marian B. Sides, RN, PhD
President, Education Enterprises, Inc.
Colonel, USAFR. NC. Office of the Surgeon
   General, Air Staff, Pentagon
Washington, DC

Nancy Korchek, RN, MSN
Associate Professor of Nursing
Purdue University Calumet
Hammond, Indiana

With 12 Contributors

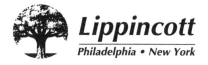

Lippincott
Philadelphia • New York

Acquisitions Editor: Susan M. Glover, RN, MSN
Coordinating Editorial Assistant: Bridget Blatteau
Project Editor: Jahmae Harris
Senior Production Manager: Helen Ewan
Production Coordinator: Mike Carcel
Design Coordinator: Doug Smock
Cover images copyright 1997 PhotoDisc, Inc.

Third Edition

Library of Congress Cataloging in Publications Data

Sides, Marian B., 1940–
    Successful test-taking : learning strategies for nurses / Marian
B. Sides, Nancy Korchek ; with 12 contributors.—3rd ed.
        p.   cm.
    Rev. ed. of: Nurse's guide to successful test-taking. 2nd ed.
©1994.
    Includes bibliographical references and index.
    ISBN 0-7817-9202-9 (alk. paper)
    1. Nursing—Examinations.   2. Nursing.   3. Nursing—Examinations,
questions, etc.   4. Reasoning (Psychology)—Problems, exercises,
etc. I. Korchek, Nancy.   II. Sides, Marian B., 1940–   Nurse's
guide to successful test-taking.   III. Title.
    [DNLM: 1. Nursing—examination questions.   2. Problem Solving—
nurses' instruction.   3. Learning—nurses' instruction.
4. Educational Measurement—nurses' instruction.   WY 18.2 S568s
1998]
RT55.S48   1998
610.73'076—dc21
DNLM/DLC
for Library of Congress   97–42752
                                                                              CIP

Care has been taken to confirm the accuracy of the information presented and to describe generally accepted practices. However, the authors, editors, and publisher are not responsible for errors or omissions or for any consequences from application of the information in this book and make no warranty, express or implied, with respect to the contents of the publication.

The authors, editors and publisher have exerted every effort to ensure that drug selection and dosage set forth in this text are in accordance with current recommendations and practice at the time of publication. However, in view of ongoing research, changes in government regulations, and the constant flow of information relating to drug therapy and drug reactions, the reader is urged to check the package insert for each drug for any change in indications and dosage and for added warnings and precautions. This is particularly important when the recommended agent is a new or infrequently employed drug.

Some drugs and medical devices presented in this publication have Food and Drug Administration (FDA) clearance for limited use in restricted research settings. It is the responsibility of the health care provider to ascertain the FDA status of each drug or device planned for use in their clinical practice.

9   8   7   6   5   4

To my Mom, Evelyn, and my Dad, Daniel,
in recognition of their constant support, interest, and encouragement
MARIAN B. SIDES

For Dennis, who has taught me much,
and for our children, from whom I have learned even more
NANCY KORCHEK

Reviewers

Michele C. Larger, RN, MS
Lecturer
School of Nursing
Indiana University
Richmond, Indiana

Arlene M. McMahon, RN, MSN
Instructor
Temple University
Philadelphia, Pennsylvania

Staff Nurse
Labor and Delivery Unit
Holy Redeemer Hospital
Meadowbrook, Pennsylvania

Contributors

Diane Black, RN, MS
Instructor
Medical Surgical Nursing
South Suburban College
South Holland, Illinois

Bette Case, RN,C, PhD
Consultant
Education for Healthcare
Chicago, Illinois

Ann Sheerer Filipski, RN, MSN, Psy D, CS
Associate Professor
Psychiatric and Mental Health Nursing
School of Nursing
Saint Xavier University
Chicago, Illinois

Patricia Chabot Hughes, RN, MSN
Lecturer/Clinical Instructor
University of Wisconsin–Milwaukee
Milwaukee, Wisconsin

Deborah Crain Kark, RN, CS, MS
Associate Professor of Nursing
Purdue University Calumet
Hammond, Indiana

Kathleen Ann Kick, RN,C, MS
Assistant Professor of Nursing
Purdue University Calumet
Hammond, Indiana

Cynthia A. Levy, RN,C, MSN
Clinical Nurse Specialist, NICU
St. Louis Children's Hospital
St. Louis, Missouri

Barbara Etling Murphy, RN, MSN
Program Manager
Perinatal Outreach Program
Stanford University
Palo Alto, California

Wayne Nagel, RN, MSN
Senior Instructor
Division of Nursing and Wellness
Palm Beach Community College
Lake Worth, Florida

Marytherese Patras, RN, MS, JD
Flight Nurse
Emergency Medicine
University of Chicago Hospitals
Chicago, Illinois

Leslie Rittenmeyer, RN, MS
Associate Professor of Nursing
Purdue University Calumet
Hammond, Indiana

Marry L. Williams, RN, BSN, SRNA
Student Nurse Anesthetist
Frank J. Tornetta School of Anesthesia
Saint Joseph's University
Norristown, Pennsylvania

1 LT
USAF, NC
Flight Nurse

Acknowledgments

The need to perpetuate thinking as the foundation for teaching and learning has fueled the formation of this third edition. Over the past four years, contributing authors have worked diligently in refining the approach to principle-centered thinking. The Education Enterprises, Inc. State Board Review has served as a powerful vehicle to field test our team approach to concept-based teaching and testing. Special recognition goes to the contributing authors of this manuscript and the faculty of the State Board Review: Diane Black, Ann Filipski, the late Karen Gousman, Patti Hughes, Kimberly Jezek-Tisch, Deborah Kark, Kathleen Kick, Nancy Korchek, Cynthia Levy, Wayne Nagel, Lori Pacura, Marytherese Patras, Leslie Rittenmeyer, Scott Sabish, Marry Williams, and Brenda Wolfe.

Many students and graduate nurses throughout the country have influenced the development of this third edition. Their unique dialogue, critical inquiry, and exploration of personal test-taking challenges have nourished the thinking in this volume. We thank them for their special contributions.

Nancy Korchek has served as the cornerstone for item writing and quality control of reasoning exercises throughout this book. A special recognition goes to Nancy for her efforts in constructing and updating items and ensuring the cohesiveness and structural integrity of test items in this volume.

A special thank you is owed to medical illustrator, Thomas L. Ingram, whose creative and skillful work adds character, spirit, and compelling humor to the powerful messages in this book.

I wish to acknowledge the wisdom and inspiration of Benjamin S. Bloom, Distinguished Service, Professor Emeritus, and mentor during my doctoral studies at the University of Chicago. His powerful teachings in the taxonomy of thinking and learning continue to influence critical thinking, problem solving, and decision making among nurses.

Lastly, I wish to extend a special appreciation to our editors, Susan M. Glover and Bridget Blatteau of Lippincott–Raven Publishers, for their support, encouragement, and guidance in the preparation of this edition.

Marian B. Sides, RN, PhD

Preface

we must not forget that
the beauty of a learned
person is
not that one's learned
but. . . . .
that one knows how
to learn!!!
Marian B. Sides

This inspirational quotation carries a powerful message to all new professionals and practicing nurses. It stresses the importance of learning as a process rather than as a product.

Through years of work with new graduates, my colleagues and I have learned that nurses find solace and comfort in clinging to facts and value concrete information as key to their future success. The practice of nursing today calls for greater sophistication in the process of critical thinking and problem-solving with less emphasis on memorization and regurgitation of facts. Likewise, the use of lecture as a vehicle for imparting information, traditionally the most common form of knowledge dissemination, must give way to more diverse and sophisticated forms of inquiry and intellectual exercises. Such reform, in shaping the minds of new professionals, will enable them to grasp key concepts and apply selected principles to the practice of nursing.

This book is written for anyone who wishes to refine his or her approach to teaching and learning. Part I focuses on patterns of learning and provides strategies to guide the mental skill development for lower level and higher level learning. Concepts include the nursing process as a decision-making model, strategies of test-taking, and personalities of test takers. A positive mental attitude is stressed as a key to success. Part II presents a concise and simple model to 20 fundamental concepts that are essential for health. Chapters on critical thinking, comfort, and child's health add special dimensions to this edition. These concepts form the foundation for nursing practice. A special feature of Part II is its simplicity and the easy manner in which it portrays the core concepts that shape wellness and balance in humans. Sometimes we tend to make learning so complex that we overlook the basic principles that shape health and its deviations. These principles are presented and illustrated in health and illness patterns. Test questions in the form of reasoning exercises follow each chapter. Based on clinical situations, these exercises challenge the nurse's use of the nursing process and levels of thinking in problem-solving and managing patient care. The rest of Part II consists of a series of specifically designed comprehensive test items to provide opportunities for the practice and refinement of decision-making and test-taking skill. In addition, this part contains rationales for the reasoning exercises.

This book is designed to bring pleasure to learning and to help new professionals meet the challenge that lies ahead.

Marian B. Sides, RN, PhD

Introduction

Since the first edition of **Nurse's Guide to Successful Test-Taking** appeared in 1989, this book, now titled, **Successful Test-Taking: Learning Strategies for Nurses,** has evolved consistent with nursing practice and nursing education. Now in its third edition, the authors frame this book as a reference not only for test-taking, but also for organizing knowledge and information. Because information is burgeoning exponentially in our current age of information, students and practitioners need to create organizational schema to store information for later use. The authors present nursing in a format that facilitates organizing knowledge and also facilitates practicing critical thinking. The questions, reasoning exercises and analyses stimulate practice of critical thinking strategies. Competent practice involves questions: posing questions, questioning assumptions and responding to questions of other colleagues, patients and their families. Nurses apply their skills with questions, answers and analyses far beyond the situations in which they take tests to earn grades, licensure, and certification or other credentials.

New graduates received the previous editions with enthusiasm. Nurse educators in schools and in health care agencies welcomed the valuable resource they found. New graduates thanked the authors for the edge of self-confidence they gained by using the book to prepare for NCLEX-RN. But before and beyond NCLEX-RN, students and nurses found the approach of the book helpful in organizing knowledge, sharpening critical thinking skills, preparing for other examinations and using knowledge in practice.

A number of books currently in print assist the new graduate with the task of preparing for the RN licensing examination. The authors of this book set their book apart by personalizing to the reader and by orienting the assistance they offer toward process and action. Part I, "Patterns of Learning," does more than simply survey cognitive strategies. Part I models concept formation, effective critical thinking, and self-assessment. More importantly, in Part I the reader finds a guide to action. Part I guides both toward test-taking success and toward success with the professional commitment of lifelong learning.

Even the inspirational message of Chapter 1 takes the form of the model for the use of ideas: concept, principle, illustration of the principle. The principles for building a successful attitude reside not only in Chapter 1, but function implicitly throughout the chapters which follow. The reader begins to experience control, freedom, and enhanced self-esteem through mastery of concepts and strategies.

Readers of previous editions have expressed growth in self-confidence after studying chapters one through six.

Self-awareness develops as the reader compares personal characteristics with the Test-Taking Personality typologies presented, and later tracks errors and corrects deficiencies in response to reasoning exercises. Imagery stimuli appear both for the test-taking situation and for nursing practice situations. The action impetus moves from general to specific, from attacking the problem of organizing knowledge, to employing alternative test-taking techniques for answering test items that represent different levels of learning. The methodology for organizing knowledge serves learners well whether they are building their knowledge bases as students, preparing for examinations, or organizing knowledge for application as practicing nurses.

Previous editions of this book greatly benefited NCLEX candidates as they faced the important challenge of the licensing examination. Everyone who has the privilege of exposure to this energetic group of beginning practitioners knows that these individuals want to be where the action is and feel ready to begin to assert control over their professional careers. The new graduate feels impatient to get out of the seat in the classroom and into the full-time practice of nursing. This book appeals to the new graduate by addressing the need to put learning to use. Of course the reader needs to read and study the book in the conventional fashion (i.e. sitting down), but the chapters demonstrate consistently how to put knowledge into action.

The action orientation evolves further in the present edition, incorporating care planning and extensive cross-referencing to provide the practicing nurse with a user-friendly reference.

The format of the book models the process it teaches. The authors stress the learner's need to organize well and then display well-organized, carefully constructed tables throughout the book. The conversational style helps concepts, principles, and nursing process to come alive. The language effectively addresses this time of transition from the academic setting to the world of nursing practice. The reader benefits from plenty of diagnostic feedback through reasoning exercises imbedded in the text as well as those assembled as practice tests in a separate section.

Nursing curricula prime their graduates to receive information about synthesizing knowledge for action and applying test-taking techniques based on levels of learning. This book builds upon readers' experiences in synthesizing and applying knowledge and in taking examinations to formulate strategies for success—success in test-taking and in lifelong learning.

The authors reveal their experience in teaching nursing and test-taking in the personalized approach they have taken. They show respect for their reader as an individual who brings knowledge and experience to the task of test preparation. They provide a readable text, complete with inspiring thoughts, memory jogs, and characterizations of Test Taking Personalities.

Readers have reported that by taking a conceptual approach and simplifying complex concepts, the book greatly facilitated their understanding. Some experienced "ah-has" such as decoding the elusive mysteries of the acid-base balance for the first time. Others found the medications information and math for meds especially useful. Readers have indicated that the approach used to present nursing process enhanced their skills in using nursing process as a problem-solving tool.

The nurse educator, whether primarily responsible for educating basic students or for facilitating professional development and continuing education with practicing nurses will find this book to be an important resource. The keystones for building a successful attitude (Chapter 1) apply to many educational and career goals toward which nurse educators assist students and nurses—goals both before and beyond success with the licensing examination.

Learners can use the strategies and techniques for test-taking throughout the nursing curriculum to help sharpen their thinking and discriminating skills as well as to improve their performance on multiple-choice tests. The "Pattern of Learning" information contained in Part I offers valuable assistance in preparing learners for examinations, in interpreting examination results with learners and discussing particular test items.

Nurse educators who develop and present review sessions for certification examinations will find applications not only for the test-taking strategies suggested, but also for the approach modeled in the text. One reader, pleased with the assistance he received in preparing for NCLEX-RN, used the book effectively to prepare for the ACLS examination.

The book provides satisfying reading for the nurse educator because it emphasizes levels of learning, developing concepts, applying knowledge and thinking critically. Nurse educators can employ the sophisticated analysis of errant responses, diagnosis, and remediation for learning errors in individual or group conferences in which they explore alternative choices of nursing action in clinical situations.

Successful Test-Taking: Learning Strategies for Nurses makes a special contribution. Readers can feel confident that while success still depends upon individual effort, this book provides an effective guide to prepare them for tests of their knowledge—whether on examinations, in discussions, or in practice. The authors present the task of organizing knowledge in a conceptual, yet practical format and provide practice materials with constructive feedback. The book helps readers identify personal priorities in learning and focus study time to maximize individual performance. The nurse educator has gained a significant adjunct to resources for refining skills in achieving goals, thinking, solving problems, forming concepts and applying knowledge as well as maximizing test performance.

In presenting their third edition, the authors have carefully reviewed and revised the second edition. They have updated sections to reflect latest scientific knowledge and practice approaches in pharmacology and other dimensions of practice. They have added emphasis to key points and incorporated timely concepts. For example, the discussions of universal precautions and oncology now delve more deeply into these concepts and related nursing implications. Principles of managing mental health alterations and alterations in children have been expanded. The book in its third edition will continue to enjoy great popularity because it offers exceptional support and assistance to readers as they face the challenge of organizing the information that forms the foundation of competent nursing practice. Readers will continue to recognize the value of the approaches which this book presents and models in supporting the professional commitment of lifelong learning.

Bette B. Case, RN,C, PhD
Chicago, Illinois

Contents

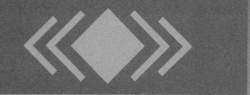

PART ONE

PATTERNS OF LEARNING

Forming the Psychology of Test-Taking Success

MARIAN B. SIDES

One's attitude is truly a vital human quality. Throughout your learning career, it will play an important role in determining how well you perform on tests. Several prominent ideas serve as keystones for building a successful attitude. This chapter will present nine important principles that embrace these ideas. If you learn them well, and modify your behavior as directed, you will feel the power, the inspiration, and the "I can" attitude necessary to achieve your ultimate goal of passing state boards.

Concept: Control

Principle

Winners set goals, establish plans, and take control

Illustration of Principle

Winners do not leave the development of their potential to chance. They find out exactly what to do to succeed, and they establish a plan to achieve that success. Remember, *you* are in control. Your future is in your own hands. How important is your future? How important are you? I hope you answer these two questions with conviction and certainty. If you do, you *will* take control.

Your mission in life, right now, is to become a professional nurse, and your goal is to pass state boards. In order to accomplish that goal, you must begin with the end in mind (Covey, 1989) and create an action plan based on clearly defined objectives and selected activities. The plan must have realistic time frames and deadlines to keep you focused and to prevent procrastination (Figure 1–1). Create a plan for each test-taking event. Execute the plan repeatedly until it becomes a habit.

WINNING THOUGHTS

*W*e are what we repeatedly do.
Excellence, then, is not an act, but a habit
(Aristotle).

**Preparation for Test-Taking Success
Sample Action Plan**

Mission: Become a professional nurse
Goal: Pass state board examination

OBJECTIVES	ACTIVITIES	DATE ACCOMPLISHED
I. Organize my knowledge around basic concepts.	1. Read Chapter 9 and 10 in review book	June 1–4
A. Describe in my own words how fluids and electrolytes work in the body	2. Form small study group and meet once a week.	May 15–July 10
B. Identify key principles in growth and development	3. Take state board review course.	June 18–25
II. Answer correctly 90% of test questions in review book and understand rationale. (Med/Surg items first)	1. Look for the key idea in test item. 2. Don't erase my answers. 3. Review test questions in review book.	Ongoing Ongoing Review 20 questions every day, except weekends, between June 1–July 1
III. Decrease my anxieties from present level	1. Establish study plan. 2. Work with someone who can help me identify and correct my weaknesses.	May 15 Once a week
IV. Establish a positive attitude about myself	1. Identify those things I do well. 2. Reward myself when I finish a task.	May 15–ongoing

Note: This plan is a model. It provides a framework that must be tailored by you to meet your specific needs. Adapt this model for all test-taking events

Figure 1-1. Sample action plan for preparation.

*A*n action plan gives you control over your immediate future. It provides organization, discipline, and a sense of direction. It helps reduce stress, anxiety, frustration, and unnecessary use of time and energy. If you don't have a plan, you may jeopardize your chance to succeed and increase your chance for failure.

A winner has a plan!

A loser has an excuse!

Your commitment to test-taking success may involve sacrifice. Climber Clara could effectively reduce her work stress on her journey to the top of the mountain if she would unload her backpack and leave behind those items that will not help her reach that goal (Figure 1–2). Likewise, if you are to be successful on your exams, you may need to temporarily give up some things that you enjoy, want, and even need, to provide more time to focus on your goal. If you work full-time, you may need to reduce your hours. If you do not work, it might be wise to delay employment until after the test. During this time, use your support network effectively. If you have children, for example, ask a friend to watch them so you can arrange an uninterrupted study time. Ask a family member or friend to assist with laundry or to shop for groceries. You can return the favor after you pass your test. Remember, you have limited time and energy to devote to this effort. Therefore, it is important that you manage your time and yourself effectively. Everything that you do or allow to have an impact on your life should contribute in a healthy way to your goal, and should not detract from it.

Balance

Remember that all work and no play reduces productivity. You need balance in your life during this important time. You must match work and study with appropriate rest, relaxation, and recreation. Set measurable goals with positive reinforcement. Reward yourself appropriately and frequently for work well done.

*T*here are those who travel, and there are those who are going somewhere. If a man knows not where he is going, any wind will get him there (Davis, 1984).

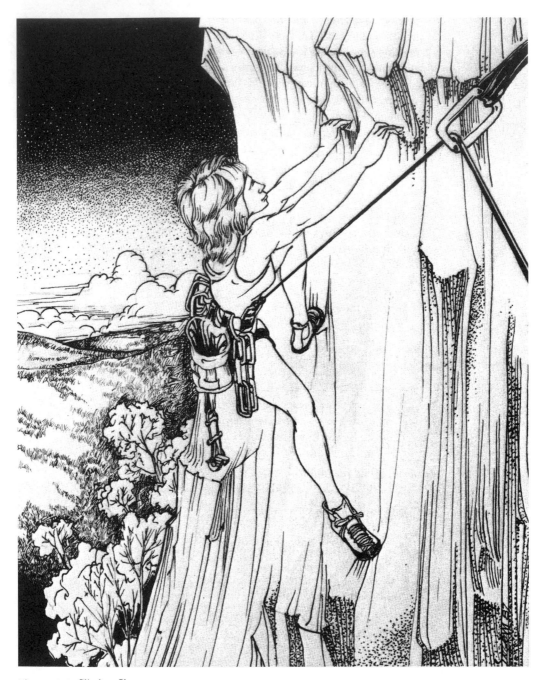

Figure 1-2. Climber Clara.

> *T*he power to achieve success is within your control. "I can pass" is power. "I will pass" is control.

Concept: Freedom

Principle

Attitude is a human freedom

Illustration of Principle

As human beings, we are endowed with the freedom to choose our attitude. Victor Frankl, a distinguished psychiatrist and survivor of a Nazi concentration camp, wrote in his book *In Search of Meaning,* "The last of the human freedoms is to choose one's attitude in any given set of circumstances. Attitude is an inner quality that can keep us free, even happy, during difficult times." A healthy attitude is one that views test-taking as an opportunity, not an obstacle. Test-taking success is a human freedom. It is not rationed. Success has no quotas—everyone can pass. Test performance is measured against a behavioral standard. That standard is the same for everyone. Attitude plays an important role in determining who meets that standard. Adopt a winning attitude: "I will pass!"

> *I*n the mind's eye lies the fulfillment of a dream. No one can give it to you. No one can take it away.

Concept: Self-fulfilling Prophecy

Principle

The outcome of your efforts is directly related to your self-expectancy and your self-image

Illustration of Principle

A powerful relationship exists between the mind and the body, in which the mind is able to produce expected outcomes. You become what you think about most. In preparing for exams, you have the choice of projecting your own performance in pass or fail terms. A winner's attitude is one that says, "I'm going to pass."

As normal human beings, we are driven to predict the consequences of our actions. Unfortunately, we often concentrate on the negative outcomes—those that we don't want to happen. Does this self-talk sound familiar to you?

> Gee, I know I'm not going to pass this test. What'll I do if I fail? I'll kill myself. I'll lose my job. I won't be able to face anyone at work. I won't be able to pass meds. What if I don't make it?

This self-talk is truly self-fulfilling. You can talk yourself into almost anything. So, why not talk yourself into passing? Expect the best; it will happen! Success is a self-fulfilling prophecy.

An effective technique used by many successful people in pursuit of important goals is guided imagery. This technique is demonstrated in the following exercise. I invite your participation.

Find a quiet spot somewhere in your home where you can concentrate for about 20 minutes without interruption. Guide yourself through this mental exercise.

Guided Imagery Exercise

Step 1. Commitment (5 minutes)

Take a journey into the future. Think for a moment: How badly do you want this RN licensure? What does it mean to you to pass state boards? How important is it to your future? What are you willing to sacrifice to get it? How much time does this goal deserve out of your busy schedule? Will it drive you to get up early some mornings, stay up late at night, and stay at home some nights when other, more exciting things are happening?

Step 2. Self-actualization (10 minutes)

Imagine for a moment what it will feel like when you finally reach that dream, when you actually achieve your success on state boards. Think about how you will feel when you open that envelope from NCLEX. In large black letters, it reads **PASS.** You are a registered nurse! Think about your new name tag with the letters *RN* after your name. You have worked hard for this. Your efforts, your determination, your hopes, and your dreams have brought you a true sense of knowing who you really are!

Think of the satisfaction you feel, the pride your family has in you. Your patients are waiting; they need you. You have a new sense of importance, a new recognition, a new kind of responsibility, and a new privilege. You have entered a rewarding and challenging profession. You are a professional nurse! Congratulations!

WINNING THOUGHTS

> *Y*ou have a choice to be your own creator. Winners make things happen. Losers let things happen!

Step 3. Mental Pole Vault (5 minutes)

In this phase of the guided imagery, you will visualize your activity. Create the details of preparing for an exam in your imagination. See yourself in the process. Let's examine some related success stories in which guided imagery has enhanced performance.

Winners All Our Lives is a film that portrays the use of imagery in cross-country marathon running and other related activities. Positive imagery has guided elderly participants, aged 75 to 80 years, to successfully run 13 miles a day. A pianist who was imprisoned in a concentration camp mentally rehearsed his skill by playing the piano over and over every day. When he left the camp, he could perform an award-wining concert immediately.

Now, bring forth your own best capabilities and rehearse them repeatedly in your mind. As you move through this book, you will become aware of some of your own barriers to success. You will encounter them courageously, and you will mentally pole vault to heightened levels of success. For example, if you have a habit of erasing answers and entering the wrong answer (second guesser), you will practice disciplining your mind to break this habit. You will visualize yourself in a test situation in which you never use your eraser.

If you are a very slow test taker, you will visualize yourself moving more quickly through the test. Of course, you must accompany this mental activity with actual practice. Select 20 test items in a review book, for example, and allow yourself 20 minutes to answer them. Practice pacing your work, both mentally and physically. Eventually the new winning behavior will become ingrained in your muscle memory, and you will be on the road to success.

A key attitude for your success comprises a belief in yourself, and a positive self-image. You must believe that you can do it. In belief you will find power. In that power is your future.

Concept: Self-esteem

Principle

The quality of your performance exists in direct proportion to your feeling of self-worth

Illustration of Principle

The person most likely to succeed is the one who has a deep sense of self-worth. You like yourself, have self-respect, and accept yourself. The easiest thing in the world to be is what you are. Your goal in life is to become the best you.

Do you feel you should pass this test? Whenever I ask this question of new graduates, I get an initial pause, a hesitancy to answer, and then some will say, "I think so," "I guess so," "I hope so," even, "I don't think so." If you don't think you'll pass, you probably won't.

WINNING THOUGHTS

> *T*hose who say I can, *will*. Those who say I can't, *won't*.

Let's ask that question again. Will you pass this test? Your answer is, "Yes, absolutely!" Now, list the reasons why you should pass. Don't stop until you've listed at least five, starting with

1. I worked hard; I deserve to pass.
2.
3.
4.
5.

A sense of self-worth means that you *are* an important person. You *can* make a difference in your chosen profession. If you don't feel good about yourself, you won't win the respect and confidence of those you plan to serve.

It's always nice to get praise and recognition from others, but you should not rely on external reinforcement alone to give you a feeling of worthiness. Self-respect and self-esteem come from within.

Concept: Self-awareness

Principle
Success begins with knowing yourself

Illustration of Principle

How well do you really know yourself? How much self-awareness do you really have? What strengths and weaknesses do you bring to this exam?

Somewhere in your nursing program you probably developed a favorite subject or a clinical practice area that you really enjoyed, or in which you excelled. You also probably can identify an area in which you performed poorly. It is important this time to sort out these differences, because the kind and amount of attention you give to each will differ.

As you identify your strengths, you can pride yourself in your skills, and perhaps guide others less skilled toward a better understanding of these concepts. Few of us enjoy hearing and learning about our weaknesses. It takes courage to recognize and acknowledge imperfection. Achievement, however, relies upon an open examination of these areas.

The wise nurse will form a network of friends or a small study group of colleagues who can provide useful, objective feedback about self-performance. One should avoid defensive behavior. Accept constructive criticism and apply corrective measures when necessary. If you concentrate on strengthening these skills in a deliberate way, you will see noticeable improvement in your performance.

> *T*ake responsibility for your errors and your imperfections. The day you stop making excuses is the day you start to the top (Davis, 1984).

WINNING THOUGHTS

Develop a self-awareness bank account. Be observant and aware of your strengths. The more strengths you bank, the stronger your sense of self and the easier it will be to acknowledge your weaknesses.

Concept: Self-confidence

Principle
Success is shaped by self-confidence

Illustration of Principle

What is self-confidence? It is an inner sense of knowing who you are—a way of thinking about yourself. How does one get self-confidence? It comes from recognizing convincing facts, and from a constant repetition of these facts. For example, when you answer a test question correctly and recognize the reasoning behind your answer, you are confident in your choice. Store this success and recycle this experience over and over. Such repetition of successful events will build your confidence.

WINNING THOUGHTS

> Success = function of (aptitude + instruction + initiative)

Success is a function of three variables: your aptitude for success, the quality of instruction you receive, and the personal effort or initiative you put forth. These three factors in concert with each other are all within reach, and in your control. For example: 1) If you didn't have the aptitude or the ability to achieve, you would not have gotten this far; 2) You can self direct the quality of instruction. Take advantage of all learning opportunities. Ask questions, seek clarification, and find a mentor—someone who will guide you and help shape your future; and 3) In doing so, you will take the initiative required to complete the success equation. Form discussion groups, and take 30 minutes after each class to reinforce the material presented. After graduation, form a study seminar group or take a state board review course. Do your best. Evaluate your progress. Validate your success. In this self-awareness, your confidence in yourself will continue to grow.

WINNING THOUGHTS

> Doing the best at this moment puts you in the best place for the next moment
> (Oprah Winfrey, 1992).

Concept: Courage/Failure

Principle

Failure is a natural consequence of a courageous person

Illustration of Principle

The only one who fails is the one who doesn't try. Most successful people fail time and time again. Have you ever failed an exam? Most of us have. How do you usually behave? How many excuses do you try to make?

> I was just getting over a fever, I wasn't feeling well. . . . Wouldn't you know, my boyfriend (girlfriend) decided to break up with me right before finals. . . . It was a bad day. . . . I knew the material, but they didn't ask what I studied. . . . The room was just too cold, and I couldn't concentrate with all the noise.

Don't make excuses. Be honest with yourself. Take full responsibility for your errors. Spend your time understanding your weaknesses and correcting deficiencies. Use the diagnostic grid in Chapter 4 to help you categorize your errors and focus on ways to correct your thinking.

If you intend to be successful, you must establish a healthy attitude toward failure. Between now and state boards, you are going to answer many questions incorrectly. Failing an exam is like hitting a pothole on the road to success. You have a temporary setback, maybe a little bruise. But you pick yourself up and move on. Failure is an opportunity to begin again more intelligently. Failure is a gift in disguise.

> *W*henever God wants to send you a gift, He wraps it up in a problem (Norman Vincent Peale, 1992).

WINNING THOUGHTS

You gain strength, courage, and confidence with every error you make if you confront each one honestly and sensibly. If you don't err, you don't grow. Remember, it's unnecessary to correct every weakness and every error. Exams are a measure of competency. You don't have to strive for perfection. Just do your best.

Concept: Perseverance

Principle

No goal is achieved without perseverance

Illustration of Principle

A powerful attribute underlying success is endurance. How many times have you thought about quitting? How often have you wished it were all over? You have recently completed a long and difficult course of study, and you probably feel physically and mentally exhausted. You still have several difficult months ahead. How will you survive?

The successful nurse recalls that the body expresses what the mind thinks. Therefore, you need to program the mind for success. Psychologists tell us that the average person uses less than 10% of his or her human potential. You realize, then, that you still have reserve energies. If you establish self-discipline and perseverance in a consistent and determined manner, you will create a positive, healthy attitude that will carry you through these next few months.

How badly do you want this success? What does it mean to you? Do you have a passion for your chosen profession? The climb to the top requires sacrifice. If you don't love WHAT you are doing in difficult moments, then love WHY you are doing what you are doing. Sacrifice for the well-being of others—those whose lives you will touch when you fully legitimize your professional status in nursing.

WINNING THOUGHTS

> *W*here there's a will, there's a way. If your WHY is strong enough, you'll find a WAY (Daniel Dimacale).

A fundamental principle to remember is that "no man is an island." The successful nurse will rely upon support networks to help maintain perseverance and a sense of direction. Create a circle of influence by surrounding yourself with positive-thinking people. The following activities will guide these efforts:

1. Work closely with one other person upon whom you can rely to lift your spirits and provide encouragement when you feel discouraged.

2. Break down your workload into manageable units of study. Completion of small, short tasks and self-made assignments will give you a sense of accomplishment and a feeling of progress. Persistence is best maintained on small tasks.

3. Openly seek feedback to obtain an objective evaluation of your progress.

4. Challenge one another's thoughts and ideas. Explore options to test questions and be able to defend your answers.

Remember, focus intensely on your goal. Maintain a strong sense of commitment. Don't give up when you're at the one yard line.

> *S*uccess is failure turned inside out. The silver tint of the clouds of doubt. And you never can tell how close you are. It may be near when it seems so far.
>
> So stick to the fight when you're hardest hit. It's when things seem worse that you must not quit (Davis, 1984).

WINNING THOUGHTS

Concept: Motivation

Principle

Motivation is the muscle behind success

Illustration of Principle

Two sources of motivation exist in relation to pursuit of an educational goal and a professional future—fear and desire.

Fear

It is human nature to fear failure, the unknown, and the discovery of imperfection. These fears are a threat to your self-image and self-worth.

Failure

No one likes to fail, especially at something as important as final exams or licensure exams. Therefore, each of us should be motivated to harness this fear by establishing a well-designed plan to succeed. First we must adopt a willingness to accept and welcome failure in performance during the early, formative stages of learning. Once we know what we are doing wrong, we can begin to correct our thinking.

Unknowns

A correlation exists between anxiety and the unknown. An increase in unknown factors causes a corresponding increase in anxiety. Therefore, your goal is to reduce fear and anxiety to a level of comfort—one that will circulate enough adrenaline to keep you alert and on your toes. What are some common unknowns? You don't know how many questions are on the exam. You don't know how the test is organized. You don't know how to pick the right option on the test question when you've narrowed it down to two answers. You don't understand the question. You don't know how to pace yourself. You don't have all the knowledge you'd like to have. You don't know the questions on the test—and many, many more. In the past nine years, through state board reviews and test-taking clinics, the faculty of *Education Enterprises, Inc.* has identified common unknowns from student nurses and new graduates across the country. Throughout this book, strategies are offered to help you reduce the number of these unknowns.

Discovery of Imperfection

The best way to deal with the fear of imperfection is to acknowledge that you aren't perfect, and then see how close to perfect you can become. The first step is to learn your imperfect ways. You may have developed some bad learning habits over the years. Glance for a moment at the caricatures in Chapter 6. Do you recognize yourself anywhere? Do you read into questions? Do you cram for tests? Are you a slow test taker? Your efforts should be directed at correcting those behaviors that will hinder your pursuit of perfection. These efforts, designed to improve yourself to avoid failure, are the intrinsic motivators that will enhance your journey toward success.

Desire

Desire is a second source of motivation. It is derived from your ambition to reap the rewards of your hard work. Rewards come in many forms. They include your licensure as an RN, the personal satisfaction of achievement, your first paycheck, power, prestige and status, and the power to help people in ways that no one but a professional nurse can. These rewards that automatically accompany success are powerful motivators.

Additional personal rewards provide inspiration and incentive to spur your efforts toward your goal. Nurses often think that the more they study, the smarter they will become. To the contrary: working harder is not always better. Your life must have balance between work and play. You should treat yourself to rewards, such as a good TV show, a movie, a night out to dinner, or a favorite dessert. Something as trite as a coffee break from a grueling itinerary can be stimulating and pleasurable. Your productivity will improve substantially with a healthy balance between study and relaxation. Anticipation of these built-in rewards is an effective motivator and should be used generously.

If you apply the nine principles discussed in this chapter in a consistent and wise manner, you will find yourself in the Winner's Circle!

> *W*hen you have done your best, wait for the results in peace (Davis, 1984).

References

Covey, S. L. (1989). *The Seven Habits of Highly Effective People.* Simon & Schuster, New York.

Davis, W. (1984). *The Best of Success.* Lombard, Great Quotations, Inc.

Peale, N. W. (1992). *The Power of Positive Thinking.* Wings Books, New York.

2 Developing Thinking Skills

MARIAN B. SIDES

Your success in test-taking is highly influenced by how effectively you think. What are thinking skills and how do you learn them?

Through years of formal and informal learning you established your own techniques and patterns of thinking. How effective are they—how well do they work for you? Effective thinking begins with an awareness of your own thinking. Unless you are consciously aware of your own thought processes, you cannot take control of what goes on in your own mind. This chapter will offer some simple and basic guidelines to improve your learning and thinking in preparation for test-taking. Attention will be focused on the common problems that learners face in developing higher level problem-solving skills.

The taxonomy of thinking consists of six levels. The first two are memory and comprehension. They form lower level thinking. The next four levels—application, analysis, synthesis, and evaluation—are higher level or problem-solving behaviors (Bloom, 1956) (Figure 2–1).

The test plan for the state board examination includes test items at the first four levels, which will therefore be the focus of this chapter. Although most of the items are written for application and analysis skills, you must have a good understanding of the basics before you attempt to master the higher level processes.

Memorization

Most new graduates, upon completion of a nursing program, have more than enough knowledge to pass state boards. Unfortunately, a substantial amount of that information is learned through memorization, and has not been incorporated systematically into higher forms of learning that can be readily used to solve prob-

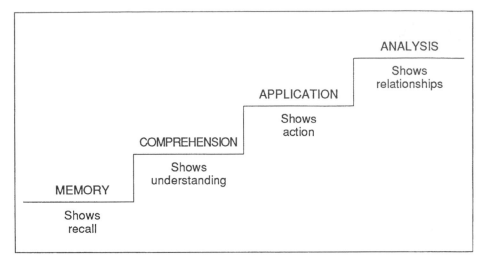

Figure 2-1. The taxonomy of thinking.

lems or to answer complex test questions. Such information exists as isolated, disjointed, and disconnected facts that simply clog and confuse the mind.

Did you ever feel overwhelmed by the amount of information you tried to learn and wonder how you would be able to retain it long enough to take the test? Student learners are often compelled to memorize everything. Consequently, they often store in memory useless data and forget the important information. Remember, you don't need to memorize a lot of detail. For example, you will never need to recite every skill a child can perform during each year of growth. Instead, you should learn key developmental behaviors for specific age categories, such as the age at which a typical child learns to walk. Remember to establish frameworks and categories of information rather than memorize details and isolated facts. Other examples include drug classifications, stages of labor, common lab tests and ranges, and the basic principles of body processes for circulation, respiration, and movement.

MEMORY JOGS

*K*now *what* to learn. Don't find security in quantity. "The more you learn, the better you'll do" assumption is false. Effective learning is selective and useful memorization.

A second problem that learners face is that they often choose short-term memory strategies like rehearsing words or repeating phrases over and over. Information learned by simple repetition usually fades as soon as the test is over, or even before the test is taken. An effective way to improve memory performance is to invent memory techniques for situations that cause memory difficulties.

Acronyms

The use of acronyms is a helpful technique often used to retrieve information from memory. The following scenario may be a *déjà vu* for you:

> Oh, I know the answer to that. . . . I learned it yesterday. I can just see it . . . it's on page 37 . . . on the top right-hand corner . . . give me a minute, I know it'll come. . . .

For important information, you want to be prepared with a retrieval tool that will trigger recall. You've learned acronyms like TLC, COPD, and PEARL that have been widely used as mental crutches to facilitate recall. Effective learners will create their own jargon or gimmicks to assist them in retrieving information.

Acrostics

This mental tool is an arrangement of words in a familiar phrase that triggers the recall of other information to be learned. An example is the familiar phrase "On Old Olympus Towering Tops a Sin in German Viewed Some Hop." The first letter of each word is also the first letter of one of the 12 cranial nerves—the mind has a tendency to recall unique and creative jingles or phrases more easily than straightforward content.

ABCs

Another strategy commonly used to facilitate retrieval is the formation of words from the ABCs. The words are intended to trigger key signs that form a vivid portrait of a classic patient problem.

> *C*linical Portrait: Emphysema
> Apprehension
> 　Barrel chest
> 　　Cyanosis
> 　　　Dyspnea
> 　　　　Engorged neck veins
> 　　　　　Frown on forehead

MEMORY JOGS

Image-Name Technique

Another effective retrieval strategy is the linkage of a name to a clinical problem that clinically portrays the patient. For example, the names *pink puffer* or *blue bloater* are used to depict patients with specific chronic obstructive pulmonary disorders.

The amount of information you should actually memorize and store is a very small percentage of the information that is available. The key to success in the first level of learning is to create and use strategies that will trigger retrieval of relevant information rather than recall isolated data. Your goals in preparing for state boards at the first level of learning are to improve memory and to reduce forgetting.

MEMORY JOGS

> *T*reat your mind like a palace with a golden gate and reserved seating. Don't let information into the gate if it doesn't belong there and if you don't have room. Ask yourself, "Do I really need to memorize this?" If you memorize without discrimination or cram carelessly, valuable information may be lost or pushed aside.

Comprehension

Effective memorization is a prerequisite to understanding. However, effective understanding requires more than simple recall or recognition. Comprehension puts memorized information into a context that gives it meaning. It bridges the gap between simply parroting information and really knowing what you're talking about.

Effective comprehension includes the ability to translate information from one form to another. This can be done by paraphrasing, summarizing, explaining, or demonstrating your understanding. For example, Mrs. Jones has a potassium level of 2.8 today. You once learned that serum potassium normally ranges from 3.5 to 5.5 mEq/L. So far you have demonstrated retrieval of memorized data. Now, interpret the meaning of the 2.8 potassium level. What is the implication of this lab value for nursing practice? The mental activity in which you are now engaged is comprehension.

In preparing for a test, you must be highly sensitive to your level of understanding and your ability to discuss relationships among important facts. Unfortunately, students and graduates often slight this level of learning, moving impulsively to the action or solution without a clear notion of how the information fits together. It's like the baker who rushes to put the cake into the oven without paying attention to whether all the proper ingredients are present or whether they are mixed together effectively. Several comprehension strategies have been effectively used by student learners and new graduates and are recommended in preparing for tests.

Small Group Work

Comprehension is most effectively accomplished by working in small groups or with at least one other person. This provides a forum for verbalizing your thought processes and critiquing each other's thinking. One way to expand your comprehension is to listen to someone else's viewpoint on selected topics of interest and to challenge customary patterns of thinking. Debate and disagreement usually provoke a deeper, richer, and more meaningful understanding of material being learned. Often a colleague will detect flaws in your thinking and can assist you in taking corrective measures to fine tune your cognitive skills. You cannot get this kind of healthy exchange and feedback when you work alone. Therefore, small group work should be used for the comprehension level of learning.

Creative Use of Questions

The use of questions in classroom teaching and testing is not a new concept. Traditionally, questions have been a useful mechanism for determining the end result of learning and for determining course grades. As you prepare to take tests, a more creative use of questions is encouraged to enhance learning at the comprehension level.

Somewhere in your nursing program you probably encountered the question, "What is the most critical sign of distress displayed by your patient who has emphysema?" You probably answered, "He's dyspneic." Now, build on this scenario by generating questions that start with the answer and work backward. List as many relevant questions as you can.

Answer: The patient is dyspneic.

Questions: Why is he dyspneic? What specifically triggered this episode of dyspnea? If he's dyspneic now, what could happen next? Can I explain the relationship between dyspnea and the pathophysiology of emphysema? What signs of improvement should I be looking for?

Use these questions in your small discussion groups. Ask for clarification, build on the original answer, and ask deeper questions until you feel you can discuss this clinical problem comfortably and all ramifications intelligently. Then you will have mastered the second level of thinking, comprehension.

Relevance of Facts

An awareness of the differences between memory strategies and comprehension strategies should help you to progress from one to the other. Memory learners digest facts. They learn, for example, that arteries are elastic. Comprehension learners try to understand the relevance of these facts. They probe more deeply into a further interpretation of the facts. For example, "Why are arteries elastic? Will they always be elastic? If not, what will cause them to lose elasticity? How will circulation occur if arteries lose elasticity? What can we do to maintain the integrity of artery elasticity?" Discussion of these questions will provide a more vivid understanding of the basic principles of circulation, a valuable and productive experience.

Imagery

A final strategic technique for fine tuning comprehension skills is the use of visual imagery, or the creation of mental pictures about your patients or the patients whom others have described to you. Fix these images in your memory. Retrieve them during test-taking to aid in answering questions correctly.

Memorization and comprehension form the lower mental processes in the taxonomy of learning. If you have mastered these skills for important concepts that frame health and its disorders, you are ready to move on to higher level problem-solving skills, application, and analysis.

Reasoning Exercises *for Lower Mental Process Items (Knowledge-Comprehension)*

1. During normal ventilation, the volume of air that does not participate in gas exchange is called
   - *A. Residual
   - B. Expiratory
   - C. Tidal
   - D. Total lung

2. A disturbance or loss of ability to use words or to understand them is
   - A. Apraxia
   - *B. Aphasia
   - C. Dysphagia
   - D. Dyskinesia

3. Mrs. James is in labor with a vertex fetal presentation. Appearance of meconium-stained fluid may indicate
   A. Abruptio placenta
   B. Normalcy
   *C. Fetal distress
   D. Premature rupture of membranes

4. Mr. Grady has emphysema. Which alteration in lung volume and capacity would you expect?
   A. Increase in tidal volume
   B. Decrease in residual volume
   *C. Decrease in vital capacity
   D. Increase in total volume

5. Sara is 18 months old. Which of the following behaviors is most typical for this stage of developmental growth?
   A. Building a tower with blocks
   B. Turning on TV by pulling the knob
   *C. Placing toys in a box
   D. Pulling a toy with a rope

6. If Mrs. Moss is given an intermediate-acting insulin at 8:00 AM, the most likely time for a hypoglycemic reaction would be
   A. 10:00 AM
   B. 12:00 PM
   *C. 6:00 PM
   D. 10:00 PM

Application

Application is the process of using information in the practice of nursing to maintain, promote, or restore health. A vital step in the application process is knowing *why* you are going to do what you plan to do. It involves the awareness and use of previously learned principles to justify your intended actions. Application *is* the implementation phase of the nursing process and is at the heart of nursing practice.

The foundation of nursing practice is built on a set of principles that explain health and its deviations. These principles are drawn from nursing and related disciplines. For our use, a principle is defined in the following way:

*P*rinciple. A basic fact or truth that can be applied in practical situations; a specific guideline that can be used to explain and support actions.

If you cannot identify the principle or provide a rationale for your nursing actions, you should not perform them.

*T*he less you know about why, the more you know about error.

The following model test item will illustrate the properties of application items and the strategies to be used in selecting the correct answer.

Application Test Item

Mrs. Miller—Depression

Mrs. Miller was admitted to the hospital with a recent history of depression. She has eaten very little since her admission. Which response to Mrs. Miller, during breakfast, would be most appropriate initially?

    A. Please start eating, Mrs. Miller; I'll be back in 10 minutes to see how you're doing.

    B. If you don't eat, Mrs. Miller, we'll have to start IVs on you or give you injections.

    C. You'll be hungry in a few hours, Mrs. Miller, if you don't eat.

    D. Let's eat just a little of everything, Mrs. Miller. I'll help fix your tray.

Properties of Application Items

Application items usually provide a brief scenario or description of the context within which the situation is based. The description is usually followed by a stem or question that leads to the four completion options or answer choices.

Selection Strategies

Before you choose an answer to this question, you must form a logical rationale based on principle to support your choice of action. Your thinking should flow something like this:

> **A** is incorrect because I cannot assume that a depressed patient will initiate appropriate behavior upon request.
>
> *Principle:* Depressed patients are not self-directed and require a guided and assertive approach.
>
> **B** is incorrect because it can be perceived as threatening and may increase anxiety.
>
> *Principle:* Nursing actions should convey respect for the dignity of the patient; nursing actions should effectively reduce anxiety.
>
> **C** is incorrect because it appeals to rational thinking.
>
> *Principle:* Nursing interventions for depressed patients should be concrete, direct, and should not seek response that relies on sound cognitive processes.
>
> **D** is correct.
>
> *Principle:* Nursing actions should show the therapeutic use of self in the form of a caring presence. Depressed patients need guidance and direction in conducting basic activities. Depressed patients consume food more effectively when served in small portions.

This item should serve as a model to guide your thinking through application questions. Repeat this mental process with each question to strengthen and refine your problem-solving skills. In a short time it will become a habit in your thinking.

Analysis

The skills involved in analysis occur at a more complex and difficult level of thought than do the skills of comprehension and application. Because analysis appears above memory, comprehension, and application in the taxonomy, the latter skills are a prerequisite to one's ability to analyze. Analysis itself can be divided into various levels of abstract thought, characterized by increasing difficulty. These skills are used frequently by scientists, scholars, detectives, and others whose jobs engage them in complex problem-solving and application of logical thinking.

It is not the intent of this discussion to make you an instant scientist. Nor is it necessary to masterfully distinguish between the levels of comprehension and analysis. It is important, however, that you recognize that differences exist, and that you know how to approach intellectually the test questions and clinical situations that require such thinking.

Therefore, this discussion will focus on the structure of the analysis question in its most simple and basic form, so that you can begin to tailor your thinking and develop efficiency in this form of thought.

No clear distinctions exist among levels of learning. Their boundaries are blurred, and the processes blend and overlap. To illustrate this phenomenon, let's examine the item about Mrs. Miller, the depressed patient, and the levels of learning upon which this item was built. This item encompasses all four of the levels that you have learned in this chapter. For example, you must be able to retrieve basic knowledge about depression as a state of the mind (Level 1). Second, you must comprehend and understand the meaning of the condition of depression, and the meaning of the communication chosen. It requires your interpretation of depression as it relates to eating and includes your ability to explain the relationship between depression and patterns of eating (Level 2).

So far the information needed to perform the lower level skills, memory and comprehension, is provided for you in the scenario or test question. In the next two levels, you must show your ability to draw upon appropriate abstract and logical forms of thought (not provided in the text) that will lead you to correct answers or conclusions. Application, for example, involves the selection of appropriate rationales or principles to justify your nursing action, as illustrated in the discussion following the test item on Mrs. Miller. These principles were not provided. You were required to supply these in the form of thinking.

Analysis is the ability to think at a level beyond comprehension and application. You may be able to comprehend the meaning of the communication used with Mrs. Miller, but you may not be able to analyze it effectively.

MEMORY JOGS

*A*nalysis emphasizes the breakdown of material into its parts and detection of the relationships of the parts to the whole (Bloom, 1956).

Analysis is an aid to greater comprehension. It requires, for example, the ability to distinguish the cause-and-effect relationships among depression, reduced appetite, and response to different forms of communication. Can you recognize and analyze the technique used to get Mrs. Miller to eat? Can you trace the traits of thought and the relationships that you must perceive to accurately answer the question? Skill development in analytic thought requires much practice.

Errors in Analysis

Learners throughout their course of study face some common problems in answering analysis questions, which often result in error.

Problem 1. Incomplete Analysis

Learners often miss important elements in the content of a communication that must be considered in analysis. For example, selecting a nursing response for a pregnant woman may be very different from selecting a response for a pregnant *diabetic* woman—which may in turn differ from selecting a response for the pregnant diabetic who is experiencing a high level of stress. The following test question illustrates this concept:

> **What effect will an unusual amount of *stress* have on the insulin requirement of an *overweight diabetic* who becomes *pregnant?***

You may be essentially on the right track in answering this question, but you may miss one of the important elements, relationships, or principles. If that occurs, you will answer the question incorrectly.

Problem 2. Overanalysis

The "philosopher" nurse goes too far in analyzing situations (see Chapter 6). This person breaks the situation up into more elements than necessary, or sometimes adds information that is not provided or is irrelevant. This person often misses important relationships and does not see the forest for the trees.

Problem 3. Quality Error

Analytic test questions often provide options that have different degrees of accuracy or completeness. The distinction is not between right and wrong but is a matter of the best response or the one that offers the highest quality.

Effective strategies for developing analytic skills comprise a combination of the methods offered in this chapter. Group work is high on the list. Working with others will enhance and deepen your familiarity with all important elements and relationships that exist in test questions.

Practice reviewing test questions and analyzing your thinking patterns. Practice with purpose; experience is the best teacher.

Reasoning Exercises *for Higher Mental Process Items (Application-Analysis)*

1. A meconium-stained vaginal discharge is noted in Mrs. Gregory during the early stage of labor. Your first action is to

    A. Determine fetal presentation

    B. Notify the doctor

    *C. Assess fetal heart tone and rate

    D. Provide information to the patient

2. Brian has been hospitalized with an acute asthmatic attack. He is receiving 2000 cc of 5% D/W with 20 mEq of KCl per day. The drop factor is 60 drops per milliliter. How many drops per minute should you administer?

    A. 48

    B. 68

    C. 76

    *D. 83

3. Mrs. Hurley continues to see "bugs" everywhere. The most appropriate response of the nurse to Mrs. Hurley's experience is

    A. "Believe me, Mrs. Hurley, there really are no bugs in your room."

    B. "I'll get rid of all the bugs so you won't see them again, Mrs. Hurley."

    *C. "I'm right here next to you, Mrs. Hurley. What you're experiencing will soon pass."

    D. "I'm going to give you some medication so you'll feel better, Mrs. Hurley."

4. Mr. Brown was admitted to the emergency room with multiple injuries suffered in an automobile accident. He has a crushed chest, abdominal trauma, probable head injury, and multiple fractures. Which of the following emergency care interventions are most appropriate and in proper order?

    A. Assess vital signs, obtain a history, arrange for emergency x-ray films

    *B. Assess breathing, control accessible bleeding, determine presence of critical injuries

    C. Conduct physical assessment, control bleeding, cover open wounds

    D. Start an IV, get blood for typing and cross-matching, assess vital signs

5. Mr. Roberts had a colon resection for removal of a malignant tumor. The day after surgery, he went into hypovolemic shock. What is an observable effect of Mr. Roberts's compensatory efforts?

    A. Level of consciousness maintained because of adequate blood flow to myocardium

    B. Cold, clammy skin as a result of peripheral vasodilation

  *C. Reduced urinary output as a result of decreased blood flow to kidneys

    D. Increased pulse rate caused by further reduction in cardiac output

Reference

Bloom B. S. (1956). *Taxonomy of Educational Objectives: The Classification of Educational Goals*, Handbook 1. New York: David McKay.

The Nursing Process: A Problem-Solving Model

MARIAN B. SIDES

The framework for exams in most nursing curricula is based on the nursing process and client needs. You will do well on "tests" and subsequently in your professional practice if you can effectively use the nursing process to meet the needs of clients with commonly occurring health problems. This chapter describes and illustrates each phase of the nursing process and provides test questions to measure your skills.

The nursing process is a diagnostic and management tool that guides the practice of nursing. It uses a scientific problem-solving approach to gather data, determine client problems, select appropriate interventions and measure outcomes.

Client needs are grouped into four categories. The weighting given to each category is illustrated in Figure 3–1. These are based on the results of a job analysis of the entry level performance of registered nurses (Kane et al., 1986). A description of client needs is included at the end of this chapter.

The five-phase nursing process model includes assessment, analysis, planning, implementation, and evaluation (Figure 3–2). Each phase is given equal emphasis in this chapter's discussion.

Assessment

The first step in the nursing process is the collection of information about the client. The purpose of this assessment is to focus on the relevant data about your client's health status to enable you to make an intelligent and valid problem statement or nursing diagnosis.

Assessment data are characterized as subjective and objective. Subjective data are obtained from the client, either through a planned interview or through

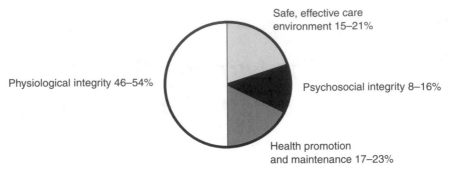

Figure 3-1. Weighting assigned to each category of client need.

incidental sharing of information by the patient. Subjective information includes symptoms such as dizziness, palpitations, pain, anger, fear, and so forth, which clearly express the patient's experience.

Objective data about the client are obtained by the nurse, the patient's family, or others who might have useful information. Data are gathered through direct observation, using the senses of vision, hearing, touching, and smelling. They include signs such as grimacing, crying, unsteady gait, vital signs, clammy skin, or bloody urine.

Data collection is done purposefully and selectively. You should seek objective information that verifies the subjective complaints or symptoms reported by the patient. These data should relate to the knowledge you have about nursing theory or about the other basic sciences. As information is gathered, it should begin to form a pattern and take on meaning. The goal of data gathering is to provide a basis for interpretation and problem definition.

Assessment: Establishing a Data Base

A. Gather objective and subjective information relative to the client:
   1. Collect verbal and nonverbal information from the client, significant others, health team members, records, and other pertinent resources.
   2. Review standard data sources for information.
   3. Recognize symptoms and significant findings.
   4. Determine client's ability to assume care of daily health needs.
   5. Determine health team members' ability to provide care.
   6. Assess environment of client.
   7. Identify own or staff reactions to client, significant others, and/or health team.

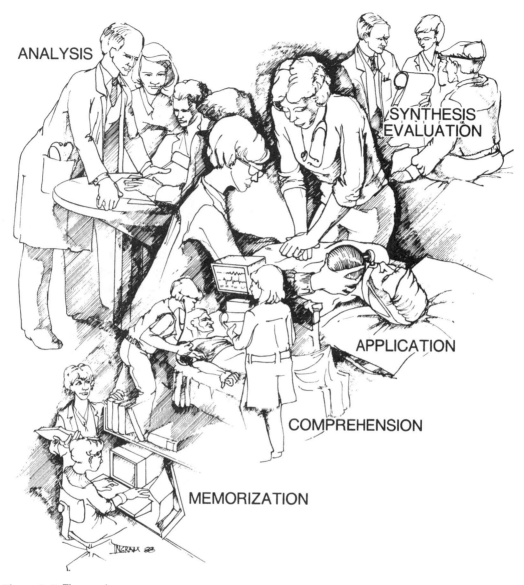

ANALYSIS

SYNTHESIS
EVALUATION

APPLICATION

COMPREHENSION

MEMORIZATION

Figure 3-2. The nursing process.

B. Verify data:
   1. Confirm observation or perception by obtaining additional information.
   2. Question orders and decisions by other health team members when indicated.
   3. Check condition of client personally instead of relying on equipment.
C. Communicate information gained in assessment (National Council, 1987).

Reasoning Exercises: *Assessment*

1. A 20-year-old female patient with a history of Hodgkin's disease was admitted through the emergency room to a medical unit. You observe her returning from the bathroom with a slightly unsteady gait. Which of the following measures would be most appropriate first?

   *A. Asking "You seem to be unsteady on your feet—are you all right?"

   B. Consulting the medical record for the latest vital signs and blood count.

   C. Re-checking her blood pressure and pulse.

   D. Putting her back to bed to protect her from falling.

In answering this question you are involved in the assessment or data collection phase of the nursing process. You know that your patient has Hodgkin's disease. You have observed her unsteady gait. This observation suggests a possible deviation from the body's normal healthy state of balance or homeostasis. Additional information should be sought to verify the presence or absence of a problem. Having analyzed the item scenario, you are now ready to look at the options. Option **D** is an implementation measure. Since you cannot determine the presence or extent of a problem from the information provided, you do not have a logical scientific rationale for option **D.** Therefore, you must withhold judgment until your data are more complete.

Each of the first three responses is a form of assessment or data gathering. The first response **A** provides the most direct lead to information about her unsteady gait. Subjective data that validate your assumptions are best provided by the client herself, and can give accurate direction for your nursing actions.

A common problem in answering assessment questions or conducting the assessment process is the inability to accurately prioritize nursing responses. Eager to take action, nurses often jump to conclusions before having the necessary information. Perhaps in choosing option **A** you will learn that she was having difficulty seeing without her glasses; logically, your action would be to get her glasses rather than to put her to bed.

MEMORY JOGS

*W*hen in doubt about the presence or nature of a problem, seek more information if time permits and if the patient's safety is not in jeopardy. Seek the most current valid and reliable information first, to rule out life threats and to expedite problem definition.

2. Johnny was admitted to the emergency room with complaints of headache and nausea. Two weeks ago he fell from a bicycle and struck his head on the cement pavement. Your first nursing action is to

   A. Obtain an order for pain medication

   __B.__ Conduct a neurological evaluation on Johnny

   C. Ask Johnny's mother to describe what led to this episode

   D. Ask Johnny if he was unconscious after he fell

In this item, option **A** is an action response and must be withheld until a problem definition is made. The last three options are assessment responses. The appropriate response is the one that seeks the most direct relevant and up-to-date information about Johnny (option **B**). It is the only response that provides useful information about his current health status, which could be life threatening.

Analysis

When all available data have been obtained or when all data that time permits have been obtained, the significance of those data must be determined. The process of interpreting the data to form a definition or statement of the problem is called *analysis.* Defining the presence of a problem and determining its characteristics are the most difficult and critical aspects of problem solving. If you err here, the rest of the process is invalid and off course.

One activity that is useful in analyzing data is discussing the assessment information with someone. Ask questions, communicate your understanding of the data, and put it into your own words. What are the possible needs and problems that could evolve from a sudden blow to the head? What are the problems that a nurse can identify? What conditions can the nurse plan to provide care for and treat?

Analysis: Identifying Actual or Potential Health Care Needs and Problems Based on Assessment

A. Interpret data:
   1. Validate data
   2. Organize related data

B. Collect additional data as indicated

C. Identify and communicate client's nursing diagnosis

D. Determine congruency between client's needs and problems and health team members' ability to meet client's needs (National Council, 1987)

Reasoning Exercises: *Analysis*

1. Mrs. Brown had an uneventful delivery of a normal, healthy baby boy three days ago. When the nurse entered her room that afternoon she found Mrs. Brown sitting up in bed, crying softly. How would you interpret her behavior?

   A. Beginning psychosis following a stressful event

   *B. Postpartum blues related to hormone changes following delivery

   C. Sadness over termination of pregnancy

   D. Normal emotional response due to exhaustion and episiotomy discomfort

Mental activity required to answer this question involves an understanding of the normal physiological changes following childbirth. Consider the information provided about Mrs. Brown in the question and make an assumption about her behavior. Option **A** is incorrect because it suggests a medical diagnosis. Although the other three opinions are stated within the parameters of nursing knowledge, option **B** is the most logical and accurate interpretation of her situation.

2. Steven, an athletic 20-year-old college student, suffered a fractured shoulder and sprained wrist in a fall at a ski resort. In developing Steven's care plan following surgery, you anticipate the following typical problem:

   A. Alteration in self concept

   B. Anxiety due to flashbacks about the skiing accident

   *C. Impairment of mobility due to immobilization of upper extremity

   D. Abnormal tissue perfusion due to swelling

Using the information provided and your understanding of patient needs following reduction of a fracture, the only problem that would normally occur is impaired mobility (option **C**). In analyzing data you first would attempt to recall and understand typical scenarios or patterns of needs that commonly occur. Validate your problem definition by incorporating specialized data or unique signs and symptoms presented by your client. These specialized data should be accompanied by a statement of cause. For example, if you noted that Steven's fingertips were cold, and that pitting edema was forming on the back of his hand, your analytic statement might be option **D,** abnormal tissue perfusion due to swelling. An accurate analysis of data provides a valid and useful framework for planning patient care.

Planning

The planning process begins with setting goals for client care and determining strategies to meet these goals. Client goals are an expression of desired outcomes that are realistic, measurable, and achievable, and that are to be accomplished within a designated timeframe. For example, an activity goal for a patient following surgery is to ambulate the full length of the room with assistance by the evening of the first day after surgery.

Planning is a complex process because it involves many variables that are interrelated. These variables include the following:

1. Locus of decision making: Who should be involved in this plan of care, and to what extent should the client, family, and others participate in this plan of care?

2. Return to normalcy: What limitations are placed on the client's potential to return to the original state of health? What impact has this illness or intervention had on the client's potential to return to normalcy?

3. Availability of resources: Are the necessary social, community, or institutional resources available to achieve the goals you plan to set?

4. Prognosis or potential for resolution of problems: What impact do the pathological, physiological, and psychological changes make on your client's potential for recovery? How great is the need for acceptance of limitations and the need to adapt to alternate states of health and balance?

5. Collaboration with health team members: Are the right people involved to provide the most comprehensive and highest quality plan of care for this client?

6. Additional data: Are more data needed to complete the plan of care, and are avenues available to obtain those data?

7. Diagnosis: Does the plan of care accurately address both medical and nursing diagnoses?

8. Intervention outcomes: Can you predict and provide reasonable assurance that the plan of care, when implemented, will lead to the expected outcomes? Are the strategies realistic and valid, and will they guide nursing actions?

Planning: Setting Goals for Meeting the Client's Needs and Designing Strategies to Achieve These Goals

A. Determine goals of care:
   1. Involve client, significant others, and health team members in setting goals.

2. Establish priorities among goals.
3. Anticipate needs and problems on the basis of established priorities.

B. Develop and modify plan:
1. Involve the client, significant others, and health team members in designing strategies.
2. Include all information needed for managing the client's care, such as age, sex, culture, ethnicity, and religion.
3. Plan for the client's comfort and the maintenance of optimal functioning.
4. Select nursing measures for delivery of the client's care.

C. Collaborate with other health team members for delivery of the client's care:
1. Identify health or social resources available to the client and/or significant others.
2. Coordinate care for the benefit of the client.
3. Delegate actions.

D. Formulate expected outcomes of nursing interventions (National Council, 1987).

Reasoning Exercises: *Planning*

Mr. Hathaway expresses his dislike of the hospital and his feelings of insecurity about being there. The nursing staff's plan to make him feel more secure should include:

  A. Allowing him to do as he pleases

  B. Providing for all of his needs

  C. Assigning specific tasks for him

  *D. Being consistent in their approach to him.

To prevent Mr. Hathaway from reacting defensively, the nursing staff should:

  *A. Be nonjudgmental and accepting of his responses

  B. Be nondefensive and provide good role models

  C. Have a matter-of-fact attitude when he has problems

  D. Make him aware of the goals to be accomplished

Both questions above have a key word in the stem that provides a focus for your thinking in answering the question. The word *insecurity* in the first stem and the word *defensively* in the second stem are keys to the intent of the questions. A common characteristic of planning items is that they provide or refer to basic principles that should guide your nursing actions.

In the first scenario, the lack of security generally comes from the presence of "unknowns" in the environment. Security comes from being able to predict the unknown and set reasonable expectations for what is going to happen. The best way for a nurse to help a patient achieve this sense of security, then, is to be consistent in one's approach to the client. Appropriate interventions include anything that shows consistency.

The same form of thinking applies to the second scenario. Discuss this scenario; exercise your thinking about planning items by using the items in the sample test in Part II.

Implementation

Once the planning phase is complete, you are ready to implement the strategies you designed to achieve the goals of care. Nursing actions span a wide range of activities, including the direct provision of care, client teaching, and the recording of information. Implementation is simply putting your plan into action.

When you answer an action-oriented item, you must first identify the rationale or principle that supports your actions. Always ask yourself the questions, "Why am I going to do this? Why should I take this action?" If you cannot answer these questions with a logical and convincing argument, you should not choose the response or take the action option. In action items, the principle and rationale are not provided. You must figure out the appropriate principle.

Implementation: Initiating and Completing Actions Necessary to Accomplish the Defined Goals

A. Organize and manage client's care.
B. Perform or assist in performing activities of daily living:
   1. Institute measures for client's comfort.
   2. Assist client to maintain optimal functioning.
C. Counsel and teach client, significant others, and health team members:
   1. Assist client, significant others, and health team members to recognize and manage stress.
   2. Facilitate client relationships with significant others and health team members.
   3. Teach correct principles, procedures, and techniques for maintenance and promotion of health.
   4. Provide client with health status information.
   5. Refer client, significant others, and health team members to appropriate resources.
D. Provide care to achieve established client goals:
   1. Use correct techniques in administering client care.

2. Use precautionary and preventive measures in providing care to client.
3. Prepare client for surgery, delivery, or other procedures.
4. Institute action to compensate for adverse responses.
5. Initiate necessary life-saving measures for emergency situations.

E. Provide care to optimize achievement of the client's health care goals.
   1. Adjust care in accord with client's expressed or implied needs and problems.
   2. Stimulate and motivate client to achieve self care and independence.
   3. Encourage client to follow a treatment regimen.
   4. Adapt approaches to compensate for own and health team members' reactions to factors influencing therapeutic relationships with client.

F. Supervise, coordinate, and evaluate the delivery of client's care provided by nursing staff.

G. Record and exchange information:
   1. Provide complete, accurate reports on assigned client to other health team members.
   2. Record actual client responses, nursing actions, and other information relevant to implementation of care (National Council, 1987).

Reasoning Exercises: *Implementation*

1. Mr. Brown has recently been told by his doctor that he has high blood pressure and should be eating a low sodium, low salt diet. Which of the following food selections provide the least amount of these substances?
   A. Hot dog with coleslaw and french fries
   B. Bologna sandwich with hard-boiled egg
   *C. Tuna salad and fruit cup
   D. Bread with split pea soup and ham

2. Mr. Brown was recently told by his doctor that he has high blood pressure. In helping him select dinner, which of the following foods would you instruct him to eat?
   A. Hot dog with coleslaw and french fries
   B. Bologna sandwich with hard-boiled egg
   *C. Tuna salad and fruit cup
   D. Bread with split pea soup and ham

What is the difference in the cognitive level of these two questions? The first item is a lower level question. The relationship between high blood pressure and a low sodium, low salt diet is provided. The nurse needs to know only which food selections are lower in sodium and salt. No action, teaching, or patient care interaction is required.

The second item is a higher level question because the role of salt and sodium is not provided. The nurse must draw upon the principle that governs the relationship of sodium and salt to hypertension, and the effects of each on the hemodynamics of the human body. The nurse must then know the relative salt and sodium content in the foods presented in order to assist the patient in making the appropriate food selections. The principles that support this item rationale come from the biological and physical sciences. Both on state boards and in clinical practice you will be expected to know the relationships among sodium and salt intake, blood pressure changes, and fluid volume precautions. You will be expected to take appropriate action in diverse situations. Therefore, it is important to challenge your own understanding of common health problems and to question the implications they have for patient care.

Reasoning Exercises: *Implementation*

Brian, 4-years-old, is sitting in the pediatric day room with Michael, another patient. He suddenly realizes that he has wet his pants and runs to the nurse, crying.

1. The most appropriate initial response by the nurse is:
    A. "Why, Brian what happened? Why did you wet your pants?"
    B. "You know better than this, Brian; next time you'll get a good spanking."
   *C. "Let's take off those wet pants, Brian, and put on something dry so you'll be more comfortable."
    D. "Wait until I tell Michael what you did. Aren't you ashamed of yourself?"

Several relevant principles come into play in selecting the correct answer to this item. A very basic principle is, "The nurse shows *respect* for the individual in treating human responses to actual or potential health problems." In other words, focus on treating the patient with respect first, and then attempt to modify wrong behavior. This principle shows an acceptable standard of nursing action.

The following describe behavior that supports unacceptable standards:

1. A rational approach to solving an emotional, psychological, or even a physiological health care problem is seldom effective (option A).
2. Punitive behavior creates anxiety and is not therapeutic (option B).
3. Imposing shame and ridicule increases anxiety and is not therapeutic (option D).

Review other implementation items in Part III. After reading the stem, before looking at the options, practice identifying the principles and rationale to support your action choices. Then read the options and select the answer that best matches your rationale.

Evaluation

The last phase of the nursing process is evaluation. It focuses the outcomes of patient care, a process that is often neglected. How effectively do *you* evaluate patient care? Let's complete the exercise in Figure 3–3 and find out how well you actually do.

The evaluation phase of the nursing process is an excellent monitor of the effectiveness of your care. It provides guidance and direction in continuing the nursing process. It validates your actions, ensures patient safety, and promotes compliance with your legal responsibilities to your patient.

Evaluation: Determining the Extent to Which Goals Have Been Achieved

A. Compare actual outcomes with expected outcomes of therapy:
1. Evaluate responses (expected and unexpected) in order to determine the degree of success of nursing interventions.
2. Determine the need for change in goals, environment, equipment, procedures, or therapy.
B. Evaluate compliance with prescribed or proscribed therapy:
1. Determine impact of actions on client, significant others, and health team members.
2. Verify that tests or measurements are performed correctly.
3. Ascertain client's, significant other's, and health team members' understanding of information given.
C. Record and describe client's response to therapy and/or care.
D. Modify plan as indicated; reorder priorities (National Council, 1987).

Reasoning Exercises: *Evaluation*

The nursing staff recognizes that Mrs. Jones is the primary support person for her husband. Mrs. Jones has identified her own problem as a role conflict—being a mother to teenage children, a wife of a hospitalized husband, and a person with rights of her own.

1. Which action by Mrs. Jones would indicate that she has analyzed her problem?
    A. She takes the children to visit her husband daily.

Directions for use: Answer each question by checking the numbered column that corresponds best to your performance in the particular care aspect described. After completion of the exercise, total your points and compare it to the effectiveness scale key.

	Strongly Agree				Strongly Disagree
	5	4	3	2	1

1. I give pain medication to my patients and always follow up to see how effective the medication was.

2. After meals I always observe what and how well my patient ate.

3. I always compare my patient's health progress with the needs and problems stated on admission.

4. I can state precisely my patient's care goals and can describe how well the goals are being achieved.

5. I know how well my patient is complying with physician and nursing orders.

6. I can describe change in my patient's status by citing the patient record and progress notes.

7. I can specifically describe the cause and effect between my patient's health status and my nursing intervention.

8. I modify the nursing care plan based on my patient's response.

Evaluation Effectiveness Rating Scale

Total Points	Effectiveness
40–37	Excellent
36–29	Good
28–21	Average
20–13	Poor
12–8	Unsafe

Figure 3-3. Evaluation tool for patient care effectiveness.

*B. She gives the children some of the home responsibilities.

C. She describes the roles of each member of the family.

D. She talks to Mr. Jones about his physical limitations.

2. The nurse approaches Mrs. Jones and states, "I see you are not staying at night with your husband anymore. Is there a problem?" What answer would indicate that Mrs. Jones is coping realistically?

*A. "I feel so angry at times. I need time to think."

B. "The children said that they needed me at home."

C. "My husband asked that I not stay anymore."

D. "The staff does everything for my husband."

Several additional evaluation item stems are presented below:

3. Which of the following comments indicate that Mrs. Turner has *accepted* her *illness?*

4. The following progress note indicates that *hemodialysis* was effective:

5. Which of the following behaviors are signs that Mrs. Brown feels *confident* in *taking care* of her 3-day-old baby girl, Melissa?

In the questions above, the italicized words are actually goals being measured. In these items as well as in your clinical practice you should be looking for evidence that these goals are being met.

The nursing process is a valuable and powerful problem solving tool. If you use it well, it will guide you successfully through state boards and will serve as a vehicle to your success as a professional nurse.

Client Needs *

I. Safe, Effective Care Environment

The nurse meets client needs for a safe and effective environment by providing and directing nursing care that promotes achievement of the following client needs:

1. Coordinated care

2. Quality assurance

*National Council of State Boards of Nursing: Test plan for the national council licensure examination for registered nurses. Chicago, 1987. Reprinted with permission.

3. Goal-oriented care
4. Environmental safety
5. Preparation for treatments and procedures
6. Safe and effective treatments and procedures

Knowledge, Skills, and Abilities. In order to meet a client's need for a safe, effective environment, the nurse should possess knowledge, skills, and abilities in areas that include but are not limited to the following: bio/psycho/social principles; teaching/learning principles of group dynamics and interpersonal communication; expected outcomes of various treatment modalities; general and specific protective measures; environmental and personal safety; client rights; confidentiality; cultural and religious influences on health; continuity of care; and control of spread of infectious agents.

II. Physiological Integrity

The nurse meets the physiological integrity needs of clients with potentially life-threatening or chronically recurring physiological conditions, and of clients at risk for the development of complications or untoward effects of treatments or management modalities, by providing and directing nursing care that promotes achievement of the following client needs:

1. Physiological adaptation
2. Reduction of risk potential
3. Mobility
4. Comfort
5. Provision of basic care

Knowledge, Skills, and Abilities. In order to meet client needs for physiological integrity, the nurse should possess knowledge, skills, and abilities in areas that include but are not limited to the following: normal body structure and function; pathophysiology; drug administration and pharmacologic actions; intrusive procedures; routine nursing measures; documentation; nutritional therapies; managing emergencies; expected and unexpected responses to therapies; body mechanics; effects of immobility; activities of daily living; comfort measures; and the uses of special equipment.

III. Psychosocial Integrity

The nurse meets client needs for psychosocial integrity in stress- and crisis-related situations throughout the life cycle by providing and directing nursing care that promotes achievement of the following client needs:

1. Psychosocial adaptation
2. Coping and adaptation

Knowledge, Skills, and Abilities. In order to meet client needs for psychosocial integrity, the nurse should possess knowledge, skills, and abilities in areas that include but are not limited to the following: communication skills, mental health concepts; behavioral norms; psychodynamics of behavior; psychopathology; treatment modalities; psychopharmacology; documentation; accountability; principles of teaching and learning; and appropriate community resources.

IV. Health Promotion/Maintenance

The nurse meets client needs for health promotion and maintenance throughout the life cycle by providing and directing nursing care that promotes achievement, for clients and their significant others, of the following needs:

1. Continued growth and development
2. Self-care
3. Integrity of support systems
4. Prevention and early treatment of disease

Knowledge, Skills, and Abilities. In order to meet client needs for health promotion and maintenance, the nurse should possess knowledge, skills, and abilities in areas that include but are not limited to the following: communication skills, principles of teaching and learning; documentation; community resources; family systems; concepts of wellness; adaptation to altered health states; reproduction and human sexuality; birthing and parenting; growth and development, including dying and death; pathophysiology; body structure and function; and principles of immunity.

References

Kane M, Kingsbury C, Colton D, & Estes C. (1986). *A Study of Nursing Practice and Roles Delineation and Job Analysis of Entry-Level Performance of Registered Nurses.* Chicago: National Council of State Boards of Nursing, Inc.

National Council of State Boards of Nursing, Inc. (1987). *NCLEX-RN Test Plan For the National Council Licensure Examination for registered Nurses.* Chicago: The Council.

Strategies for Effective Test-Taking

MARIAN B. SIDES

An important objective in preparing for exams is to develop and refine your test-taking skills. Competence in test-taking requires mastery of both content and process skills. You might have a good knowledge base for the practice of nursing, but if you can't take a test, you won't be able to demonstrate what you really know.

The purpose of this chapter is to examine your strengths and weaknesses in test-taking. Common problems and errors in performance will be presented. You will evaluate your own intellectual practices to determine patterns or trends in your thinking that may lead you to the correct or incorrect answers. This is an exercise in getting to know yourself better so you can develop and refine your skills.

The first step in developing test-taking wisdom is to learn as much about the examination and the condition of testing as possible. This chapter will focus on the development of specific strategies for effective test-taking.

Computerized Adaptive Testing (CAT)

Computerized adaptive testing (CAT) is the new method of testing for the National Council Licensure Examination (NCLEX). CAT is an interactive testing experience that is individually tailored to the candidate's knowledge and skills. The number of items on the test will vary between approximately 75 and 265, depending upon the candidate's pattern of testing. The CAT advantage significantly reduces the amount of time needed to complete the exam—from the traditional two days to a matter of hours. Participants in CAT testing view the experience as better, easier, and less stressful than the traditional paper and pencil test. Instructions are provided to the candidates prior to the examination, and candidates are given a practice exercise designed to teach them how to take the CAT exam. Candidates do not need prior computer experience to take the CAT exam (National

Council, 1992). Test-taking templates in most nursing programs are designed in accordance with the CAT system. Computer labs on campus provide opportunities for computerized test-taking throughout the program.

Although the modality and procedures for taking the NCLEX have changed, there are no substantial changes in the test plan. Although the CAT test design may include more single or individual items than found in the previous exam, the traditional item sets built around a particular patient scenario are still the format. Therefore, the cognitive strategies that are used to develop effective test-taking skills will be similar for all forms of test-taking, including certification exams, other forms of paper and pencil tests, and computerized testing.

Basic Rules for Test-Taking Success

In the following paragraphs, ten basic rules for test-taking will be presented. These rules evolved from strategies used in helping new graduates overcome common, recurring test-taking problems in preparation for the licensure examination.

Rule 1. Know the Parts of a Test Question and How to Read Them

A multiple choice test question consists of three main parts: a background statement, a stem, and a list of options. The background statement is a brief scenario that provides information necessary or useful in answering the question.

The stem is the element that contains the specific problem or intent of the item. It can be presented in the form of a question or an incomplete statement, and is formed by a subject and a verb. These components are shown in the following chart.

Stem Forms of a Test Question

A young woman arrived at the hospital in early labor.	**Background statement**
Which of the following signs is the best indicator that labor is progressing?	**Stem in question form**
The best indicator that labor is progressing is	**Stem form in incomplete statement**

The background statement does not always provide information essential to answering the question. It may be included to provide a framework for the stem, or to flavor the test with interest and personality. It may be included to determine how effectively you can sort through data and select pertinent information. The chart above, for example, provides a background statement that is not needed to answer the question. The background statement in the chart, however, is critical to answering the question correctly. In developing test-taking skills, you will learn how to discriminate essential from nonessential information in the background statement and in the stem.

A 41-year old, at term and a diabetic, arrived at the labor and delivery suite in early labor. **Background statement**

Which of the following assessment data should the nurse obtain upon admission? **Stem in question form**

The assessment data that the nurse should gather include **Stem in incomplete statement form**

The options are a list of possible answers to the question or solutions to the problem. The correct answer is called the *keyed response*, and the other options are called *distractors*. The words option, distractors, response, and answer are used interchangeably in this text. A question is usually followed by four single-option choices.

In answering the test question you will select the option that best completes the question or statement. In the chapters to follow you will have many opportunities to work with options and develop your skill in selecting the correct one.

Rule 2. Read the Question Carefully Before Looking at the Options; Identify Key Words in the Stem

The stem is the heart of the item. It provides the focus and directs your thinking. Your key words will be found in the stem. Read it carefully and grasp the complete thought before looking at the options. Then, read each option and select the one that best solves the problem or answers the question. If you don't read the entire stem, and gloss over words or misread them, you will misinterpret the question. A common error is to miss the word *except*, as shown in the following question:

1. All of the following behaviors are typical of a 3-year-old except
    A. Putting on make-up and playing grown up

*B. Reciting address and telephone number

C. Throwing a ball about 5 feet

D. Identifying animals from a picture book

The word *except* in the stem directs you to look for the response that is not typical of a 3-year-old child. If you miss the word, you will select the wrong answer.

MEMORY JOGS

> *H*aste makes waste! Read each word in the stem carefully before looking at the options. Look for key words such as *first, primary, initial, early, most important, except.*

A 3-year-old child was admitted to the emergency room after being rescued from a fire in his home. He is having difficulty breathing.

2. An early sign of respiratory distress that you might observe is

*A. Increased pulse rate

B. Cyanosis

C. Decreased pulse rate

D. Clammy skin

If you missed the word *early* in the stem, you might have chosen cyanosis as the answer. Although cyanosis is a sign of respiratory distress, it's a late sign rather than an early sign.

Other key words commonly used in test stems are *primary, initial, best, except*, and *most*. These words will not be highlighted or emphasized in any way on the test. You must be alert and read each word carefully to extract the true meaning of the stem.

Rule 3. Identify the Theme of the Item, and Base It on Information Provided in the Stem; Don't Assume Information That Is Not Given

Each test question is designed to measure a specific unit of knowledge or process skill. When you read the stem you need to identify the precise idea it intends to convey. Confine your thinking to the information provided and don't add to it. A common error is to choose a response that might have been appropriate for a patient you previously cared for, or a response that worked in another situation. Remember, each person is different; what's appropriate in one instance may not apply for the patient in your test question.

A husband was admitted to the emergency room in delirium tremens (DTs). This admission is his third visit in 2 weeks. While waiting to see her husband, the wife said to the nurse, "What in the world can I do to help my husband get over this drinking problem?"

1. The best initial response for the nurse is
    A. Don't feel guilty; I know this must be difficult for you.
    B. Let's go into the lounge, so we can talk more about your concern.
    C. You need to convince him to seek professional help.
    D. How long has your husband been drinking?

If you chose Option **A,** you are reading into the question and adding a factor that was not provided—that the wife is feeling guilty. Perhaps you know of someone who did feel guilty in a situation like this, or perhaps you thought she should feel guilty. Because this background statement does not tell you how she feels, you can't make this assumption (option **A**).

Option **C** is incorrect because you don't have enough information about the situation to offer this advice. You should be in the assessment or data collection phase of the nursing process. Option **D** is not the best choice because it focuses on his problem and channels the interaction specifically, rather than encouraging her to express her concerns. Since she is concerned about what *she* can do to help her husband, the correct response is one that first encourages her to verbalize how she is feeling (option **B**).

Rule 4. Answer Difficult Questions by Eliminating the Obviously Incorrect Responses First; Then Select the Best of the Remaining Options

If you can reduce your options on a difficult question to two choices, you can sharpen your focus, and the task will seem more manageable. Eliminate the obviously wrong distractors, then reread the stem. Identify rationales for each of the remaining answers, and select the strongest option. This process can take several minutes at first, but you will develop speed as you gain skill through practice.

If you cannot eliminate any of the options, take a wild guess and select any answer. You are not penalized for guessing, and you will have a 25% chance of getting it right. In CAT testing, you cannot return to previous questions, so you must answer them as you go. In traditional paper and pencil tests, however, you may wish to skip the question and return to it later.

Rule 5. Select Responses That Are Therapeutic, Show Respect, and Communicate Acceptance; Eliminate Responses That Are Bizarre, Inappropriate, and Punitive

Your actions should always be guided by the basic principles of interpersonal relationships. The intent to respect others should underlie every interaction. In school you were taught to "accept the patient as he is." Therefore, you can automatically eliminate distractors that violate these principles, because they are always inappropriate. The use of basic principles to guide your thinking can help you select the correct response even if you don't understand or recognize the item idea or condition described in the stem. The following question illustrates this concept.

A patient is recovering from a colon resection for removal of a malignant mass in the large bowel. Following breakfast one morning, she tells the nurse, "I'm tired of waiting, I want my bath now. You're never here when I need you."

1. Which of the following responses by the nurse is most appropriate?
    A. "What do you mean, I'm never here? I spent 3 hours with you yesterday."
    B. "I'm sorry you've been waiting. Let's get you comfortable now, and I'll be back in 20 minutes to give you a bath."
    C. "I'm doing my best. You know I have three other patients to take care of today, besides you."
    D. "I must see another patient right now. She's really sick today. I'll be back as soon as I can."

The only appropriate response is option **B.** Acknowledge her feelings and give her a clear, factual response to her concern. Never challenge a patient's statements, and don't be defensive (option **A**). Do not reprimand the patient unnecessarily or talk about the needs of the other patients (options **C** and **D**). In this case you did not need to know a lot about colon resections to answer this question. You did need to have skill in basic communication and human interaction.

Rule 6. Know the Basic Principles That Guide the Practice of Nursing

The best preparation for test-taking success is to know your professional discipline, nursing. Know your subject matter. Part II presents the basic principles that underlie the practice of nursing. Focus on learning principles and broad concepts for client problems that are prevalent in our society. Recognize and learn common needs and aspects of care of high-volume patient populations. You may become skilled in recognizing familiar illness portraits even if you don't recognize the medical disorder described in a item. Consider the following two items:

A 48-year old woman was brought to the Sunny Manor Nursing Home in a debilitating state with Helsink's disease. Her husband says that she has become very unstable on her feet; her motor skills have become very spastic. She is becoming increasingly irritable and is having difficulty eating by herself. The couple appears very depressed.

1. Following the initial assessment, the best action for the nurse is to
   A. Give them a few hours of privacy so they can gather their composure
   B. Introduce them to other clients in the day room so they won't feel so isolated
   C. Get her settled in her room; give them a basic orientation to their immediate surroundings
   D. Assist her to ambulate in the corridor to regain her strength

2. Activities that would be appropriate for her are those that would allow her to
   A. Compete with others
   B. Succeed at a task
   C. Engage in social interaction
   D. Tax her thinking skills

The answer to question 1 is option **C**. The answer to question 2 is option **B**. Did you answer those questions correctly? Did you recognize the disease, Helsink's? If not, did you proceed to answer the questions anyway, or did you panic and wonder what you should do because you never learned this disorder—or at least you don't remember learning it?

The purpose of this demonstration item was to expose you to an exercise with a fictitious disorder (*Helsink's disease*) to see if you could answer the question correctly by interpreting the information provided and recognizing the familiar clinical portrait described. Whether you knew Helsink's disease or not, you probably did recognize these behavior patterns.

The patient's complaints and symptoms are typical of a degenerative neurological condition. Persons with this type of problem sense a loss of independence and control. The important implication for nursing is to assist the client to gain control over the environment and to achieve a sense of autonomy and independence whenever possible. These individuals are not ready to socialize or spend time in day rooms with other people. They are focused on their own personal needs. These problems and care needs are very fundamental, regardless of whether the client has Huntington's chorea, Parkinson's disease, CVA, or Helsink's disease.

*W*hen you confront strange or unfamiliar background statements or vignettes, don't panic. Proceed with the question. Look for behavior patterns or clinical portraits that will provide clues for nursing action.

Rule 7. Look for Patterns in Your Performance and Flaws in Your Thinking. Analyze Your Test-Taking Behaviors, Then Establish Strategies to Correct These Problems

Typically students and new graduates learn by trial and error. Seldom is learning well designed and led by a systematic plan. Even more seldom do students evaluate their performances and analyze their learning strengths and weaknesses.

The test-taking grid diagrammed in Figure 4–1 is a tool that will assist you to track your patterns of thinking and identify flaws in your practices. It will help you establish a mental mechanism for higher level thinking and problem solving. This tool can be used to answer test questions in Part III of this book.

Rule 8. Manage Your Time Effectively During Test-Taking

Although timing is not a critical factor in CAT testing, you should make every effort to pace yourself sensibly to avoid unnecessary expenditure of time and energy. CAT testing is primarily an untimed, self-paced testing experience.

For exams that are timed, you should allow approximately one minute per item. Pace yourself accordingly so you can complete the exam during the designated time allowance. When you feel you have mastered the content for a particular aspect of nursing, start timing yourself in the practice tests. If you are a slow test taker, practice reading at a faster pace. Pay attention to your comprehension. If you are making more errors when you pick up speed, perhaps your knowledge base is weak for the content you are reviewing. Familiarity and mastery of the material certainly will enhance your speed in test-taking.

The quality of concentration during test-taking can also affect your pacing and your speed. Try to block sound and motion interference during test-taking. Don't be distracted by nurses coming to or going from the test site. You shouldn't care what others are doing, how soon they finish, how far they are, or whether you're the last one done. You are not competing with them. Concentrate on your own test, your time, and yourself. CAT testing is easier because you are not in a room filled with a large number of candidates. You are seated at a computer in a more private environment. You will feel like you are the only one there and you can focus on the task at hand.

Error Categories	PRACTICE TESTS						Items Wrong Per Error Category
	1 Test	2 Test	3 Test	4 Test	5 Test	Integrated Exams	
1. Did not recognize or remember subject matter							
2. Did not understand subject matter							
3. Did not recognize item idea							
4. Did not recognize principle or rationale for correct answer							
5. Missed key word							
6. Did not read all distractors carefully							
7. Did not understand question							
8. Read into question							
9. Used incorrect rationale for selecting response							
10. Changed the answer							
11. Other							
TOTAL ITEMS WRONG PER TEST							

Figure 4-1. Directions for use of diagnostic grid for recording test-taking errors.

The purpose of this grid is to display your errors in test taking. The form consists of a column for each of five tests and one for an integrated exam. These columns can be used in reviewing items from any source. Categories of test-taking errors are listed in the left margin.

When you miss an item, place a mark in the square that you think best describes errors in thinking. Make sure you place the mark in the appropriate test column.

Once you have listed all your errors, look for patterns in your thinking. Begin to analyze the thoughts that led to the wrong answers. Do you frequently miss key words? Do you read into the question something that isn't stated? Make appropriate corrections in your thinking by applying the principles and ideas presented in this book.

Continue to practice test-taking. Your weakness should gradually decline, and you should see fewer errors.

Don't spend too much time on one item. In traditional testing, if you cannot eliminate any distractors, skip the question and return to it later, if time permits. If you can eliminate two options, but can't decide on the answer, take a guess. You may not have time to return to the question. On CAT testing, eliminate options in a systematic and timely manner. Then, make your selection, because you cannot return to the question once you proceed. If you progress in a timely fashion, you will feel confident about your performance, and you will maintain control and composure in the testing situation.

Rule 9. Do Not Change Answers Without Good Reason or Sound Rationale

Your first attempt at answering a test question is usually accomplished with an orderly and well-disciplined thought process. Your thinking is logical and systematic. When you decide to change an answer, your behavior is often driven by anxiety and nervousness rather than sound, rational thought. On CAT testing, you will not have a choice of changing the selected answer. However, you can change answers mentally before making the final selection, so this rule applies for CAT as well as traditional test-taking methods.

In traditional paper and pencil test-taking, if you are a *second guesser* and have a habit of changing answers, you should not review your entire test. Review only those questions about which you were unsure or those you did not answer. Do not change answers you have marked unless you have a good reason and can provide a defensible rationale. If you are a *second guesser,* refer to Chapter 6 for further discussion of this test-taking personality.

Rule 10. Choose Options That Are Within the Realm of Nursing; Be Able to Differentiate the Need for Nursing Judgment from the Need for Physician Judgment

Test questions that are action-oriented are based on clinical situations that require nursing judgment. Occasionally distractors will be used that call for physician action. The nurse may inappropriately call the doctor and refer to physician judgment when the situation really calls for nursing judgment. Such behavior can result in negligence.

A 58-year-old is recovering from a suprapubic prostatectomy. His urinary output in the past 2 days has been satisfactory; however, the nurse now notices that it is becoming increasingly bloody.

1. The initial action of the nurse should be to
    A. Irrigate the Foley catheter

    B. Notify the physician

    C. Take vital signs

    D. Empty the drainage bag

Your immediate goal is to determine whether the increase in bleeding is causing a life threat to the patient and whether it is threatening his stability. Taking the vital signs (option C) is the only action that will give you information on the patient's physiological status. The nurse should not notify the physician until she can provide further assessment of the patient's condition.

A patient is receiving Dilantin to stabilize his seizure condition. One morning when he is taking a walk in the corridor, you, his nurse, notice his gait is extremely ataxic and that he complains of dizziness.

  1. Which of the following nurse's notes indicates that appropriate nursing action was taken?

    A. Very unsteady gait, probably owing to Dilantin toxicity. Notify physician.

    B. Complaining of dizziness while walking. Gait unsteady, returned to bed, blood pressure 110/70, pulse 112, respiration 32. Physician notified.

    C. Gait very unsteady. Returned to bed. Physician notified.

    D. Gait unsteady. AM dose Dilantin withheld. Blood pressure 110/70, pulse 112, respiration 32.

Options A and D are not within the realm of nursing judgment. You don't know that Dilantin is causing the unsteady gait, and you should not withhold the medication without proper assessment. Option C is appropriate but not sufficient. The nursing notation in option B provides factual information related to appropriate assessment and provides a data base for physician analysis.

Reducing Stress and Anxiety

Stress is simply the wear and tear imposed on the body by the normal or abnormal events of life. The environment in which we live surrounds us with stressors that affect our ability to maintain a sense of balance and equilibrium. The activities of walking, breathing, eating, and talking all stress the body in different ways to keep us alive and healthy.

    Stress related to test-taking can produce unusual demands upon the body. The key to success during this particular time lies in the ability to control and balance the stressors in your life. See Chapter 1 for guidelines and inspirational tips on managing these stressors.

Remember to create a plan that will realistically blend this additional responsibility with other stressors in your life. Preparation for exams should be systematic and well spaced to allow for the natural assimilation and digestion of information. Adopt and use stress reduction and relaxation exercises to assist you in managing stress. Relaxation tapes are available from local book stores and can be purchased from textbook publishing companies.

Anxiety related to test-taking is often a major impediment to effective test performance. Have you ever noticed that the first question on the test is often one you can't answer. That's because your anxiety is high and anxiety interferes with clear thinking. Although anxiety and stress are related phenomena, anxiety differs from stress in several ways. Whereas stress is a generalized state of tension resulting from many different life events, anxiety is a specific state of uneasiness produced by a particular stressor. Anxiety related to test-taking can result from lack of information, lack of skill, or the presence of unknowns surrounding the test-taking situation. Strategies to decrease anxiety should focus on these three areas—that is, gaining information, developing skill, and decreasing unknowns. A reduction in anxiety will effectively reduce stress.

State Board Review Course

As you progress through your nursing program, you will begin to think about the final preparation for the state board exam. Many new graduates benefit from state board reviews. Others do well without them.

Benefits

A well-designed state board review will assist you to

1. Organize your knowledge for the practice of nursing
2. Improve your understanding of the basic principles and concepts that form the practice of nursing
3. Strengthen problem-solving skills
4. Improve test-taking skills
5. Reduce anxiety and stress
6. Establish confidence
7. Formulate a positive attitude
8. Develop wisdom and insight into your own strengths and weaknesses

A good state board review will offer you a support network of instructors and colleagues who share a common interest. It will also share some of the decision making that you otherwise would be making independently in preparation for state boards. Many graduates gain a sense of security in this experience.

Limitations

Be aware that a state board review is not a crash course in nursing and is not intended to offer you an entire nursing curriculum in a few days. It will not perform miracles, nor will it bridge the gap between a life-long deficit in learning and success on state boards. You must enter the review with an adequate foundation in the nursing discipline. A review will help you put the finishing touches on your learning. It is wise to realize that the best preparation for boards begins when you enter your nursing program. Cultivate good test-taking skills from the start and you will refine these skills as you progress through the program.

References

National Council of State Boards of Nursing, Inc. (1992). *Computerized Adaptive Testing (CAT)*. Chicago National Council of State Boards of Nursing, Inc.

Critical Thinking

MARIAN B. SIDES

Principle

Critical thinking is embedded in everything we do.

Illustration of Principle

Critical thinking is essential in all domains of nursing practice. The art of critical thinking is rapidly becoming a key organizing concept in educational reform today. The National League for Nursing (NLN) requires the integration of critical thinking in the nursing curricula. The Joint Commission for Accreditation of Healthcare Organizations (JCAHO) likewise requires the active participation of nurses in the quality improvement process and higher order thinking.

So what is critical thinking? Critical thinking is a process that has many dimensions. It involves the mysterious way of the mind, about which we know so little. Some aspects of our thinking we will never really know about, because they have been so deeply rooted in our past and simply brought forward as traditions by our ancestors. They are known as values, habits, and paradigms that were part of growing up. They are so integral and intertwined with self that they can no longer claim a separateness. In this reality lies the danger of imposing our own point of view on others, rather than accepting them as they are. In this reality, too, lies the challenge of looking beyond the parameters of our thinking and viewing situations as others do.

On the other hand, critical thinking is a process that can be masterfully cultivated through a disciplined effort, in accordance with universal intellectual standards and elements of reasoning (Paul, 1993).

> *C*ritical thinking is a mental process that uses elements of reasoning to shape choices and make sound judgments.

MEMORY JOGS

*E*lements of Reasoning
- Purpose
- Question or Central Problem
- Point of View
- Evidence
- Concepts
- Assumptions
- Implications
- Inferences (Paul, 1993)

MEMORY JOGS

*S*pectrum of Universal Intellectual Standards
- Clear
- Precise
- Relevant
- Accurate
- Deep
- Significant
- Consistent
- Broad
- Logical
- Realistic
- Sufficient
- Appropriate
- Justifiable
- Reasonable
- Rational
- Fair
- Insightful (Paul, 1993)

In order to learn and understand the core concepts and principles that shape the discipline of nursing science and nursing practice, we must concentrate on these elements and standards of reasoning as we try to figure things out and solve problems. They form the framework by which we assess the reasoning process of the learner. To determine whether you are reasoning well, ask these questions: How precisely and deeply can you explain the problem or question at hand? How realistic is your plan of action? How fairly are you judging the patient's point of view? How accurate are your calculations? How relevant is your assessment to the central problem? How sufficient is your evaluation of the outcome or consequences? Clarity in expressing and applying these universal standards and elements is the hallmark that anchors effective thinking in nursing practice. Part II in this book displays simply and clearly the conceptual foundations for nursing practice that shape health and selected alterations. Assess your own thinking and reasoning as you progress through these chapters.

Critical thinking can be defined in many ways. Simply defined, it is a mental process that uses elements of reasoning to figure things out. It is a disciplined and structured use of the mind that generates thought processes based on intellectual standards to help us shape choices and make sound clinical judgments.

Whenever we reason, we are trying to answer a question or solve a problem. We reason toward some goal. Stephen Covey says, "We must always start with the end in mind" (Covey, 1989). We reason with a point of view and within a subject domain. We make assumptions, draw inferences, and create implications from our findings.

The cognitive process model (Figure 5–1) structures thinking and maps the flow of thought processes to ensure effective outcomes. This framework integrates three models of thinking—the nursing process (Yura, Ozimek & Walsh, 1976), taxonomy of thinking (Bloom, 1956), and elements of reasoning (Paul, 1993)—into a single model, and charts the flow of these processes. In this book, we do not fully master its depth and complexity, but examine several elements of the model as they relate to thinking in test-taking and the nursing discipline.

For our purposes, a simple demonstration of thinking, using a single phenomenon (headache), will guide us through the steps. The model portrays thinking in two dimensions. One is very basic and simple, and the other, multifaceted and complex. Let's begin at the top of the model. Your patient complains of a headache. A headache is simply pain or discomfort that can occur in different sections of the head. You have gathered the data, made an assessment, and processed the definition of headache (memorization). The next step is comprehension. What does headache mean to you? In order to proceed in the thinking process, you must understand the logic of headache. What alteration exists in the human anatomy and physiology to cause headache? Comprehension simply means understanding the anatomy and physiology behind the scenes. You have now reached a decision juncture in the model (Figure 5–1)—the first small triangle. If your patient tells you he has a mild headache and you assess no other symptoms, you will move with the arrow to the left of the small triangle, and follow the arrow down to application/intervention, thereby sidetracking the assessment, analysis, and synthesis processes. Treatment protocol will probably consist of two Tylenol or the equivalent.

The next step is to evaluate the effectiveness of your actions. Did the Tylenol relieve the headache? If so, what implications do you draw for future actions? If not, what are the consequences? You have a choice here (Figure 5–1, second small triangle), to end or to go back to the beginning and to reassess and revise your plan, if necessary.

Let's return to the top of the model and again examine a scenario featuring the phenomenon headache. Your patient complains of a headache. Once again, you ask yourself, "What alteration exists in the human anatomy and physiology to cause headache?" During your initial assessment, your patient becomes drowsy and starts to vomit. You immediately proceed to intervention and give the patient Tylenol, as ordered. This time the Tylenol does not relieve the headache. Two hours later your patient becomes nauseated and restless, and the headache continues to worsen. Further assessment at this point reveals elevated blood pressure, widening pulse pressure, and unequal pupils—clearly signs of increased intracranial pressure (ICP). Your thinking was patterned to give Tylenol for headache, from rote memorization. You did not recognize the ICP dynamics that were operating here. Your initial assessment was incomplete, and you took the wrong decision path.

Many learners never cross the threshold from memorization to comprehension before making decisions and taking action. This is a key reason students fail tests.

CRITICAL THINKING – DECISION MAKING – PROBLEM SOLVING

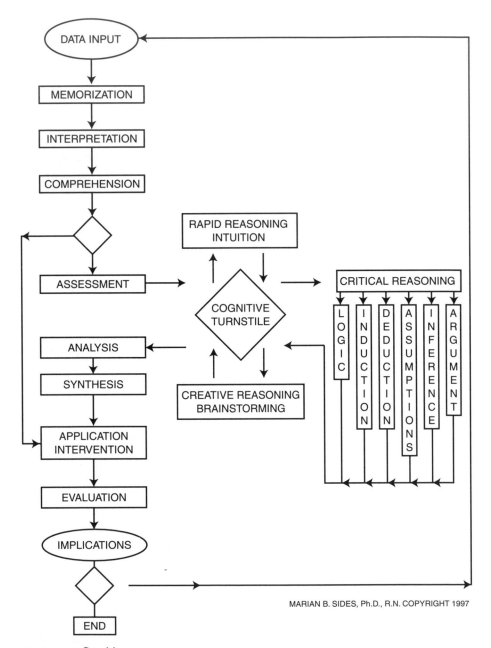

Figure 5-1. Cognitive process map.

A thinking person thinks for himself, and does not memorize someone else's thinking. A thinking person crosses the threshold from
memorization to comprehension before implementation.

**MEMORY
JOGS**

Instead of choosing the intervention path, you should have continued the assessment process, asking questions that would have provided a more complete
history. Analysis of data in this second scenario unveils signs of a severe neurological problem. Now the interventions are based upon a clear and complete understanding of ICP. Instead of pain relief, the immediate purpose of intervention is to
reduce the ICP.

*O*ne who memorizes acts blindly and errs. One who comprehends
acts purposefully and suceeds.

**MEMORY
JOGS**

In patient situations, when the problem is not instantly available or obvious,
the assessment process will move into the cognitive turnstile (Figure 5–1). The
thought processes within the turnstile will vary according to the situation. You will
incorporate thinking that is appropriate to the situation. For example, if the patient with ICP suddenly stops breathing, you will not choose the brainstorming,
creative reasoning path. You will use critical reasoning and apply the logic that
accompanies respiratory arrest. Quickly review what it means not to breathe. Exit
the cognitive turnstile to intervention. Here you would confirm that the patient
was not breathing, check the pulse, and if pulse was present, you would start pulmonary resuscitation.

*T*he cognitive turnstile is a junction or station along the thinking continuum where higher order reasoning takes place.

**MEMORY
JOGS**

Your lifesaving protocol in this situation will also include deductive thinking
based on the principle that all body cells need oxygen to survive. You will also
use inferential reasoning. If I don't provide oxygen to the brain within a few minutes, the brain cells will die.

When the reasoning process within the cognitive turnstile is complete, exit the turnstile. The outcome is analysis. The reasoning process has brought forth a synthesis of ideas and thoughts that has transformed separate pieces of information into a new whole. A simple headache is now a life-threatening neurological problem. Intervention is now based on removing a life threat. Next, you evaluate the effectiveness of your intervention. Draw implications, reassess, and revise the plan if necessary (Figure 5–2).

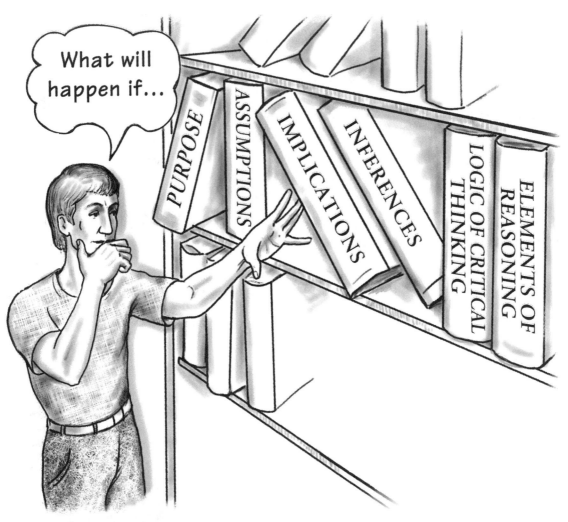

Figure 5-2. The reasoning process.

Principle

Effective use of questions will guide the learner in the critical thinking process.

Illustration of Principle

Questions, not answers, are the driving force in critical thinking. Too much emphasis is placed on answers, which unfortunately bring thinking to a deadly halt. Every answer should generate another question (Figure 5–3).

Many learners progress through their studies without ever understanding the mechanisms in altered health states. Furthermore, they are seldom challenged to examine the logic of their own thinking. Consequently, they merely dust the surface of a subject and achieve only a superficial understanding of the situation at hand.

The intellectual standards we discussed earlier provide a framework for assessing the quality of reasoning. The following scenario will demonstrate how thinking can fail to comply with these standards and how effective questioning can guide thinking to higher levels. The interaction occurs between the teacher who questions and the student who responds.

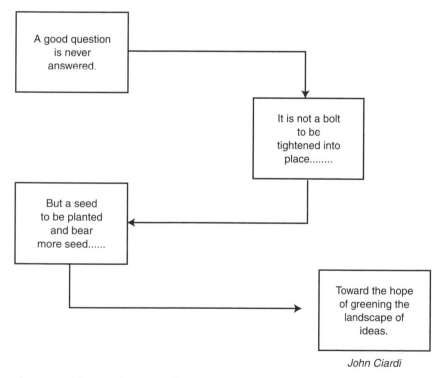

John Ciardi

Figure 5-3. The question-generating process.

Teacher:	What is the relationship between thirst and diabetes?
Student:	Diabetics who are hyperglycemic show signs of polydipsia.
Critique:	This response glosses over the surface of the issue and demonstrates memorization.
Teacher:	That's correct. But can you tell me why the patient is thirsty?
Student:	Yes, high blood sugar causes thirst.
Critique:	This response demonstrates memorization with no understanding.
Teacher:	OK. That's correct, but let's expand your thinking. Can you explain the mechanism of water distribution and how high blood sugar affects it?
Student:	I can't really explain it, but I know you must always watch for the three P's—polydipsia, polyphagia, & polyuria.
Critique:	Again, this thinking shows only memorization.
Teacher:	Let's think this through. In the hyperglycemic state, the blood contains a high level of glucose and is more concentrated than the fluid within the body cells. Fluid moves between the cells and the blood stream by the process of osmosis. Can you tell me what osmosis means, and in what direction water will move, given this hyperglycemic state?
Student:	Yes, osmosis means that water moves across a semipermeable membrane from a solution of lesser concentration of solute to one of higher concentration of solute. Therefore, the fluid will move out of the cells and into the blood stream.
Critique:	This response shows understanding of the process of osmosis.
Teacher:	If fluid moves out of the cells, what will happen to the cells?
Student:	The cells will shrink up like prunes.
Teacher:	Now can you tell me why the patient is thirsty?
Student:	Because of intracellular dehydration.
Teacher:	Excellent! Now let's answer this test question.

A middle-aged woman, admitted to the unit this morning, complains of excessive thirst and frequent urination. She is a diabetic with a blood sugar level of 350 mg/dL. What is an accurate interpretation of these data?

    A. Poor circulation in the diabetic results in a low blood volume, causing an alteration in thirst.

B. Thirst occurs because of the process of osmosis, which moves water out of the blood stream and into the tissues.

C. A decrease in concentration in extracellular fluids results in cell dehydration and thirst.

D. Thirst results from intracellular dehydration that occurs when blood glucose levels rise and water is drawn out of the cells.

Student: The only correct answer is **D.** Water moves from the cells, which contain solution of lesser concentration, and moves to the blood stream, which contains a high level of glucose and thus a solution of higher concentration. Responses **A, B,** and **C** are incorrect because these dynamics do not occur as described.

Teacher: Yes, **D** is the correct answer, and your reasoning is accurate.

Critique: This response demonstrates understanding and comprehension of the relationship between hyperglycemia and thirst. The instructor used the technique of questioning to coach the student's thinking to a deeper level of understanding. The student can now cross the threshold from lower order thinking to higher order thinking and perform nursing actions safely and with a clear purpose and sound rationale. The level of comprehension has been mastered.

> *T*ell me and I will forget
> Show me and I will remember
> Involve me and I will understand
> (Confucius).

MEMORY JOGS

Principle

Test items are tools that can be used to assess and enhance student reasoning, and to measure compliance with the universal intellectual standards.

Illustration of Principle

The state board examination for nurses is written in a multiple choice item format. Its purpose is to test minimal competence and safe practice. Because it is the format of choice on NCLEX, it is commonly used for teaching and testing the learner in the nursing curricula. The multiple choice question, however, cannot fully challenge critical thinking skills, nor will the test results themselves provide insight into the critical thinking process of the learner.

MEMORY JOGS

> *C*reative use of the multiple choice item can enhance higher order thinking.

If used as a teaching and learning strategy, the multiple choice item can serve as an effective tool in enhancing thinking skills. Several strategies can contribute to this skill development. Learners can be asked to provide a rationale for their answer of choice and provide reasoning that explains why they did not select the other options. Following a test, learners can be divided into small groups. Through group discussion they will debate, argue, and analyze test situations and reach consensus on an answer. They will then construct a group answer key. The groups will compare their keys and continue the process until they reach agreement on a single answer key. One person from each group will serve as leader in this process. This activity will exercise many of the elements in the thinking template, will shape new points of view, trigger more questions, and force a deeper understanding of the content, principles, and concepts.

Small group discussion is an excellent strategy for lifting learning from a mechanical mode to an independent thinking mode. In this transition, the learner crosses the threshold from memorizing other people's thinking to embracing the skills of independent thinking. Retention increases manifold, confidence grows, and learning becomes purposeful and rewarding.

Consider the following test question. Using the rules of test-taking, answer the question by selecting the best response from the information provided in this situation.

A 44-year-old woman cut her finger on rusty gardening shears. The cut required three stitches. You discuss the need for a tetanus shot, because she has not had one for 10 years. She says frantically, "NO, NO, NO. I don't want a shot. I do have a right to refuse, you know." Your initial response is:

    A. You need the shot to prevent infection. It's for your safety.

    B. Yes, you do have the right to refuse. Tell me why you don't want the tetanus shot.

    C. If you refuse, we are not liable if you develop an infection.

    D. You haven't had a tetanus shot in 10 years. You really need this protection against infection.

Now, let's use this test item as a tool to exercise our reasoning skills in the cognitive turnstile of our thinking template (Figure 5–1). What assumptions did you make in answering this question? What inferences can you draw? What implications and consequences can you foresee for this patient? Does creative reasoning come into play? Write several new questions, using short-essay format. For example, describe in approximately 150 words how one's point of view or frame of reference can be used as an element of thought in the reasoning process for this test item.

Effective communication is very important in this situation. Effective communication requires putting yourself in the patient's paradigm of thinking, the patient's frame of reference, and getting inside the other person's head and seeing it from her point of view. Your point of view may be faulty, may be based on erroneous assumptions, and may not connect with your patient's thinking. Effective communication requires critical listening. The only choice that satisfies this line of thinking is choice **B.** In selecting this option, you are acknowledging her perceived right rather than contradicting her. You are also entering her point of view by asking her why she does not want a tetanus shot.

This assessment will provide additional insight into her thinking to guide you in your next step. In this stem, you don't have enough information to know whether the other options might be appropriate. If her refusal is a matter of not understanding the purpose of a tetanus shot, option A might be a follow-up action. However, at the moment, your patient is apparently frantic and highly emotional, and a reasoning approach (options **A** and **D**) would not be an effective first action. Option **C** is a last resort action and would be selected only to inform the patient of a liability status if she ultimately refused the tetanus protection.

The next example features clarity and accuracy and relevancy as essential intellectual standards by which we maximize our ability to skillfully use inferential thinking. When you read a test question, you must clearly and accurately recognize the purpose and intent of the question before you attempt to answer it. Response options must have relevance to the situation. Consider the following question:

A 32-year-old man presents with a headache. He complains of no energy and weakness for the past two days. He has no upper respiratory infection.

All vital signs are normal. Which of the following assessment data would you seek next?

A. Blood glucose
B. Throat culture
C. Drug screen
D. White blood count

As a nurse, if you ask the right questions during your assessment and gather all pertinent data, you can structure and organize information to facilitate an accurate diagnosis and to clearly define the problem. Your inferential thinking would be: if he has a headache, is weak, and has no energy, he could be hypoglycemic. Therefore, a blood glucose level would be helpful **(A)**. A throat culture is not indicated, because there are no signs of infection, sore throat, or elevated temperatures. A drug screen and white blood count have no relevance to the situation. The logical answer is **A.**

The purpose of this question is to determine whether you can recognize a specific clinical portrait or set of symptoms, and whether you can then accurately use inferential thinking to reach a logical conclusion. That conclusion would be a determination of which additional data are relevant and would be most useful in assisting the physician in making an accurate diagnosis and in clearly defining the patient's health care problem.

The following test item demonstrates the use of assumptions based on fragmented rather than complete information. Assumptions are the starting points of our thinking—that which we take for granted. Assumptions can be based on what we know is true and accurate. But they can also be based on faulty reasoning. Here's an example:

An elderly man with advanced stage emphysema has a CO_2 level of 75. He is aware of the CO_2 level and asks the nurse what it means.

Before you respond to the question, state your interpretation of this patient's condition. This question was posed individually to three nurses. Each nurse responded, "He can't possibly live with a CO_2 level that high." This response suggests a lack of understanding of acid-base dynamics and a faulty assumption that the CO_2 level can be interpreted separately from other values. An appropriate response would be a question, such as "What is the pH value and bicarbonate (HCO_3) value?" It is not possible to make an accurate interpretation without these values. Each nurse's response was based on faulty inferential reasoning—that if the patient has a very high CO_2 level he will not live. The patient's blood gas values were:

$$pH\ 7.35;\ CO_2\ 75;\ HCO_3\ 49$$

His body is compensating at this time. The HCO_3 rises to bring the pH into normal range.

Let's look at this question again with four options this time:

An elderly man with advanced stage emphysema has a CO_2 level of 75. He is aware of the CO_2 level and asks the nurse, "What does this mean?" How will you respond?

A. How do you feel now?
B. Let's see first what your other blood gas values are.
C. We'd better start your oxygen to bring that CO_2 down.
D. Your CO_2 is quite high. It really concerns me.

You do not have enough information in this stem to make an accurate interpretation. You cannot assume information that is not provided. So the correct response is **B**—seek more information. Option **A** will not provide the necessary information. Choice **C** is incorrect—in fact, it could be harmful. Choice **D** is not an effective response and is not a therapeutic response.

Test items are effective tools to use in discussion groups to promote higher level thinking. Learners can debate, discuss, and defend their thinking in discussion with each other to enhance understanding and promote retention.

Critical thinking is a skill that can be cultivated. Simply pay attention to your thinking patterns, carefully examine the choices you make, and always evaluate the results you get. Ask questions regularly and your intellectual skills will soon soar to new heights. Welcome to the network of independent thinkers!

References

Covey, S. (1989). *Seven Habits of Highly Effective People.* New York: Simon & Schuster.

Paul, R. (1993). *Critical Thinking, How to Prepare Students for a Rapidly Changing World.* Foundation for Critical Thinking.

Porth, C., & Erickson, M. (1992). *Physiology of Thirst and Drinking.* Heart & Lung, 21–23; 273–284.

Yura, H., Ozimek, D., & Walsh, M. (1976). *Nursing leadership, Theory and Process,* New York, Appleton-Century-Crafts.

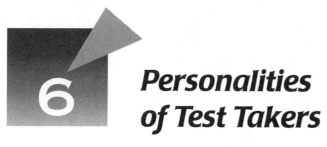

Personalities
of Test Takers

NANCY KORCHEK

Throughout our lives, demands to obtain and process knowledge, develop skills and insights, and synthesize solutions and strategies are placed upon us as growing individuals. As young children, we are challenged by the intricate handwork of tying a shoe lace. At school age, we are at first baffled by the complexity of long division. Approaching adulthood, we attempt to conquer the intangibles of geometry, theology, or a foreign language.

Learning that occurs in the very early years tends to occur on a continuum with maturation. If a child has difficulty learning to balance on a bicycle and ride independently at the age of four years, it is most likely because he or she has not yet achieved the developmental or maturational level required. However, after frequent falls and multiple attempts, the child at the age of five years will acquire the skill of bike riding and then maintain that skill throughout life. Learning, then, occurs over a period of time, on a continuum with the maturation and development of the growing child. There is no mandate—no timeframe—limiting the learning period.

In the academic environment, mandates such as timeframes *do* exist. Learning is often quantified for measure by framing a set of chapters, a period of weeks, or a series of lectures, and by means of regularly scheduled examinations. The adult student in the academic environment becomes acutely aware that tests mandate achievement and accomplishment within a set period of time. It is easy to understand, then, that students may come to fear examinations or to view them as hurdles in the learning process that must be overcome in order to continue onward through the chosen course of study.

Nursing educational systems not only mandate accomplishment of specific concepts and content within preset timeframes, they require *application* of the newly acquired knowledge almost immediately. The nursing student is expected to utilize new knowledge of nursing principles and actions gathered in the classroom to make decisions about patient care in the clinical setting. The transfer of practice in the laboratory to practice in the clinical setting is most often a very rapid one for the student nurse, mandating a rapid processing of newly acquired knowledge. An additional stressor is placed upon the student nurse by the realization that errors in practice could well be harmful to a human patient. The learner, then, naturally begins to identify testing in nursing as a potential barrier or as a possible threat, and test-related anxiety is a natural consequence of that perception.

Since the national licensure examination is that series of tests by which the student nurse verifies his or her achievements and abilities as a professional nurse, and thereby receives licensure to practice in the health-care setting, the examinee must face and cope with an unyielding timeline—the few weeks between graduation from a program of nursing and the dates for the licensure examination. The purpose of this chapter is to explore some typical reactions to the stresses of testing that students might use in order to cope with test-related anxiety. Suggestions for controlling undesirable testing behaviors are identified. The reader should attempt to identify how he or she *personally* copes with testing by relating his or her own behaviors to those of the test-taking personalities discussed in this chapter. With new insight into testing behaviors, the reader may practice more successful or appropriate testing behaviors, which will ultimately result in better performance on the licensure examination for nursing.

"The Rusher"

The Rusher is an individual who hurries through the entire process of taking an examination in a desperate rush to complete the test before essential facts that have been studied are forgotten. The Rusher arrives at the testing room one-half hour early, waits anxiously outside, and mumbles tidbits of information that are rapidly becoming confused and jumbled. "Let's see . . . if the pH goes up, the CO_2 goes down . . . or is it the other way around? Well then, what does the HCO_3 do? Up? Down? Left? Right?" The anxiety that the Rusher experiences as she readies for the examination causes her body to tighten up, and she prepares to begin the test while entwining her legs around the base of her seat and taking a vicelike grip on her pencil. While most students are just completing the first few items, the Rusher is already one third of the way through with the exam.

He or she flies through each item and circles a chosen response as quickly as possible, prompted not only by his or her fear of forgetting information, but also by the physiological forces that take hold when anxiety occurs—racing pulse, rapid respirations, and neuromuscular excitement. It's a sure bet that the Rusher will be the first person to complete the exam and will hurry out of the testing room as quickly as he or she entered. Once away from the testing situation, the test-related anxiety decreases, and the Rusher experiences feelings of exhaustion, both physiological and mental.

The problem that the Rusher experiences while racing through the examination is that he or she is unable to read carefully and completely each situation and question. He or she is at high risk for misreading, misinterpreting, and mistaking, because the focus of attention is on getting *through* the test—finishing it—rather than accepting and *taking* the test. If the Rusher encounters a difficult item that he or she is not readily able to answer, anxiety to complete the examination is heightened, and he or she is likely to quickly pick a guessed response to the question simply to continue moving through the exam.

The Rusher should employ two techniques to alter rushing behaviors in testing situations. First, he or she should practice progressive relaxation exercises while preparing for the scheduled examination, in order to reduce feelings of increasing anxiety as the test time approaches. Secondly, the Rusher should develop a plan of study prior to the examination that will allow ample time for the review of important concepts and content, thereby eliminating the need to "cram" just prior to the test, and reducing testing anxiety significantly. The Rusher may also find it helpful to practice test-taking strategies at home by taking sample test questions and attempting to slow down the pace of reading and answering them (Figure 6–1).

"The Turtle"

The Turtle, in contrast with the Rusher, does nothing fast when it comes to testing. Often fearful of missing important points or necessary details in items on an examination, the Turtle moves slowly, methodically, and deliberately through each question—reading and then rereading, underlining important points, scratching out unwanted responses, and then rereading the item to check over the selected response. Although it might seem at first that this careful process would help the examinee to perform better on the test, such may not be the case. Turtles often are the last to finish an examination, *if* in fact they are able to complete the examination at all. Typically the Turtle has far too many questions to complete in the limited time period left, and thus must hasten through a last series of items and quickly jot down an answer, any answer, for each. Turtles, then, tend to score much better in the first section of a test than in the last, having taken undue time and caution in the first section and leaving insufficient time for the last section.

The average multiple choice examination is designed to allow 1 minute per item. Simple, straightforward items will require 20 to 30 seconds, leaving a bit of extra time to answer more difficult or complex items. Turtles may take up to 60 or 90 seconds simply to read the questions, however, needing additional time to select the correct responses. Turtles, then, tend to have great difficulty finishing the entire examination within the set time limitations, and thus their scores suffer, not from lack of knowledge or poor preparation, but from lack of time and inability to complete all of the examination items.

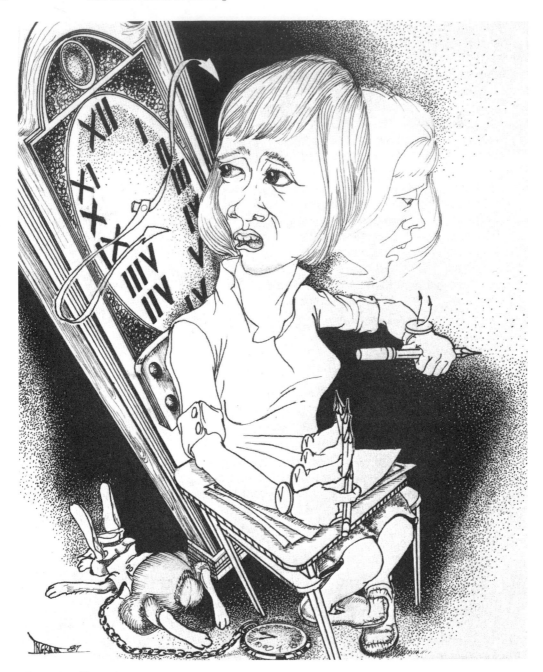

Figure 6-1. The rusher.

Turtles can best overcome the tendency to test too slowly by taking practice tests at home, focusing on the time spent on each item. With continued practice in reading and answering items, the Turtle should note an increase in speed and comprehension in reading. He or she would also benefit by wearing a watch with a large face and easy-to-read numbers, in order to remain aware of the passage of minutes during testing. To reduce wasted time in moving the wrist to glance at the watch, he or she should place the watch on the desk. Finally, the Turtle should make a mental note of the total number of items on the examination in conjunction with the total time allotted for the examination, and mark on the test sheet approximately where in the test he or she should be halfway through the test period. This will allow adequate time to complete all the questions on the test in an unhurried and relaxed manner.

"The Personalizer"

The Personalizer is most often an older, more mature graduate who has gained personal knowledge and insight more through undergoing life experiences than through formal, structured education. Although experiential learning is indeed valuable and often leaves a more lasting impression than classroom or laboratory settings may provide, there is an inherent risk in relying upon what one has learned through observation and experience only. The graduate nurse preparing for the licensure examination who attempts to understand broad concepts and applications based upon experience with a limited population in practice faces a great risk for developing false understandings and stereotypes about larger populations. Personalizers can easily err in testing situations, because their personal beliefs and experiences may not, in fact, be the norm, the standard, or the expected.

The national licensure examination for registration of nurses maintains set standards of nursing practice in its questions for the examinee. The focus is placed on an expected duty of care owed to selected patients, and the examinee must be able to choose appropriate measures to provide that expected duty of care. The Personalizer who relies upon personal exposure to patients and clinical situations may have significant difficulty in identifying the expected measures for meeting the standard or the duty of care owed to a selected patient.

Consider the following example: An examination item requires the reader to identify an appropriate nursing intervention for the patient undergoing detoxification from alcohol toxicity. The Personalizer's thought process might be:

When I was in my Psych rotation at County Hospital, I had a patient who was going through alcohol detox, and I remember that he became very agitated and combative, and the staff was really worried that he would become violent. They didn't want him to hurt anyone—they put him in restraints—that's the right answer, then! It's **C.** Place the patient in leather restraints.

What appears in this example to be a process of deductive reasoning based upon life experiences and personal clinical exposure is in reality faulty thinking and even stereotyping. The Personalizer relied upon personal exposure to the detoxifying patient rather than on the standards for care for that type of patient. It is *not* considered standard or expected practice to place the detoxifying patient in restraints, because this may serve only to agitate the patient more. In this example, the Personalizer reflected upon an experience she had as a student. Unfortunately, the care delivered to the remembered client was incorrect and inappropriate, in violation of a standard practice for that type of patient. In selecting responses in the examination based upon personal experience and exposure, the Personalizer erred and thus selected the incorrect response.

The Personalizer can best alter this pattern of test-taking by focusing on the broad principles and standards that guide and support nursing actions. The Personalizer should avoid making mental connections between patients in case situations included on an examination and individual patients whom she may have met in practice. Even though the experience of illness is unique for each individual, many generalities occur among certain types of patients, thus allowing health care givers to predict patient needs and anticipate care requirements. The Personalizer should focus on the generalities about the type of patient, and formulate decisions in testing situations based on standards of care established for nursing practice.

"The Squisher"

The Squisher is an individual who views an examination as a hurdle to jump, a barrier to cross, and a threat to self-esteem, rather than as a natural and expected event in a course of study. Squishers tend to be very preoccupied with grades, placing great value on personal accomplishment and fearing personal failure. Since a testing situation may result in less than desired achievement, or even worse, in failure, the Squisher attempts to avoid the responsibility and accountability associated with the testing experience, thus reducing anxiety over failure to reach a personally determined level of achievement (Figure 6–2).

Rather than pursuing a plan of ongoing study and preparation for an examination, the Squisher faces an upcoming test with an attitude of "I'll worry about it tomorrow." The defense mechanism of suppression (placing an anxiety-causing event out of the mind and away from immediate thought) is overused by the Squisher, resulting in the development of "mental lists" for test study and preparation that are never fully actualized.

Typical mental lists of the Squisher personality include the following thoughts:

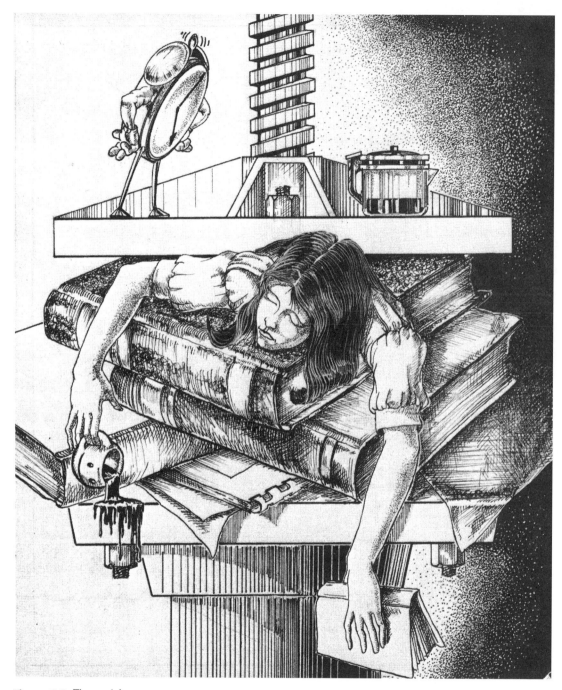

Figure 6-2. The squisher.

> The test is in 2 weeks. I'll do the required readings this weekend.
>
> Well, I can always read the textbook during the following week.
>
> I'm sure I won't need to do the readings if I review my class notes very thoroughly.
>
> I'll take a peek at the class notes this weekend before the exam, so the material will be fresh in my mind.
>
> I'll probably remember the material even better if I study the morning of the test.
>
> Gosh, the test is in 2 hours! What should I do? I'll flip through my notebook and hope for the best!

The pattern of avoidance behavior exhibited by the Squisher in the above scenario clearly demonstrates this individual's inability to cope with the uncertainties of examinations and the associated feelings of performance anxiety. The Squisher spends excess time and psychic energy in planning avoidance *of* the examination, rather than simply preparing *for* the examination. Unfortunately, pretest anxiety increases as the actual examination approaches, and the ability of the human mind to absorb facts, organize knowledge, and correlate information markedly decreases. The Squisher thus attempts to "squish" knowledge into his or her mind just before the examination, when the mind's ability to learn and process new knowledge is at its lowest level. The feelings of anxiety prior to the test are thus actually exacerbated by the increasing anxiety and guilt generated by avoidance behavior that inhibits the ability to learn, perform, and succeed.

The Squisher can best correct these inappropriate, personally hazardous behaviors by setting a plan for progressive, disciplined study. A prescription for study and test preparation should be devised, with defined timeframes identified for completion of a unit of study. The Squisher consequently will not view the process of test preparation as an overwhelming one, but rather, as a step-by-step process that can be readily accomplished and completed. Just as an Olympic athlete must train for competition through consistent and progressive practice, so too the Squisher can "train" for the testing experience through consistent and progressive study.

"The Philosopher"

The Philosopher is typically a talented, thoughtful, intelligent student who has enjoyed a successful academic career, mainly as a result of persistent, disciplined, and well-structured study. The Philosopher places a high value on understanding, or at least on recognizing the complexities of a situation, but somehow never really believes that he or she knows *enough* about a topic or subject. Thus, when placed in a testing situation, he or she tends to "pore over" selected questions with great intensity and concentration, looking for underlying, hidden meanings of the items. The Philosopher studies an item with undue care and caution, searching for an unstated intent or "trick" in the question. It is quite likely that she has been told by her faculty or colleagues that she "reads into" the questions on examinations, yet has great difficulty reading items for the obvious content and intent of the questions.

Philosophers are easy to recognize in a testing situation, because much of the philosophic, "searching" process is evidenced in their outward behavior. They have a tendency to stroke their chins while studying an item, calling to mind images of a famous statue, *The Thinker.* Often, they will look all around the test room or stare upward toward the ceiling, deep in thought, unaware of others around them. Inevitably, they begin to lose sight of the actual intent of an item, overanalyzing even simple or straightforward questions, and reading information *into* an item that does not exist. They answer questions, then, with their own additional information added, rather than according to the intent of the original question.

The mental process of a Philosopher answering the question "What pancreatic hormone does a diabetic patient lack?" would be as follows:

> Okay, well, the patient with diabetes does not manufacture insulin in his pancreas. So, it seems reasonable that the answer is insulin. But that seems so *obvious.* Maybe this is a trick question. I wonder if this question is really talking about the adult onset or Type II diabetic. Then the answer would not be insulin. Maybe the diabetic could be managed on diet alone, and wouldn't need insulin. Of course, the pancreas also manufactures glucagon. Glucagon raises blood sugar. Does the diabetic manufacture glucagon? Well, since his pancreas does not function correctly, he probably doesn't. It *was* a trick question! The answer is *definitely* glucagon!

The obvious answer *is* insulin. The *correct* answer is insulin. The Philosopher chose the correct answer at first, but after overstudying the item, eventually chose an incorrect response. In the effort to allay anxieties over not knowing *everything,* or not understanding completely enough, the Philosopher actually developed a misconception about the intent of the above question, and will inevitably end up feeling even greater anxiety upon discovering that the chosen response was, in fact, an incorrect one.

The Philosopher can best correct this inappropriate testing behavior by progressively developing self-esteem and self-confidence so that there will be less tendency to question initial responses to test questions. The Philosopher must learn to focus on the items *as they are written,* and avoid the tendency to read an item over and over, adding information or meanings unintended by the test authors. Continued practice with sample test items included in this book should help the graduate preparing for the State Board Examination to overcome "Philosopher" behavior (Figure 6–3).

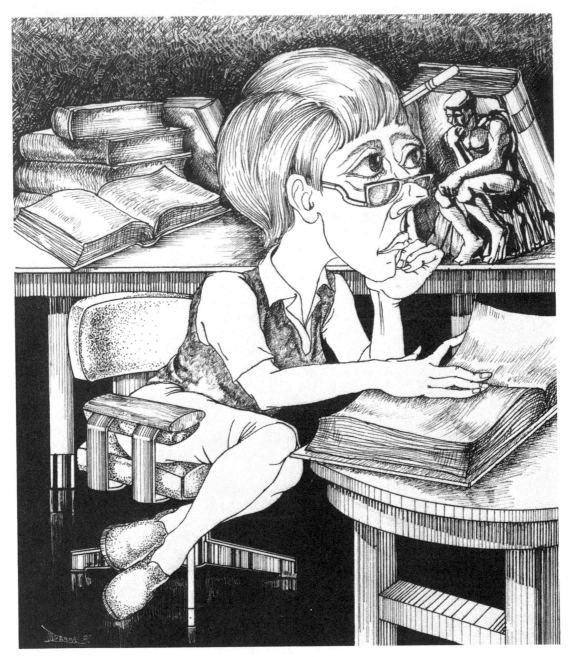

Figure 6-3. The philosopher.

"The Second Guesser"

The Second Guesser attempts to forestall feelings of anxiety in testing situations by playing the roles of both student and teacher, examinee and examiner. First, the Second Guesser carefully answers each question on the examination, taking the role of examinee. Then, however, he or she assumes the role of examiner and grades her own examination. This individual believes that a second look at each answered question will allow him or her to "catch" any possible error, and so the individual proceeds through the completed examination, changing initial responses throughout. In a sense, this person is "grading" his or her own test, playing the role of examiner.

Of course, the Second Guesser cannot with certainty know each answer to each question. But erasing the believed incorrect response and filling in a second, supposedly correct response gives the individual a sense of control, thus reducing testing anxiety. Unfortunately, the examinee is far more likely to respond correctly to a question with a first answer than after repeating the item and altering the initial response. When a human experiences anxiety, the perceptual field narrows, and the ability to think clearly, logically, and reasonably wanes. For this reason, the Second Guesser, experiencing increasing levels of anxiety while progressing through the examination, is likely to have greater difficulty processing information and formulating correct responses when going through the examination the second time and "correcting" it. The pencil eraser that seems to be his or her greatest ally in "fixing" responses on a test becomes in fact the biggest foe. Invariably, the Second Guesser will comment after receiving a graded examination, "Gosh! I had it right, but then I changed it to the wrong answer. I did that on about five of my questions!"

Second Guessers likewise court danger in testing by changing selected responses because they "seem" wrong—they don't fit into a pattern, or there is too much repetition of the same response. This individual becomes ill at ease when, rereading the examination answers, he or she notes six **B** responses in a row, or too many *True* answers. Convinced that it is an error to have so many answers in one pattern, he or she randomly changes one or two initial responses, forming a new pattern of response that seems more acceptable.

The Second Guesser can easily alter this nonproductive behavior by rereading *only* the few items he or she is very unsure of, and avoiding erasing or changing any initial response unless absolutely necessary. The examinee should focus on moving through the examination progressively and carefully, without setting aside the end of the examination period for rereading and "grading" behaviors (Figure 6–4).

"The Lawyer"

The hallmark characteristic of a good attorney is the ability to carefully formulate questions in order to get the most valuable and informational responses. An attorney will attempt to get at the truth of a situation by following a successive series of

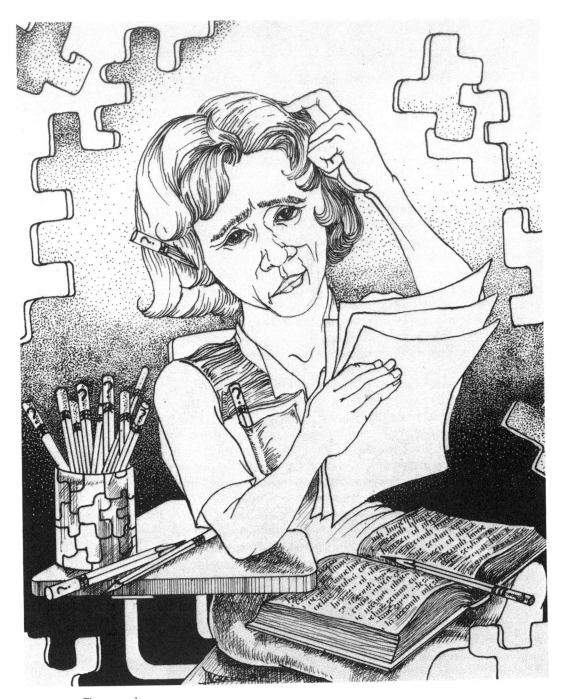

Figure 6-4. The second guesser.

questions that ultimately lead to the needed or desired answers. When the lawyer oversteps appropriateness in his questioning and attempts to place ideas or words into the witness's responses that the witness did not intend, the lawyer will be called upon for *leading the witness.*

It seems that communication questions, especially when placed in psychosocial settings, bring the "lawyer" out in many test takers. When presented with a situation of nurse-patient or nurse-family interchange that requires selection of the most appropriate nurse response, examinees often veer away from obviously appropriate responses and select responses that place words or ideas into the patient's statements that were not really intended. The examinee who attempts to get at the truth or reality of what a patient is saying by choosing a "leading the witness" response is only *providing his own view* of the truth.

Consider the example below:

> *Patient:*   Life has been so difficult since my husband's death. I can't seem to get involved in anything. I feel so empty and lifeless.
>
> *Nurse response:*   Have you thought about suicide?

In this example, the nurse, in an effort to get at the reality of the patient's feelings and thoughts, oversteps appropriateness in her questioning, placing meaning into the patient's words that may not have been intended. Simply, the nurse in this example is "leading the witness," as a *lawyer* might, rather than seeking to help the patient to express herself, as a *nurse* should. The nurse did *not* verbalize the implied, because the patient never alluded to a desire to end her own life. Rather, the *nurse provided her view* of the patient's reality.

Let's try another example:

> *Patient:*   I'm nervous about this open heart surgery tomorrow. Do you think I'll be all right?
>
> *Nurse response:*   You seem terribly frightened. Perhaps you should talk with your surgeon about your fears.

Wow! If the patient wasn't frightened at first, he sure is now! The patient simply states his nervousness about impending surgery and seeks reassurance from the nurse. The nurse, however, oversteps the real meaning of what the patient is saying and "leads the witness" to feelings of being "terribly frightened." Exaggerating the patient's feelings into intense fear may well cause the patient considerable emotional upset, an undesired effect of communication, especially just prior to a major surgery.

The Lawyer needs to focus on listening to the patient and hearing his or her thoughts and feelings, rather than on formulating responses targeted at getting certain information. Reflecting the patient's remarks is often a very effective way to encourage greater and fuller expression by the patient. Likewise, sharing observations made about the patient by the nurse can facilitate communication and ideally foster greater interaction between patient and nurse. Several helpful tips and examples of strategies that may be used by the examinee in answering communication questions are offered under the heading of "Communication" in a Chapter 18 of this book.

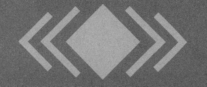

PART TWO

CONCEPTUAL FOUNDATIONS FOR NURSING PRACTICE

A Conceptual Model for Learning: Essentials for Health

MARIAN B. SIDES

The framework for the organization of this nursing review is based on the conceptual foundations of nursing practice. It applies the philosophy that human beings constantly aspire to achieve an optimal state of health. This state of being requires internal harmony among all the processes that contribute to human functioning.

Health occurs along a continuum from wellness to illness. Each of us falls somewhere along this continuum. Optimal health depends upon our ability to maintain a delicate internal balance while relating to the environment around us.

This section presents 16 core concepts that frame health and common deviations from health. Chapters are organized around the model illustrated in Figure 7–1.

Each chapter focuses on a fundamental health concept, such as oxygenation or acids and bases. Key principles for each concept are identified and illustrated in the text. Throughout, you will be led into thinking about how these concepts are acted out in the human body. Who is at risk for development of disease or illness? How are these manifested? What interventions are appropriate for regaining balance? How do you know when the balance has occurred? This strategy for reviewing nursing will make you an active, thinking participant in the nursing process. It guards against the rote memorization of materials and encourages the understanding and application of principles to new and different situations.

This review does not include detailed descriptions of every illness or disease. Certain broad concepts and principles are common to many disease and illness states. Once you become familiar with them, through use of this book, you will possess the skills that can be used to answer questions about most health situations.

Reasoning exercises in the form of test questions are provided to give you practice in mastering these concepts and applying the nursing process. If you

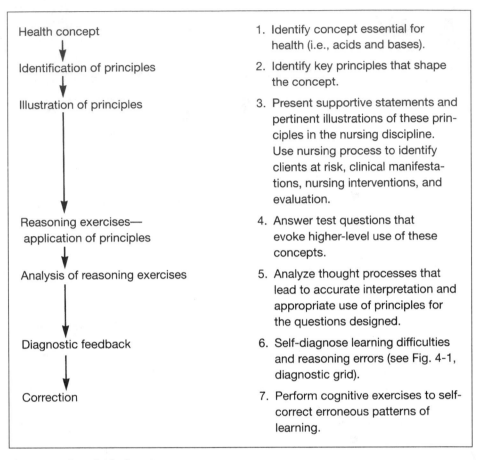

Figure 7-1. A model for learning.

have difficulty understanding the content in these chapters, you may need to consult a textbook to strengthen your knowledge base in these areas.

Be sensitive and alert to your strengths and weaknesses as you review. Analyze your performance by using the diagnostic grid to detect patterns.

A systematic and logical approach to this learning challenge will gradually bring you to mastery. It has worked for hundreds of nurses. It *will* work for *you!*

8

Oxygenation

MARYTHERESE PATRAS

Principle

To maintain oxygenation, the body requires a constant supply of O₂ and CO₂

Illustration of Principle

In order for the body to function, it is necessary that atmospheric oxygen (O_2) be inhaled and absorbed through the respiratory system. To understand this process, the nurse needs to be familiar with the structures involved in the respiratory system (see Figure 8–1).

The nose is the respiratory system's air filter and humidifier. Atmospheric oxygen (O_2) enters the respiratory system and passes through the larynx. The larynx is at the top of the trachea and includes the vocal cords. When breathing occurs, the vocal cords open, allowing the free passage of O_2 through the larynx into the trachea. The trachea branches into two mainstem bronchi that direct O_2 into several bronchioles, which then branch off into millions of sac-like alveoli. It is at this point, where alveoli meet blood capillaries, that gas exchange occurs. Oxygen is transported from the respiratory system to the circulatory system by this process for use by the body's cells. By a reversal of this process, carbon dioxide (CO_2) moves out of the cells into the respiratory system, and excess CO_2 is exhaled.

Respiration is the process that enables the exchange of O_2 and CO_2. During inspiration, contraction of the diaphragm and intercostal muscles occurs. The rib cage expands, creating a partial vacuum in the lungs. Because the pressure outside the body becomes greater than the pressure inside, air is drawn into the lungs.

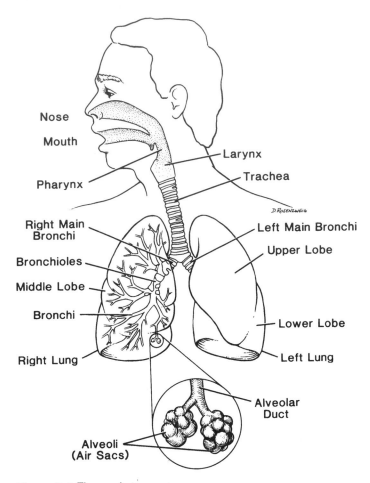

Figure 8-1. The respiratory system.

When the body is in a state of equilibrium and is disease-free, the amount of O_2 in the cells is balanced by the amount of O_2 transported by the blood to the tissues. The CO_2 transported out of the lungs matches the volume produced by the tissues. This exchange of gases is necessary to maintain optimal body functioning and oxygenation.

MEMORY JOGS

*I*n the healthy patient, adequate O_2 is inhaled, and excess CO_2 is exhaled.

This gas exchange can be measured by a blood gas sample that will indicate the patient's blood pO_2, pCO_2, and pH. Both acid–base abnormalities and respiratory abnormalities can be demonstrated by blood gas values, which are covered in detail in Chapter 11.

Principle

Oxygenation may be impaired when airways are affected by airway obstruction

Illustration of Principle

Airway obstruction can pose a threat to a patient's oxygenation. Airway obstruction is characterized by an increased resistance to flow in the airways of the lungs. This can result in variable degrees of dyspnea (difficulty breathing), easy fatigability, wheezing, and often a cough producing sputum. A disruption of oxygenation can occur upon acute airway obstruction (e.g., asthma) or during chronic airway obstruction (chronic bronchitis or emphysema). Nurses must always be aware of the patient's oxygenation and how it is affected by airway obstruction.

> *A*irway obstruction can be fully reversible in acute asthmatic attacks, but may not be reversible in chronic bronchitis or emphysema.

MEMORY JOGS

Bronchial asthma is characterized by intermittent airway obstruction and narrowing. This obstruction involves constriction of bronchial smooth muscle and mucosal edema that results in bronchospasm. When this occurs, oxygenation can become impaired.

Asthma can be either intrinsic or extrinsic. Intrinsic asthma is generally considered to be the result of the autonomic nervous system's response to an inhaled irritant, weather changes, infection, emotion, or exercise. Intrinsic asthma is thought to result from an imbalance in the actions of the sympathetic and parasympathetic nervous systems. Sympathetic stimulation relaxes bronchial smooth muscle; parasympathetic stimulation constricts bronchial smooth muscle. Increased parasympathetic stimulation results in hypersensitivity of the airways, which can trigger an asthma attack.

MEMORY
JOGS

*I*ntrinsic Asthma
Parasympathetic stimulation causes airway sensitivity and can trigger
an asthma attack.

Extrinsic asthma can be caused by external factors such as allergens. Pollen, dust, and feathers can often precipitate an asthma attack. In many asthmatic patients, the attack begins with a nonproductive cough, wheezing, chest tightness, and shortness of breath. Wheezing may be prolonged during expiration, as a result of airway obstruction. In severe attacks, wheezing may decrease as dyspnea increases. This is a dangerous signal that complete airway obstruction may occur. The nurse must be constantly aware of the physical signs of hypoxia, which can include the use of accessory respiratory muscles, such as the sternocleidomastoid in the neck and the intercostal muscles between the ribs. Because O_2 to the brain may be diminished, symptoms of acute restlessness, anxiety, and confusion may occur. A sedative should never be given to an asthmatic patient to alleviate anxiety. The administration of a sedative could lead to further depression of the patient's respiratory status.

MEMORY
JOGS

*N*o sedatives during asthmatic attacks.

Nonpharmaceutical measures should be taken by the nurse to reassure the patient. Asthmatic patients often become afraid that they will stop breathing and "need a tube to help me breathe." This is a genuine fear because many asthmatic patients can require intubation and may have been intubated previously for severe asthmatic attacks.

Nursing care of the asthmatic patient will often involve the administration of aminophylline, a bronchodilator. Aminophylline relaxes smooth muscle and dilates the bronchial tubes. This allows the patient to breathe easier, and oxygenation is improved. Aminophylline also stimulates the cardiac muscle and the central nervous system and can irritate the gastric mucosa. Palpitations, anxiety, restlessness, nausea, and vomiting are side effects of aminophylline and may indicate a higher-than-therapeutic level.

MEMORY
JOGS

*A*minophylline dilates the bronchioles and improves oxygenation.

The nurse must be continually aware of the patient's oxygenation status. An ongoing assessment of the patient's respiratory function should occur. The nursing assessment should include the degree of shortness of breath, the duration and severity of the attack, and the duration, severity, and frequency of past attacks. The general appearance of the patient must be assessed to determine the presence or absence of respiratory distress, inspiratory or expiratory wheezing, and accessory muscle use. Auscultation of the lungs should reveal the severity of the attack. In severe attacks, many patients may be moving so little air through their lungs that they have barely audible breath sounds and may be unable to speak in complete sentences. Another clinical sign that can be easily identified by the nurse is pulsus paradoxus. A pulsus paradoxus of greater than 10 millimeters (mm) of mercury (Hg) indicates a severe attack. It is present when the systolic blood pressure during inspiration is more than 10 mm Hg above that of expiration.

MEMORY JOGS

---

*S*evere Attack

Use of accessory muscles

Barely audible breath sounds

Pulsus paradoxus of greater than 10 mm Hg

All patients with asthma must be carefully observed by the nurse to detect any decrease in oxygenation and worsening of hypoxemic signs and symptoms. The nurse's ongoing assessment can be invaluable in recognizing and preventing the progression of asthma attacks.

Principle

Oxygenation may become impaired when the respiratory system is affected by disease, resulting in damage to lung function

Application of Principle

In order for the cells and the tissues they comprise to function effectively, they must have adequate O_2. The adequacy of oxygenation, or the process by which O_2 is delivered to the cells and tissues, depends on three interrelated factors: O_2, hemoglobin, and cardiac output. The presence of O_2 requires sufficient cardiac output to deliver oxygenated blood and an adequate amount of functional hemoglobin.

*N*eeds
Adequate oxygenation depends on:
Cardiac output
Hemoglobin
O_2

In chronic respiratory disease, a permanent alteration in O_2 delivery occurs. Chronic diseases of the respiratory system generally limit the O_2 supply to the tissues, creating a state of chronic hypoxia. Chronic hypoxia occurs slowly and continues over a long period of time. The body is able to adjust to this limited O_2 supply—to a point. In most cases, there are no obvious symptoms of chronic hypoxia. When acute exacerbations of chronic respiratory disease occur, however, signs and symptoms result. There may be fatigue, shortness of breath on exertion, and a general feeling of being less able to carry out the activities of daily living.

Chronic obstructive pulmonary disease (COPD) is the most common chronic respiratory condition in which chronic hypoxia occurs. COPD refers to a group of diseases (chronic bronchial asthma, chronic bronchitis, and emphysema) that are characterized by increased airway resistance. These result in varying degrees of dyspnea, easy fatigability, wheezing, and a productive cough. These symptoms may be the same as in acute obstruction, but are much more ominous in chronic disease. The nurse must be alert for underlying chronic illness when confronted with acute symptoms.

*C*OPD is characterized by:
Increased airway resistance
Dyspnea
Fatigability
Wheezing
Productive cough

Chronic bronchitis is a continual inflammation of the lining of the respiratory bronchioles. Normally, the bronchioles are open and elastic. They allow and aid O_2 to move in and out of the lungs, ensuring proper oxygenation.

In chronic bronchitis, diseased bronchioles are narrowed by chronic inflammation. As a result of the inflammation, airway obstruction and excessive mucus production develop. Mucus replaces surfactant, a substance manufactured by respiratory cells that is necessary to decrease the surface tension of the airways. Without surfactant, these airway passages lose their stability and tend to collapse easily. One of the first symptoms of chronic bronchitis is a recurrent productive cough. Shortness of breath on exertion progresses over years. Chronic airway narrowing and obstruction are the end results (see Figure 8–2).

Emphysema is another chronic lung disease in which patients experience chronic hypoxia. Emphysema is defined in anatomic terms. It is present when

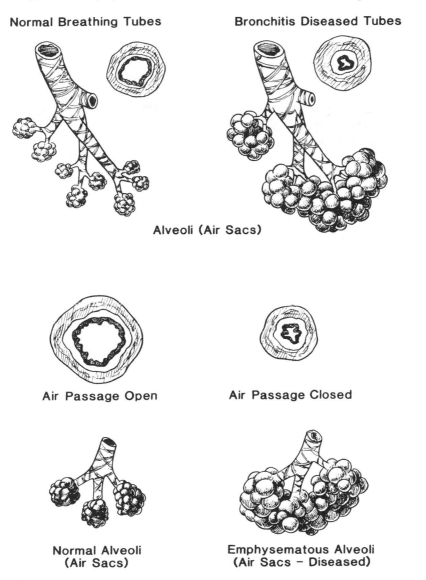

Figure 8-2. The bronchi (breathing tubes).

there is a permanent abnormal enlargement of any part or all of the alveoli. Their many thin elastic walls are destroyed, leaving much larger air sacs and less surface area through which to exchange gases (see Figure 8–2). The result is that the lungs cannot deflate and expand as they should normally, and air trapping occurs. Patients are forced to breathe through pursed lips to try to eliminate the excess air. It becomes more difficult to blow air out than to breathe it in. Constant shortness of breath is the end clinical result.

Cigarette smoking is thought to be a major contributor to the development of chronic bronchitis and emphysema. Tobacco irritates airways and produces excess mucus and airway obstruction. Air pollution and occupational exposure also may be contributing factors.

While caring for the patient with chronic respiratory disease, nurses can take several therapeutic roles. First, they can encourage patients to stop smoking. Second, because nicotine in cigarettes is addictive, nurses must be aware of the signs and symptoms of withdrawal: headache, nausea, anxiety, and restlessness. These symptoms can parallel symptoms of hypoxia; therefore, a good history and evaluation of the patient's respiratory status must be obtained. Third, nurses must understand and teach that smoking itself is an addiction for which the patient should not be blamed, but instead is an addiction which he or she, with the help of health professionals and loved ones, can fight against and win.

Nursing management must include an assessment of the patient's ability to remove secretions. Adequate hydration and mobilization of secretions, by suctioning, by chest physical therapy, or by encouraging the patient to cough are all essential. Continual evaluation of the patient's vital signs and identification of the signs and symptoms of pulmonary infection are necessary for the patient with COPD. Frequent assessment of the rate of respirations, their pattern, and their depth should be noted. Any changes in breathing must be continually assessed.

Principle

Oxygen therapy is necessary to restore oxygenation when oxygenation is impaired

Illustration of Principle

Oxygen is essential for life. All cells require adequate oxygenation to remain viable. The purpose of O_2 therapy is to increase the percentage of O_2 gas in the alveoli and pulmonary capillaries. Goals of O_2 delivery should be to prevent or reverse cellular hypoxia, to decrease the work of breathing, and to decrease the myocardial workload. Oxygen is a drug that MUST be administered carefully, properly, and safely. Too much O_2 can cause damage to the body. In patients with COPD, too much O_2 can eliminate the patient's drive to breathe (*hypoxic drive*) and allow CO_2 retention and respiratory depression.

Too much O_2 = decreased hypoxic drive

MEMORY JOGS

Nurses must have an adequate understanding of frequently used O_2 terms and modes of O_2 therapy.

Fraction of inspired O_2 (FiO_2) equals the percent of O_2 delivered to the lungs. Room air is a constant 21% O_2; therefore, room air is an FiO_2 of 21%. When patients require additional O_2, they can receive an FiO_2 from 24% to 100%. A blood-gas should always be obtained prior to O_2 administration unless it is a life-threatening situation.

High-flow O_2 is a system of O_2 delivery in which the total gas flow delivered to the patient is the only gas the patient is breathing. The advantage of high-flow O_2 systems is that they are reliable in delivering a precise amount of O_2. These systems cannot be influenced by the patient's breathing pattern.

Low-flow O_2 is a system that can deliver any O_2 concentration from 21% to 100%. These systems lack the accuracy and dependability of a high-flow O_2 system.

Nasal cannula is a low-flow O_2 system. Nasal prongs are placed in the nares of the patient. One to six liters of O_2 may be delivered to the patient. Oxygen delivery by nasal cannula should never exceed 6 liters because of nasal mucosal drying. The nurse must remember that because the patient also inhales room air, the precise fraction of inhaled O_2 is unknown. Therefore, the exact FiO_2 delivery cannot be determined when O_2 is given through a nasal cannula.

Simple O_2 mask is a low-flow system. A simple mask is placed over the patient's nose and mouth to deliver an FiO_2 at a range of 24% to 60%. This is the most common low-flow O_2 system.

Venturi mask is a high-flow system—a mask that fits over the patient's nose and mouth. It mixes O_2 and room air prior to delivery to the patient. It is the only mask available in which the exact amount of FiO_2 can be determined. This mask is indicated for the COPD patient.

Oxygen mask with a reservoir bag is a high-flow system. This mask can deliver 70% to 90% O_2 for the patient with severe hypoxia that cannot be corrected by other O_2 systems. This system is used most commonly in patients with smoke inhalation and CO_2 poisoning.

Endotracheal tube is a high-flow system. This requires that a tube be inserted into the trachea to the lungs to deliver as high as 100% O_2. Any concentration of O_2 can be delivered to the patient. In addition, intubation is the most effective method of O_2 administration for the severely hypoxic patient. Benefits of intubation include the prevention of aspiration and a direct route to suction patients.

Nurses must administer O_2 carefully because its effects can be damaging. It is critical that the nurse be knowledgeable as to the amount of O_2 that is appropriate for a given patient, depending on the clinical situation. Accurate O_2 delivery can correct hypoxia and assist the patient's recovery.

Reasoning Exercises: *Oxygenation*

1. Which of the following patients would correctly be placed in an orthopneic position?
   A. A patient having edema of the lower legs and ankles
   B. An elder patient who has fluid accumulation in the lungs
   C. A patient having a decubitus ulcer on the coccyx and buttocks
   D. An immobilized patient who has calf tenderness due to a thrombus

Intended Response: **B.** The suffix "pnea" refers to respiration and the prefix "ortho" refers to position. An orthopneic (Fowler's) position is used when individuals are unable to breathe unless in a sitting position. Persons with fluid accumulation in the lungs will have less dyspnea and respiratory difficulty if positioned upright in a sitting position.

2. Which of the following is a correct action of a nurse performing nasopharyngeal suctioning?
   A. Suction is applied during insertion of the catheter
   B. Suction is limited to 5–10 seconds duration
   C. Suctioning intervals are repeated every 5 minutes until clear
   D. The suction catheter is resterilized in alcohol after use

Intended Response: **B.** Oxygenation may be impaired when airways are affected by obstruction. Accumulation of respiratory secretions potentiates airway obstruction, causing a need for suctioning. In order to avoid removing excess oxygen while suctioning, suction is applied only upon removal of the catheter **A**, limited to 5–10 seconds duration, and repeated in as few intervals as possible **C**. As the trachea, bronchi, and lungs are considered sterile, use of a new, unused sterile catheter is required for this procedure.

3. While providing nasopharyngeal suctioning, the nurse hears the patient's pulse oximeter alarm sound. The pulse oximeter indicates the

patient's oxygen saturation reading is 86%. Which of the following actions should the nurse take?

   A. Continue suctioning for 10–15 more seconds and then withdraw suction catheter

   B. Keep the suction catheter inserted and wait a few seconds before beginning suctioning again

   C. Withdraw the suction catheter and instruct the patient to cough several times

   D. Discontinue suctioning and administer oxygen to the patient

Intended Response: **D.** A pulse oximeter provides patient data regarding oxygenation status. The drop in oxygen saturation from the expected range of 95–100% may indicate that the suctioning procedure has removed excess oxygen. The nurse should immediately discontinue suctioning and administer oxygen to resaturate arterial blood.

4. The chest x-ray of a patient with congestive heart failure indicates accumulation of fluid in bilateral lung bases. Which of the following acid–base imbalances is the patient at risk of developing?

   A. Metabolic acidosis

   B. Respiratory acidosis

   C. Metabolic alkalosis

   D. Respiratory alkalosis

Intended Response: **B.** Fluid accumulation in the bases of the lungs will interfere with gas exchange in the alveoli, causing a decrease in oxygenation and retention of carbon dioxide. As CO_2 mixed with H_2O creates carbonic acid, the patient is at risk for developing respiratory acidosis, and should be monitored for evidence of this acid–base imbalance.

5. The nurse is preparing to discharge home a patient with emphysema on oxygen therapy. Which of the following instructions regarding oxygen therapy should be included in the discharge plan?

   A. "It would be best for you to maintain a steady rate of flow of your oxygen using a nasal cannula."

   B. "You should rinse your oxygen tubing in sterile water once weekly."

   C. "Increase the flow rate of your oxygen to 4 or 5 liters if you are feeling short of breath."

   D. "Limit your intake of oral fluids to a minimum."

Intended Response: **A.** As the patient with emphysema experiences chronic hypoxia, it is important for oxygen therapy to be maintained at a steady low flow rate. Increasing the rate of flow of oxygen **C** is contraindicated, as alveolar air sacs will further overinflate and thus reduce or eliminate the stimulus to breathe (hypoxic drive). Oral fluids **D** are encouraged to liquify accumulated secretions in the respiratory tract, making it easier for the patient to cough and clear the airway. Oxygen tubing should be changed or replaced at regular intervals to prevent acquired infection of the respiratory tract.

6. A patient is admitted to the emergency room with suspected left pneumothorax secondary to a motor vehicle accident chest trauma. Which of the following clinical manifestations would correlate with this suspected diagnosis?
   A. Diminished breath sounds on both sides of the chest
   B. Congested respirations in the right mid-thoracic region
   C. Absent breath sounds on the left side of the chest
   D. Bilateral wheezes upon inspiration

Intended Response: **C.** Deflation of a lung in pneumothorax prevents air from entering the lung, resulting in the absence of breath sounds over the affected area.

7. The nurse is counseling a mother of a child with laryngotracheobronchitis (LTB) regarding care of the child in the home. Which of the following instructions to the mother would be most effective in dilating the child's airway?
   A. Place the child in a hot, steamy shower stall
   B. Position the child for sleep sitting up in a comfortable chair
   C. Place a cool, moist humidifier in the child's room
   D. Administer an over-the-counter cough suppressant

Intended Response: **C.** Cool, moist humidification of room air is the ideal method of dilating airway passages; correspondingly, heated air has not proven effective. Positioning the child in an upright position will have little effect on ventilation, as it has no effect on airway constriction. A cough suppressant could worsen this condition by increasing airway congestion.

8. The nurse is counseling a mother providing care in the home to an infant with laryngotracheobronchitis (LTB) regarding signs and symptoms of respiratory distress. The nurse should instruct the mother to monitor for which of the following?

A. Use of accessory muscles and nasal flaring

B. Frequent crying and frantic sucking motions

C. Generalized muscle weakness and serous nasal discharge

D. Fever and respiratory congestion

Intended Response: **A.** Both use of accessory muscles and nasal flaring indicate the body's effort to increase intake of oxygen in respiratory distress. An ability to cry **B** indicates that the child has oxygen intake through the tracheal airway, and is thus not a sign of respiratory distress. Neither serous nasal discharge ("runny nose") nor fever are indicative of distress; respiratory congestion **D** is expected in LTB and does not indicate distress.

9. The nurse is caring for a newly ventilated patient receiving 40% FiO_2. Which of the following laboratory values would be most important for the nurse to check in determining the effectiveness of this intervention?

A. Red blood cell count

B. Arterial blood gases

C. Platelet count

D. Serum electrolytes

Intended Response: **B.** Arterial blood gases will indicate the effectiveness of oxygenation interventions by means of pO_2 and oxygenation saturation values. If the FiO_2 setting of 40% was an inadequate percentage of oxygen for the patient in this situation, the patient's arterial blood gases would reveal continued inadequate oxygenation by means of low oxygen and saturation values.

10. A patient with chronic obstructive pulmonary disease (COPD) complains of feeling short of breath. Which of the following interventions would be most beneficial?

A. Place the patient in Fowler's position

B. Instruct the patient to take full, deep inhalations

C. Increase flow of oxygen per nasal cannula to 6 L/min

D. Use a Venturi mask at a 32% FiO2

Intended Response: **D.** A Venturi mask which delivers a set FiO_2 percentage is ideal for the patient with COPD and would be most beneficial in relieving the sensation of shortness of breath. Oxygen per nasal cannula **C** must be at a low rate of flow (2–3 L/min) to prevent depression of the hypoxic drive stimulus to breathe.

A patient with COPD is unable to take full deep respirations because of the patho-physiologic changes of this disease. Instructing a patient with COPD to sit up and lean over A a bedside table allows for better oxygenation with less respiratory effort.

Reference

Cahill S, Balskus M. *Intervention in Emergency Nursing: The First 60 Minutes.* Rockville, MD, Aspen Systems Corp, 1986.

Circulation

NANCY KORCHEK

Principle
All human cells require O₂ for life

Illustration of Principle

A basic essential for cellular viability and function is O_2. Regardless of type, structure, or role of the cell, O_2 is *critical* to life. When cells are deprived of a ready and adequate supply of O_2, even for a brief period of time, cellular integrity and viability are compromised.

> *J*ust as an automobile engine, even if in prime condition, cannot function without adequate input of gasoline as fuel, the human cell cannot function without adequate input of O_2.

MEMORY JOGS

Thus, nurses must always be concerned with the adequacy of the patient's oxygenation and be constantly aware of any factors that could interrupt O_2 transport by the extensive circulatory system. Such factors can range from prolonged placement of a forearm tourniquet during IV insertion to the more complex congestive heart failure with secondary circulatory collapse.

*I*nterruption of O_2 supply to body tissues will result in cellular damage or death.

The principle that all human cells require O_2 for life can be applied in a virtually limitless number of clinical situations. For example, the patient on complete bed rest, who cannot turn and reposition himself or herself, will develop circulation-related complications, perhaps most obviously in the skin layers. Prolonged pressure on the patient's sacral or gluteal areas will result in an impairment of oxygen-rich blood flow. As the tissues of the skin layers are deprived of adequate O_2, degenerative changes and cellular damage occur, progressing from *ischemia* (temporary anemia) to eventual *necrosis* (tissue death). The formation of *decubitus ulcers* is evidence of circulatory impairment.

*D*ecubitus ulcers are caused by prolonged pressure to an area of the body, which impairs circulation of O_2.

The same tissue death that occurs in decubitus ulcers occurs in *myocardial infarction*. The human heart uses O_2 at a greater amount and rate than any other organ in the human body. Any factor that interrupts oxygen-rich blood flow through the coronary arteries, then, will result in damage or even death to cells of the cardiac muscle. Similarly, brain cells deprived of essential O_2 as a result of thrombosis or rupture of a cerebral vessel will infarct, as in cerebrovascular accident. Thus, even though most signs and effects of cerebrovascular accident are *neurologic*, the process itself is very much *circulatory*.

A final illustration of this principle is the dependence of a developing fetus on the adequate circulation of oxygen and nutrients by way of the maternal placental system. Should umbilical cord compression occur during labor, O_2 delivery by the placenta will be impaired, with resultant changes in fetal heart tones, indicating fetal distress or hypoxia. A prolonged decrease in fetal–maternal circulation can result in fetal cell damage, as in the various syndromes of cerebral palsy. Awareness of this principle guides the nurse to closely monitor both the progress of the mother through her labor and the response of the fetus to uterine contractions that might cause a decrease in fetal circulation or oxygenation.

*I*mpairment of the circulation of O_2 results in tissue damage.
Skin: Decubitus ulcer
Heart: Myocardial infarction
Brain: Cerebrovascular accident
Placenta: Fetal cell damage

MEMORY JOGS

Principle

The human heart is a two-sided or "double" pump generated by electricity

Illustration of Principle

The heart serves as the mechanical pump for blood flow in the human body. Activation of the pumping of fluid by way of ventricular contraction occurs in response to electrical stimulation of the muscle fibers of the ventricles by the sino-atrial (SA) node (pacemaker of the heart). The two sides of the heart, each composed of an atrial chamber and a ventricular chamber, allow blood flow from the body to progress through the oxygenation process in the lungs and then to be redistributed to the cells through simultaneous but separate phases of filling (diastole) and contraction/ejection (systole). The right heart receives blood from the body by way of the venous system, and then sends blood to the lungs for oxygenation. At the same time, the left heart receives blood from the lungs by the pulmonary vein, and then sends oxygen-rich blood back to the body through the aorta. The heart, then, is a "double" pump, allowing for two separate but simultaneous pumping actions to occur.

The atrium of the heart essentially serves as a "waiting area" for incoming blood, analogous to a waiting room in a busy physician's office. As more and more patients enter the waiting room, with fewer chairs available, congestion occurs. This congestion is much like the pressure that increases in the atrium as blood fills this chamber. When the waiting room becomes too crowded, patients are allowed through a door connecting the waiting room to the treatment areas, where the actual work with patients occurs. Similarly, when the atrium fills and pressure rises, a door between the atrium and ventricles opens to allow blood to leave one chamber and enter the other. These "doors" are termed *valves*; they open and close to facilitate passage of blood in a continuous direction through the cardiac cycle. In our analogy, the treatment areas of the office, where the work is carried out, are like the ventricles, which receive the blood, and after attaining adequate filling, do the "work" of systole (contraction), causing blood to move either to the lungs or to the aorta.

For the average adult patient with a heart rate of 70 beats/min, the above cardiac events occur in less than 1 second. It is very apparent, then, that each structure within the heart must function correctly in both its action and timing in order for the patient to maintain adequate cardiac output. *Cardiac output*, the volume of oxygenated blood ejected from the left ventricle every minute, is normally between 5 and 6 liters/min. Disease conditions or degenerative changes that interrupt the series of events occurring with each cardiac cycle will result in a compromised cardiac output, with subsequent loss of circulation of O_2 to the cells of the body.

For example, if the SA node malfunctions or fails, regulation of the mechanical or pumping action of the heart is affected. Since the SA node generates the electrical impulse that ultimately stimulates the muscles of the ventricles to contract, a deficit of SA node function will result in decreased excitation of the cardiac muscle with a subsequent decrease in cardiac output.

Likewise, valves within the heart that are *stenosed* (narrowed and inflexible) or *insufficient* (unable to fully open and close) will impair the full filling and emptying of the chambers of the heart, influencing cardiac output. Narrowing or stenosing of the mitral valve, for example, will result in a decrease in the volume of blood leaving the left atrium, with subsequent reduced filling of the left ventricle. With less blood filling, the left ventricle will contract, but less blood will be ejected, resulting in a decrease in cardiac output.

Finally, myocardial infarction provides another excellent example of how disease-related changes can negatively influence the critical activities of the heart.

Myocardial infarction muscle damage occurring secondary to impaired oxygenation reduces the ability of the muscle to contract forcefully enough to eject blood effectively. The infarcted muscle is weakened and loses strength of contraction, resulting in a decreased stroke volume, or volume of blood ejected from the left ventricle with each heartbeat (or stroke). The reduced stroke volume results in a decreased cardiac output.

Since the heart pumps oxygenated blood to all tissues of the body, a decrease in cardiac output results in a decreased O_2 supply to the body's tissues. Since all human cells require O_2 for life, the effects of cardiac impairment can be noted in virtually every system of the body. For example, the kidneys are dependent upon an adequate perfusion of blood in order to sustain their activities of filtering, cleansing, and eliminating. When cardiac output is significantly decreased, blood flow to the kidneys is decreased, with subsequent loss of kidney function that ultimately may result in renal failure. Likewise, a decrease in cardiac output of oxygen-rich arterial blood will result in inadequate oxygenation of brain cells. Evidence of such impairment includes changes in mental status, with a patient becoming more disoriented, combative, and restless. As O_2 deficit continues, the patient will slip into unconsciousness and may suffer irreversible brain damage secondary to cardiac insufficiency.

$$\uparrow CO_2 \rightarrow \downarrow O_2 \rightarrow \downarrow \text{ function of organs}$$

MEMORY JOGS

It is obvious from this discussion that cardiac impairment can cause many undesirable and potentially life-threatening effects in the body. The nurse must always be conscious of the patient's status of circulation and oxygenation and should use ongoing assessment strategies to ensure adequate circulatory function (see Assessment Guidelines in this chapter).

Principle

Veins and arteries are the passageways for circulation of O_2 to the cells of the body

Illustration of Principle

Adequacy of O_2 transport through the body's circulatory system is dependent upon the integrity of the veins and arteries—structures that serve as the passageways for blood flow. Thus, even though cardiac function may be adequate and cardiac output may be within normal parameters, circulation of O_2 may *still* be inadequate if these structures of blood flow are not functioning properly. The nurse, then, must be aware of any impairment of blood flow in veins or arteries, because these structures must function *with* the heart to ensure adequate circulation of O_2.

*A*rteries carry oxygenated blood away from the heart to the body's cells. Veins carry deoxygenated blood back from the body to the heart and lungs.

MEMORY JOGS

Veins are thin-walled structures that carry blood toward the heart under low pressure. Each vein has a series of valves, which serve to prevent back-flow or pooling of blood in the structure as the blood courses through the body. Failure of these valves to function correctly will result in a pooling of blood in the vein, increasing pressure within the structure and resulting in the eventual development of *varicosities*—swollen, bulging, engorged veins with weakened walls. Such veins cannot support adequate circulation, resulting in notable signs of peripheral edema, extremity coolness, and aching or tenderness of the extremity. Blood that pools in the structures may form clots, or *thrombi*, which will further decrease blood flow within the structure and blood flow to the tissues the vein supplies. Thrombus formation within the venous passageway, then, causes an impairment of circulation, even though cardiac function may be entirely adequate.

Changes within the structure of the arteries likewise can compromise oxygenation. Deposits of *plaque* (accumulated fats, cholesterols, and other elements) will cause an impairment of arterial blood flow to the cells of the body. Plaque deposits cause a narrowing of the arterial lumen, with a subsequent decrease in blood flow and increase in pressure within the artery. The plaque formation in *atherosclerosis* may lead to hypertensive disease and impairment of oxygen transport to body tissues supplied by the arterial structure. Since all cells require oxygen for life, the effect of this disease becomes obvious. Atherosclerotic changes in the arteries that supply brain cells, for example, will cause decreased oxygenation of those cells, resulting in impaired mental acuity and ability—as in organic brain syndrome. Thus, the degeneration of mental processes noted in some elderly patients, which was once attributed to old age and termed "senility," is more accurately attributed to impairment of cerebral blood flow and a decrease in cerebral oxygenation secondary to changes within arterial structures.

**MEMORY
JOGS**

*D*eposits of plaque (atherosclerosis) narrow arterial lumen.
Rigidity of arterial walls (arteriosclerosis) increases arterial pressure.
Both degenerative changes reduce arterial blood flow.

Similarly, arteriosclerotic changes in the arteries will result in an impairment of circulation or of oxygenation. In arteriosclerosis, the arterial wall loses its flexibility, becoming less and less able to expand and contract with corresponding changes in pressure from blood flow. As the artery becomes increasingly rigid, pressure within the structure rises, resulting in hypertension and decreased arterial perfusion. Because the heart consumes O_2 at a very high rate, circulatory impairment from athero- and arteriosclerotic changes within the arteries becomes the number one cause of *myocardial infarction*, necrosis, or death of myocardial tissue secondary to cessation of arterial oxygen supply to the heart. Alteration in arterial blood flow, then, presents a hazardous, potentially life-threatening condition for the patient, and must be considered by the nurse as important a concern as alteration in cardiac output.

Principle

Delivery of O_2 to the cells is dependent upon microscopic blood cells, which "carry" O_2 gas

Illustration of Principle

Essential to the delivery of O_2 *to* the cells and the removal of CO_2 *from* the cells are an adequate number and function of certain microscopic blood cells, principally erythrocytes or red blood cells (RBCs) and hemoglobin (Hgb), which serve to "carry" these gases in the blood stream. A reduction in the numbers of these circulating blood cells, or defects in the structures of the cells, may result in decreased oxygenation of the cells of the body. Thus, even though cardiac output of oxygen-rich blood may be adequate, and arterial perfusion may be unrestricted, oxygenation can *still* be compromised by altered blood cell functions.

Microscopic blood cells, such as RBCs and Hgb, carry O_2 to the cells and remove CO_2 from the cells. The heart pumps the blood, the veins and arteries are the passageways for blood, and the blood cells "carry" these gases through the passageways.

MEMORY JOGS

Patients with decreased numbers of these blood cells, such as those experiencing significant blood loss, will show signs of impaired oxygenation: pallor, dyspnea, shortness of breath, and fatigue. Other patients at risk for decreased numbers of RBCs and Hgb include those with poor dietary intake of iron, hematopoietic diseases such as polycythemia vera and leukemia, or bone marrow depression secondary to cancer chemotherapy and radiation therapy.

Nursing Management

The numbers of these blood cells are assessed routinely in certain patients to ensure adequate transport of O_2. The nurse should note depression of RBC and Hgb blood values that might suggest an impairment of O_2 transport. Patients experiencing surgical intervention, traumatic injury with blood loss, or labor and childbirth should be considered at risk for impaired oxygenation secondary to decreased numbers of these essential O_2 carriers.

MEMORY JOGS

> *A*ny disease condition or clinical situation that involves loss of blood likewise will cause a loss of RBCs and Hgb, essential oxygen carriers in the blood. The nurse should monitor such patients for evidence of hypoxemia.

Patients with decreased RBC and Hgb values may require nursing intervention in order for adequate oxygenation to be maintained. Such supportive measures include:

- Working in conjunction with medical intervention to arrest source of blood loss
- Administering transfusions of blood or blood products to increase the numbers of circulating RBCs and Hgb
- Maintaining the patient on bed rest to reduce O_2 need
- Administering O_2 therapy to increase cellular oxygenation (see oxygenation, Chapter 8, for discussion of oxygen therapy)
- Continuing to monitor blood values of RBCs and Hgb, oxygenation status, mental status, and orientation

Defects in the *structure* of oxygen-carrying blood cells will also influence cellular oxygenation. In sickle cell anemia, for example, the shape of the red blood cell changes from its usual round shape to that of a sickle, with an elongated, hooked shape. Such misshaped cells cannot traverse easily through the circulatory passageways, resulting in impaired O_2 transport. Thus, symptoms of sickle cell anemia are very much like symptoms displayed by patients with a decreased number of oxygen-carrying blood cells—fatigue, shortness of breath, and so forth. It is apparent that both the number and the structure of oxygen-carrying blood cells significantly influence cellular oxygenation.

With the last few principles, then, we have reviewed the many structures of the circulatory system and their interrelated roles in the process of cellular oxygenation. In order for oxygenation to be adequate, the human body must have proper cardiac function and output, adequate and unrestricted venous and arterial blood flow, and sufficient number and function of oxygen-carrying cells in the blood.

Principle

Because the circulatory system provides essential O_2 to all cells in the human body, alterations in cardiovascular function are evidenced by many systems

Illustration of Principle

It is apparent that the cardiovascular system supplies O_2 and nutrients to all cells in the human body in order to maintain their viability and function. Thus, impairments of circulation may be evidenced in a variety of ways and in a variety of systems, depending upon the source and nature of the circulatory impairment. For example, chest pain would certainly be a typical cardiovascular symptom indicating a circulatory impairment. Pain in the lower extremities associated with intermittent claudication *also* would indicate cardiovascular impairment, with both chest pain and extremity pain suggesting decreased oxygenation of that particular area of the body. Therefore, the nurse must observe carefully for symptoms suggesting cardiovascular impairment that would result in decreased circulation.

The nurse may find it easier to conduct assessments of cardiovascular function by examining for signs and symptoms of alterations *vis-a-vis* the following specific cardiovascular functions:

Cardiovascular Function	Associated Signs and Symptoms
Oxygenation	Pain (such as chest pain, extremity pain) Loss of function of body part or parts (i.e., hemiplegia following CVA) Rate, depth, and ease of respirations Color, warmth, and moisture of skin Abnormalities in arterial blood–gas values Presence of abnormal findings, such as pallor, mottling, cyanosis, shortness of breath (SOB), dyspnea, syncope
Fluid circulation	Alterations in blood pressure Alterations in urine output Alterations in central venous pressure Rate and adequacy of apical and peripheral pulses Presence of abnormal findings, such as edema, distended jugular veins, lung congestion, decreased urinary output
Cellular nutrition	Presence and distribution of body hair Integrity of skin layers General physical vitality, energy, strength Presence of abnormal findings, such as body alopecia, decubitus ulcers, persistent fatigue, fatigue upon exertion

Principle

The characteristic features of normal sinus rhythm signify cardiac events occurring in a timely and rhythmic manner

Illustration of Principle

Electrical impulses are conducted (transmitted) through the cardiac musculature in an organized and rhythmic manner. The heart contains specialized conductive tissue capable of initiating and conducting an electrical impulse that causes the heart to contract. This group of conductive tissues is called the conduction system and consists of the SA node, the AV node, the bundle of His, the bundle branches, and the Purkinje fibers. *All* of these components are capable of *conducting* an electrical impulse, but normally only the SA node, AV node, and Purkinje fibers have the ability to *initiate* or generate an impulse.

The SA (sinoatrial) node normally initiates the electrical impulse, and therefore is called the *pacemaker* of the heart. Impulses initiated from the SA node are transmitted down the conduction system. The SA node is located in the upper portion of the right atrium and has the inherent rate of 60–100 beats per minute. The impulses are conducted to the left atrium and down to the AV (atrioventricular) node. Located in the lower right atrium, the AV Node itself does not have the capability to originate an impulse, but the surrounding junctional tissue does (see Figure 9–1).

MEMORY JOGS

*B*ecause the SA node initiates impulses at an inherent rate of 60–100 beats per minute (bpm), the normal adult pulse is likewise 60–100 beats per minute.

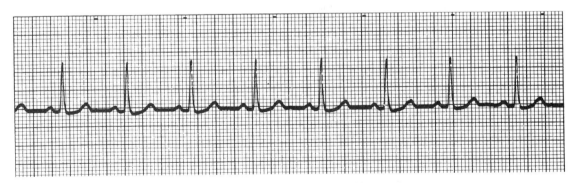

Figure 9-1. Example of normal sinus rhythm. (From Huff J, Doernbach DP, White RD: ECG Workout: Exercises in Arrhythmia Interpretation (2nd ed.), p. 40. Philadelphia, J. B. Lippincott Company, 1993).

Junctional tissue can serve as a backup pacemaker capable of initiating an impulse at the rate of 40–60 beats per minute. (This pattern on the electrocardiogram (ECG) would be called a junctional rhythm because the junctional tissue initiated the impulse.) Once the impulse reaches the AV node, it is delayed briefly to allow the atria to contract and the ventricles to fill. The impulse is then transmitted to the bundle of His, which bifurcates into the right and left bundle branches. The right bundle conducts the impulse to the right ventricle and the left bundle conducts to the left ventricle.

The impulse is then transmitted down to the Purkinje fibers. These fibers reach down into the myocardium and ultimately cause the heart muscle to contract. The Purkinje fibers are also capable of initiating an electrical impulse, but at a much slower rate of 20–40 beats per minute (see Figure 9–2).

In review, the synchronized rhythmic contraction of the heart is caused by the initiation of the electrical impulse in the SA node. The impulse is normally conducted to the AV node, and travels down the bundle of His, the bundle branches, and the Purkinje fibers, causing contraction of the heart muscle. When electrical conduction occurs in this sequence and is regular, at a rate of 60–100 beats per minute, the electrical activity seen on the electrocardiogram is designated normal sinus rhythm (normal conduction of the impulse originating in the SA Node). (See Figures 9–3, 9–4, and 9–5.)

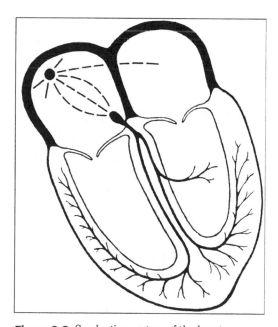

Figure 9-2. Conduction system of the heart.

Components of the ECG

P Wave: Represents stimulation and contraction (depolarization) of the atria. The electrical impulse has traveled from the SA node throughout the atria.

QRS: Follows the P wave and represents ventricular depolarization (contraction). Atrial repolarization (relaxation) is buried in the QRS on the ECG.

T Wave: Indicates ventricular repolarization. No cardiac activity is occurring.

Principle

Disturbances of impulse conduction secondary to ectopic foci result in a decrease in cardiac output

Illustration of Principle

Electrical impulses initiated in the SA node and transmitted in a normal manner through the conduction system produce a synchronized heart muscle contrac-

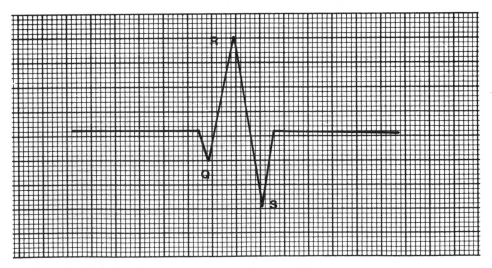

Figure 9-3. QRS wave complex on the ECG.

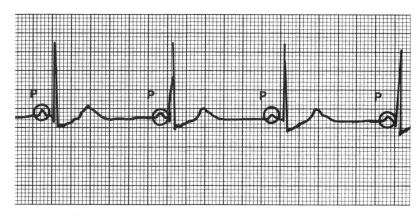

Figure 9-4. Normal P waves are upright and rounded. One P wave for each QRS.

tion. Synchronized contractions maintain an adequate cardiac output to meet the body's demands (normally 5–6 L/min). Impulses originating from a site other than the SA node are called ectopic beats. Ectopic beats are variations in the site of impulse origination, and conduction of these can jeopardize cardiac output. Manifestations of decreased cardiac output include decreased blood pressure (BP), altered pulse rate, and decreased level of consciousness.

Principle

Ventricular dysrhythmias indicate a lethal disturbance or interruption in the cardiac cycle, with a profound decrease in cardiac output

Illustration of Principle

Acutely ill patients are at risk for developing ventricular dysrhythmias, which may be fatal and which require immediate recognition and intervention. Lethal ven-

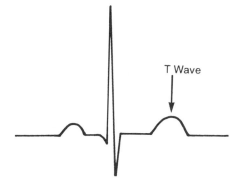

T Wave

Figure 9-5. Normal sinus pattern on ECG with normal T wave.

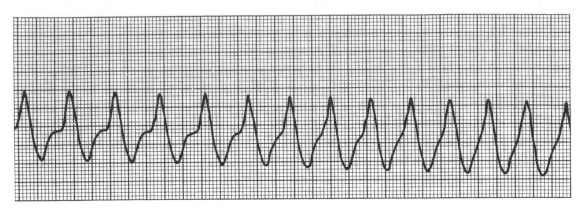

Figure 9-6. Example of ventricular tachycardia.

tricular dysrhythmias are ventricular tachycardia (VT) (Figure 9–6) and ventricular fibrillation (VF) (Figure 9–7). In both dysrhythmias, the electrical impulse is initiated from the ventricles, with loss of synchronized contraction of both the atria and ventricles. This loss of synchronized heart contraction causes a decrease in the time the ventricles have to fill with blood from the atria. Because there is less blood in the ventricles, there is less blood available to be ejected during ventricular contraction. A decrease in the amount of blood ejected causes a decrease in cardiac output.

If cardiac output is adequate, the patient with VT may still be awake and have a stable blood pressure and pulse. The ECG pattern shows a wide QRS at a rate of 100–250 beats per minute, without visible P waves. Therapy depends on the patient's condition.

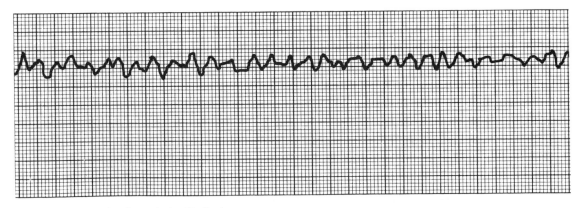

Figure 9-7. Example of ventricular fibrillation.

If a pulse is palpated, the patient should receive an antiarrhythmic drug—for example, lidocaine (Xylocaine), IV push, followed by a continuous infusion drip. Procainamide (Pronestyl) or bretylium (Bretylol) may also be given if the lidocaine does not convert the VT. If the patient is in VT and pulseless, a cardiac arrest situation exists and cardiopulmonary resuscitation (CPR) must be initiated. The patient should be defibrillated immediately. Defibrillation delivers an electrical shock by means of two paddles to the anterior chest wall. The current goes through the heart, stopping the ventricular tachycardia and restoring a normal sinus rhythm.

Ventricular tachycardia can rapidly deteriorate to ventricular fibrillation. In VF there is no organized heart muscle contraction. The heart is fibrillating or "quivering"; therefore, there is no cardiac output. Death is imminent unless the fibrillation is stopped. The patient in VF will be unconscious and pulseless. On the ECG, no discernible QRS complexes are identified. The rhythm almost resembles "scribbles" with a wavy baseline. The rate is too fast to count. CPR must be started immediately and the patient must be defibrillated to stop the "quivering" and to restore normal rhythm and cardiac output. Immediate recognition and defibrillation are essential for the treatment of this lethal dysrhythmia.

Another lethal dysrhythmia is asystole. Asystole is also known as ventricular standstill (Figure 9–8). On the ECG monitor asystole is characterized by a flat line. This indicates that there are no ventricular contractions; therefore, there is no cardiac output. This is a life-threatening situation and CPR must be initiated immediately. Epinephrine and atropine may be given via IV push in an attempt to increase contractility and heart rate. An artificial pacemaker may be considered. This involves inserting an electrode into the right ventricle by means of a large vein to electrically stimulate the heart muscle to contract.

Ventricular tachycardia, ventricular fibrillation, and asystole are life-threatening dysrhythmias that require the nurse's immediate recognition and intervention to restore normal rhythm and cardiac output.

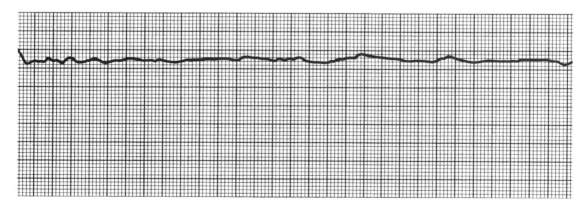

Figure 9-8. Example of asystole.

Reasoning Exercises: *Circulation*

1. Which of the following clinical manifestations would alert the nurse that a patient in prolonged bradycardia was experiencing decreased cardiac output?

   A. Increase in blood pressure

   B. Decrease in respiratory rate

   C. Increase in pupillary dilation

   D. Decrease in urinary output

Intended response: **D.** A decrease in urinary output indicates decreased renal perfusion secondary to decreased cardiac output. Blood pressure decreases as respiratory rate increases in conditions causing decreased cardiac output. Changes in pupillary dilation are more often associated with neurologic disorders; however, change in pupillary response related to decreased cardiac output would occur relatively late, indicating a profound and potentially irreversible decrease.

2. A patient evidences extreme bradycardia (heart rate = 2 bpm) on the cardiac monitor. In addition to administering the appropriate medication to increase heart rate, which of the following actions would be most appropriate for the nurse to take?

   A. Elevate the head of the bed to a semi-Fowler's position

   B. Position the patient on his or her left side

   C. Apply a pulse oximeter and begin nasal oxygen administration

   D. Prepare equipment for endotracheal intubation and mechanical ventilation.

Intended response: **C.** Cardiac Output equals Heart Rate multiplied by Stroke Volume ($CO = HR \times SV$). If heart rate drops significantly, so too will cardiac output, compromising cellular oxygenation. Because medication to increase heart rate (e.g., atropine) has been administered in this situation, a secondary intervention is to support oxygenation via the administration of O_2 therapy. The outcome of both medication and O_2 administration can then be measured via pulse oximeter readings.

3. The nurse is caring for a patient in early hypovolemic shock whose cardiac output is decreased secondary to hemorrhage. Which of the following pulse findings would correspond to this patient's status?

   A. Bradycardia

   B. Pulse full and bounding

   C. Pulses 3+ bilaterally or moderate strength, bilaterally

   D. Rapid, thready pulse

Intended response: **D.** As circulating fluid volume is decreased in hemorrhage, cardiac output likewise decreases. Pulse rate increases in response to the body's effort to compensate for decreased fluid volume. Decreased fluid volume pressure exerted on arte-rial walls causes the pulse to become thready.

4. Which of the following changes in laboratory values, outside of normal limits, would indicate renal impairment secondary to decreased cardiac output?

    A. Decrease in blood urea nitrogen (BUN)

    B. Increase in hematocrit (Hct)

    C. Decrease in potassium (K^+)

    D. Increase in creatinine (Cr)

Intended response: **D.** Loss of kidney function secondary to decreased cardiac output can be recognized by increased creatinine levels. BUN may increase in renal impairment, but it is too affected by fluid volume status to be definitive for renal disease. As potassium is excreted by the body in urine, serum potassium values increase in renal impairment. Hematocrit may indicate fluid volume status and has no role in determining renal function.

5. Which of the following clinical manifestations is most indicative of decreased coronary oxygenation secondary to atherosclerotic plaque deposits?

    A. Complaints of chest pain and tightness

    B. Edema of lower extremities

    C. Complaints of dizziness with position changes

    D. Exertional dyspnea

Intended response: **A.** Chest pain (angina) is a hallmark manifestation of impaired myocardial oxygenation secondary to decreased coronary artery blood flow. Although the patient may also experience edema of the lower extremities **B** or exertional dyspnea **D** in heart disease, these symptoms are not definitive for or limited to coronary artery atherosclerosis. Complaints of dizziness with position changes suggest orthostatic hypotension.

6. Which of the following classes of drugs is indicated most for the management of symptoms associated with coronary artery atherosclerosis?

    A. Nitrate

    B. Vasopressor

    C. Salicylate

    D. Thrombolytic

Intended response: **A.** Chest pain (angina) is a hallmark manifestation of impaired myocardial oxygenation secondary to decreased coronary artery blood flow. Nitrate medication (e.g., nitroglycerin) causes vasodilation of coronary vessels, enhancing arterial blood flow and thus reducing the frequency, intensity, and duration of anginal episodes. Vasopressor medication causes arterial constriction, potentially worsening anginal pain. Salicylates (e.g., aspirin) are used in a daily low dose to reduce the risk of clot formation that might precipitate myocardial infarction. Thrombolytics are indicated for clot lysis, as in acute myocardial infarction.

7. Which of the following clinical manifestations would a nurse expect to note in a patient whose hemoglobin value is below normal?

    A. Reddened, flushed facial appearance

    B. Slow, shallow respirations

    C. Fatigue and weakness

    D. Slow and bounding pulse

Intended response: **C.** As hemoglobin is an essential oxygen carrying blood cell, a value below normal would indicate impaired oxygen transport to body cells. Clinical evidence of decreased cellular oxygenation includes pale (fair-skinned) or ashen (dark-skinned) color, rapid pulse, palpitations, fatigue, weakness, dizziness, and transient confusion.

8. Which of the following is characteristic of normal sinus rhythm (NSR)?

    A. QRS complex is peaked, narrow, and smaller than P or T waves

    B. Atrial and ventricular rhythm is variable

    C. Each QRS complex is preceded by a T wave

    D. Atrial and ventricular rates range from 60–100 bpm

Intended response: **D.** Because the sinoatrial node ("pacemaker") has an intrinsic rate of 60–100 beats per minute (bpm), atrial and ventricular rates in normal sinus rhythm must occur within that range. The QRS is tall, peaked, and larger than any other waveform in the ECG complex. Rhythm is constant and regular in NSR. T waves follow the QRS, indicating the diastolic phase.

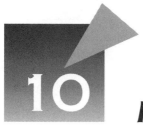

10

Fluids and Electrolytes

NANCY KORCHEK
DIANE BLACK

Principle

Where sodium (Na^+) goes, water (H_2O) goes

Illustration of Principle

Sodium is an electrically charged ion (electrolyte) that has an intimate relationship with water or fluid in the human body. This basic principle is critical to one's understanding of fluid and electrolyte balance, because it helps to explain the processes and results of Na^+ excesses and losses that may result from inadequate Na^+ intake or Na^+ loss. Therefore, when planning care for the client with an Na^+ imbalance, it is necessary to review the client's *fluid* status as well, because presentation of the Na^+ imbalance also will be evidenced in changes in the client's *fluid* balance.

*A*lthough Na^+ as an electrolyte influences central nervous system (CNS) function, its primary action is on fluid balance in the body. Thus, when the patient experiences an Na^+ imbalance, the nurse must also anticipate an alteration in fluid balance.

MEMORY JOGS

127

Principle

Na⁺ is well stored in the human body

Illustration of Principle

Because a large percentage of the body is composed of fluid, and Na^+ and fluid are interrelated, there is usually ample storage of Na^+ in the human body. Additionally, the hormone aldosterone plays a role in Na^+ retention and excretion by its action on the kidneys.

The human body requires approximately 4 g of Na^+ per day, supplied principally by dietary intake. However, because the body stores Na^+ so well, a decrease in dietary intake of Na^+ will not immediately result in an Na^+ imbalance, because reserve stores of Na^+ are available.

Food sources rich in Na^+ can be easily remembered by the use of this simple acronym:

Prevent **M**ore **S**odium

The *P* in *Prevent* stands for *processed* foods, because Na^+ is often used as a preservative for such foods. Examples of processed foods include:

- Frozen foods (e.g., vegetables, dinners)
- Canned foods (e.g., soups, gravies, fruits)
- Boxed pastry mixes (e.g., cakes, breads)
- Prepared cereals and breads
- Processed meats (e.g., bologna, sausage, corned beef, franks)

The *M* in *More* stands for *Moo* food, that is, dairy products. This group includes:

- Milk and cream
- Cheese
- Butter
- Ice cream

Finally, the *S* in *Sodium* stands for *salty* foods, that is, foods with an obvious salty taste. These foods are rich in Na^+ because salt is used in the manufacture of the products. This group includes:

- Potato chips and pretzels
- Pickles and olives
- Nuts
- Bacon
- Ham

The nurse should be aware that restrictions of these food groups will depend on the type of sodium-restricted diet ordered for the patient. Whereas some Na⁺ restrictions only call for the avoidance of table salt, others will restrict salt in cooking and in the foods in these groups. Regardless of the type of restriction, the most common indication for Na⁺ restriction is *fluid* imbalance. Patients placed on Na⁺ restrictions are most often those suffering from conditions that involve fluid problems, such as congestive heart failure or renal disease. Once again, the intimate relationship between Na⁺ and fluids in the body is emphasized.

> *S*odium-rich foods can be best categorized as belonging to one of three groups: processed foods, dairy products, or salty foods.

MEMORY JOGS

Principle

Hypernatremia (Hyper, "too much" or "excess")
            (Na, symbol for sodium)
            (Emia, "serum" or "blood")
is an excess of Na⁺ concentration in the blood, characterized by a shift of fluid from the cells into extracellular fluid, causing a shrinking of the cells

Illustration of Principle

Although hypernatremia can be caused by either an increased concentration of serum Na⁺ or an excess loss of body fluid, the symptoms of this imbalance are the same. The hallmark feature of hypernatremia is *dehydration,* because the high concentration of serum Na⁺ "pulls" fluid from the cells, resulting in cell shrinkage. The classic symptoms of dehydration, and thus, of hypernatremia, include the following:

- Hot, dry, flushed skin with poor turgor
- Thirst
- Dry mucous membranes
- Absence of tears (particularly in children)
- Soft, sunken eyeballs
- "Doughy" abdomen
- Increased body temperature

The vascular effects of hypernatremia cause fluids to shift from intracellular to extracellular compartments, thereby initially raising pressure in the arteries (increasing blood pressure) and causing tachycardia and increased urinary output. The body then compensates for fluid shift and loss with oliguria and decreased blood pressure (BP) in an effort to retain needed fluid. Because Na^+ as an electrolyte influences the transmission of nerve impulses, CNS symptoms may also appear, including irritability, excitability, restlessness, and convulsions.

Laboratory data will evidence hypernatremia with an elevated serum Na^+ value greater than the normal range of 132 to 142 mEq/L.

Patients at risk for hypernatremia are principally those experiencing a decreased intake or excess loss of fluid. For example, in the disease diabetes insipidus, excessive loss of fluids in urination may result in a hypernatremic state. Likewise, patients experiencing severe diarrhea have an excessive loss of fluids, which may result in hypernatremia. Patients experiencing kidney failure, congestive heart failure, or shock can experience hypernatremia owing to reduced glomerular filtration.

The primary treatment for a patient with hypernatremia is the administration of fluid replacement therapy and the continuation of fluid maintenance therapy. Supportive measures are needed, with continued close assessment of the patient's condition in terms of fluid balance.

Principle

Hyponatremia (Hypo, "too little" or "decreased")
       (Na, symbol for sodium)
       (Emia, "serum," or "blood")
is a less than normal concentration of sodium in the blood

Illustration of Principle

Hyponatremia may result from two causes: excess loss of Na^+ from body serum or excess retention of body fluids.

In hyponatremia, there is a low serum level of Na^+, 132 mEq/L or lower. Because Na^+ is an electrolyte that influences the transmission of nerve impulses, decreased serum Na^+ will cause symptoms of headaches, abdominal cramps, and muscular weakness. Because of excess fluid accumulation, nausea and vomiting are common symptoms.

Clients at risk include those who experience loss of Na^+ through the skin from excessive sweating as a result of increased environmental temperature, fever, or muscular exercise. Great quantities of Na^+ are also lost through burn wounds, postoperative wound drainage, bleeding, a combination of a low-Na^+ diet and po-tent diuretics, and excessive plain H_2O intake. With adrenal cortex dysfunction, hyponatremia can present itself as Addison's disease, with loss of Na^+ across renal tubules caused by decreased mineralocorticoid production. Hyponatremia can result from SIADH (syndrome of inappropriate antidiuretic hormone), which causes excessive H_2O to be absorbed and extracellular fluid to become diluted.

The goal of therapy for hyponatremia is to restore normal sodium levels. If there is an excess of fluid with a decrease of Na^+ levels, therapy is aimed at restricting fluids. If fluid balance is normal with decreased Na^+ levels, an isotonic saline solution is given.

Principle

Overhydration is an excess of H_2O in the extracellular compartment with a normal amount of solute or a deficient amount of solute

Illustration of Principle

Water is the primary body fluid. It serves many functions, from the transport of nutrients and temperature regulation to the removal of waste products.

The adult human body is approximately 55% to 70% fluid, while an infant body is 70% to 80% fluid. Therefore, the infant and young child are at risk for fluid imbalance problems because of the large percentage of body weight that is H_2O. Likewise, the elderly are also at risk, because they have less fluid reserve; their body H_2O content averages 45% to 50%.

When discussing hydration, our assessment of clients pertains to extracellular fluid composition, which consists of interstitial (fluid between cells or in tissues) and intravascular (plasma) fluid.

Many terms have been identified for excess extracellular fluid volume, such as overhydration, H_2O excess, and hypervolemia. In essence, there is an excess of fluid volume, which causes the following symptoms:

- Weight gain and edema
- Dyspnea
- Cough —————————————— **Fluid congestion in lungs**
- Moist rales
- Puffy eyelids
- Increased central venous pressure
- Bounding pulse ————————— **Fluid excess in vascular system**
- Neck vein engorgement

- Bulging fontanelles
- Decreased hemoglobin and decreased hematocrit (hemodilution)
- Nausea, vomiting

Many types of clients are at risk for the development of overhydration, particularly kidney failure caused by the retention of Na^+ and H_2O, and congestive heart failure (clients have a back-flow of fluids as a result of a weakened pump). Cushing's syndrome can create fluid overload because of increased production of adrenal corticoid hormones.

Massive generalized edema may also be called anasarca, which is fluid retention for an extended period of time, usually of cardiac or renal origin.

The primary goal of treatment is to restrict fluids to lower fluid volume. Diuretics or hypertonic saline may be used. The nurse is cautioned to make continuous skin assessments to prevent skin breakdown and to record daily weights to assess progress of treatment.

Principle

Dehydration is a loss of body fluids, particularly from the extracellular fluid compartment

Illustration of Principle

Water moves from an area of lesser concentration to an area of greater solute concentration until both are equal. With dehydration, the excess loss of body fluids occurs in the extracellular compartment, thereby creating a hyperosmolar dehydration. The signs and symptoms of dehydration are, then, closely related to those of hypernatremia.

Signs and symptoms include:

- Thirst
- Dry mucous membranes
- Sunken eyeballs
- "Doughy" abdomen
- Dry skin with poor turgor
- Elevated temperature
- Body weight loss

As dehydration progresses, vascular effects become noticeable. The hyperosmolar dehydration causes a state of hypovolemia, leading to tachycardia, increased respiratory rate, and decreased blood pressure. Behavioral changes lead to:

· Restlessness, irritability
· Disorientation and delirium
· Convulsions
· Coma evolves with fatal dehydration of 22% to 30% loss of body H_2O

Loss of body fluids can occur from fever or insufficient water intake, as with clients that are NPO or comatose. Dehydration can also occur from losing body fluids from the gastrointestinal system (diarrhea, vomiting), renal system (excess urine output from diabetes insipidus or diuretics), or integumentary system (excessive perspiration, burns). Clients in hypovolemic states may have a great loss of body fluids from hemorrhage, shock, or metabolic acidosis.

The treatment for dehydration is primarily the administration of fluid replacement therapy and continued fluid maintenance therapy. This fluid replacement is especially crucial in children because their bodies are approximately 70% to 80% H_2O. The formula to follow in infants is 100 cc/kg of body weight every 24 hours.

Principle

Potassium (K^+) is an essential electrolyte in body fluids whose primary function is to irritate. Potassium serves to irritate nerve cells, which ultimately influences muscular function

Illustration of Principle

As an electrically charged ion, K^+ plays a critical role in neuromuscular function through the excitation, or *irritation,* of nerve cells, resulting in muscular contraction. Both smooth and skeletal muscle, and especially the human heart, are dependent upon K^+ for proper and regulated contraction and function.

Unlike sodium, K^+ is poorly stored in the human body, with approximately 90% being excreted in urine. Therefore, imbalances of K^+ can occur rather quickly when an insufficient supply of K^+ is ingested or an excessive loss occurs, such as in potassium-wasting diuretic therapy.

Because K^+ is poorly stored, the human body requires a daily intake of potassium-rich foods in order to maintain adequate K^+ levels and thus maintain proper neuromuscular function. Food sources rich in K^+ are perhaps most easily remembered by the word *fruit,* because many fresh fruits are potassium-rich.

Fruits rich in K^+ include:

Peaches

Figs

Bananas

Oranges/orange juice

Strawberries

Pears

Prunes

Raisins

Watermelon

Dates

Cantaloupe

Apricots

Although many may mistakenly believe that tomatoes are vegetables, they are, in fact, fruits, and tomato juice is likewise potassium-rich. Finally, instant coffee and many salt substitutes currently on the market are relatively high in K^+. The human body requires approximately 40 mEq of K^+ per day, and this need is usually met with dietary intake alone.

Principle
Where Na^+ Goes, K^+ doesn't

Illustration of Principle

Sodium and K^+ have an inverse relationship in the human body. Thus, when an imbalance of Na^+ occurs in the serum, the opposite imbalance of K^+ frequently occurs. For example, if excess Na^+ is retained, as in *hyper*natremia, a corresponding excess of K^+ will be excreted, resulting in *hypo*kalemia. This principle illustrates the fact that electrolyte imbalances will occur infrequently in isolation, and therefore the nurse should monitor *all* electrolyte values of a client experiencing a single electrolyte imbalance.

MEMORY JOGS

*P*otassium (K^+) is an electrolyte whose primary action in the body is excitation of nerves, which influences muscular function. Potassium is poorly stored in the body, and dietary intake of potassium-rich foods such as fruits must meet the need for 40 mEq of K^+ per day.

Principle

Hyperkalemia is an increase in serum K⁺ levels characterized by muscular irritability and tension

Illustration of Principle

In hyperkalemic states, increased levels of serum K^+ circulate to body cells, resulting in an increased irritability of nerves and muscles. The symptoms of hyperkalemia, then, are those of *hyperexcitability* of the target body system. For example, when the gastrointestinal tract is overstimulated by excess K^+, symptoms of gastrointestinal hyperexcitability, including nausea, colic, and diarrhea, result. Muscular cramping, pain, and weakness are evidence of overstimulation of muscle cells by excess K^+. As with hypokalemic states, the impact of K^+ imbalance on the function of the human heart is *most* critical and thus the priority concern for the nurse. Because hyperkalemic states lead to increased irritation of the cardiac muscle, tachycardia and potentially life-threatening dysrhythmias (which may ultimately lead to cardiac arrest) can result.

Treatment of hyperkalemic states must be prompt in order to forestall alterations in cardiac function and possible cardiac failure. If the patient evidences a serum K^+ in excess of normal parameters (3.5 to 5 mEq/L), the nurse, in conjunction with the physician, must take aggressive steps to achieve the goal of reducing serum K^+ levels. These steps include:

· Withdrawal of all potassium-rich foods, supplements, or IV additives
· Administration of IV fluids, and Lasix diuretic therapy to "flush out" excess K^+ through urine (only *if* the hyperkalemic patient has adequate renal function)
· Administration of Kayexalate solution (most often via rectal instillation) to hasten removal of excess K^+

The nurse should monitor serum K^+ values carefully for evidence of efficacy of treatment measures, and assess cardiac function by electrocardiograph tracings. Safety measures, such as placing side rails in an upright position and having someone in attendance with the hyperkalemic patient, should be employed to reduce the risk of injury to the patient in a hyperexcited state.

> *H*yperkalemia results in *hyper*excitability of nerves and muscles. The nurse should place greatest priority on cardiac function, because the heart is overstimulated and may evidence life-threatening changes in rate and rhythm.

MEMORY JOGS

Principle

Hypokalemia is a decrease in serum K^+ levels characterized by muscular weakness and fatigue

Illustration of Principle

In hypokalemic states, there is an insufficient supply of K^+ to body cells, causing insufficient stimulation or irritation to nerves and muscles. Therefore, muscular weakness is a cardinal feature of this electrolyte imbalance.

Because K^+ is poorly stored in the human body, reserves of K^+ are limited. Patients who are unable to take in adequate amounts of K^+ (40 mEq/day) by mouth are at risk for hypokalemia. Additionally, patients who are experiencing K^+ loss, secondary to taking oral diuretics or having severe diarrhea, may also be at risk for this imbalance.

MEMORY JOGS

*P*atients need a daily intake of K^+. Those with limited or restricted oral intake of foods and fluids should be monitored for hypokalemia. These patients include:

- Surgical patients with NPO status

- Patients with pronounced anorexia (cancer chemotherapy)

- Patients with impaired chewing or swallowing (post-CVA)

- Patients undergoing gastric suction or surgery

Because hypokalemia results in decreased irritation to nerves and muscles, symptoms of this imbalance are related to neuromuscular function. Symptoms include:

- Muscular weakness
- Fatigue
- Decreased muscle tone
- Decreased cardiac rate
- Dysrhythmia

It is important to note that the end result of either K^+ deficit or excess is cardiac arrest, or asystole, in response to changes in stimulation of the cardiac muscle. Thus, the effects of either potassium imbalance on the human heart can best be summarized as "K^+ kills," underlining the critical effects of K^+ imbalance.

Serum K^+ levels below the normal range of 3.5 to 5 mEq/L indicate hypokalemia. Because hypokalemia may be related to either an insufficient intake or an excess loss of K^+, K^+ *replacement* is the key to management of this imbalance. Potassium may be administered orally via potassium-rich foods or K^+ supplements, such as K-Lyte or K-Lor. If K^+ is to be added via an intravenous route, it *must* be added to an IV drip, and never by direct IV route, because this route will cause rapid irritation of cardiac muscle with potential dysrhythmia and asystole.

Supportive nursing measures include careful monitoring of the IV insertion site, if IV drip route is being utilized, because K^+ infusions may cause venous irritation and subsequent extravasation. The nurse should closely monitor the client's cardiac function, which is best observed via a continuous ECG monitor. Because the client's muscles are weak and fatigued, the nurse should monitor client safety and prevent accidental falls by keeping the bed rails up and the call light within easy reach of the client. Finally, the nurse must monitor the client's urinary output carefully, because K^+ supplements are being administered and must be excreted to avoid a potential K^+ excess from therapy.

Reasoning Exercises

1. The nurse caring for a patient with dehydration should expect to note which of the following clinical manifestations?

   A. Hypertension

   B. Hot, flushed skin

   C. Bradycardia

   D. Peripheral edema

Intended Response: B. As body fluid serves to cool body tissues, a classic sign of dehydration is hot, flushed skin. Blood pressure decreases in dehydration **A** as heart rate increases **C** in the body's effort to maintain effective circulation in fluid volume deficit. Edema **D** is associated with fluid overload.

2. Which of the following changes in the laboratory values of a patient receiving fluid replacement for dehydration would indicate to the nurse that therapy has been effective?

   A. Increase in blood urea nitrogen (BUN)

   B. Decrease in hematocrit (Hct)

   C. Increase in creatinine (Cr)

   D. Decrease in hemoglobin (Hgb)

Intended Response: **B.** The hematocrit value represents the ratio of blood cells to plasma. As dehydration is reversed with fluid replacement, the percentage of plasma will increase, lowering the Hct value, and indicating that therapy has been effective. BUN value **A** should lower with hemodilution. Creatinine values should remain constant in fluid volume disturbances. Hemoglobin, if affected by fluid replacement, would decrease with hemodilution.

3. Which of the following classes of medication is indicated for the management of dilutional hyponatremia related to fluid volume excess?
   A. Loop diuretic
   B. Broad spectrum antibiotic
   C. Vasopressor
   D. Plasma expander

Intended Response: **A.** A loop diuretic such as Lasix is indicated to draw off excess fluid and thus restore normal sodium levels in the serum. Vasopressor agents are contraindicated, as blood pressure is elevated in fluid volume excess. A plasma expander will increase circulating fluid volume, an undesired effect in fluid volume excess. Broad spectrum antibiotics would serve no purpose in correcting a fluid disturbance.

4. A patient receiving intravenous fluids at a flow rate of 150 mL/hour develops a moist cough and dyspnea. Which of the following actions should the nurse take initially?
   A. Elevate the head of the bed to semi-Fowler's position
   B. Encourage the patient to cough and deep breathe
   C. Administer oxygen per nasal cannula at a low flow rate
   D. Decrease the rate of flow of IV fluids

Intended Response: **D.** The patient is demonstrating classic signs of fluid volume excess. The rate of flow of IV fluids should be decreased to prevent further fluid overloading.

5. A patient is receiving diuretic therapy for fluid volume excess. Which of the following observations would indicate to the nurse that therapy has been effective?
   A. Increase in blood pressure
   B. Decrease in body weight
   C. Increase in central venous pressure
   D. Decrease in pulse

Intended Response: **B.** Diuretic therapy will draw off excess fluid, resulting in a loss of weight. Thus, daily weight measurement is an important assessment of patients receiving diuretic therapy for fluid volume excess. Blood pressure **A** and central venous pressure **C** should decrease; pulse **D** should correspondingly increase and stabilize as excess fluid is excreted in urine.

6. A patient is placed on a low-sodium diet. Which of the following meals would be appropriate?

   A. Tuna fish sandwich, potato chips and dip, lettuce salad, glass of iced tea

   B. Veal parmesan, broccoli, baked potato, milkshake

   C. Breast of chicken, peas, lettuce salad, 1 slice of bread, glass of 2% milk

   D. T-bone steak, cauliflower with cheese sauce, green beans, instant chocolate pudding, cup of hot tea

Intended Response: **C.** C contains no processed foods or salty foods. A contains salty foods, such as potato chips, and processed foods such as tuna fish. **B** contains dairy food, such as cheese and tomato sauce on the veal parmesan, and the milkshake. **D** contains high Na^+ concentration in the cheese sauce and the instant chocolate pudding.

7. A newly admitted patient has a serum potassium value of 3.1 mEq/L. Which of the following questions would be important for the nurse to ask the patient during the admission history?

   A. "Do you have any difficulty sleeping at night?"

   B. "Have you had any surgeries in the past?"

   C. "Have you developed any new symptoms in the past few days?"

   D. "Are you presently taking any medications?"

Intended Response: **D.** Hypokalemia is often induced by medications such as diuretics or corticosteroids. The nurse should identify any medication the patient may have been taking that could have induced the hypokalemia, and closely monitor medication therapy until the hypokalemia has been reversed.

8. A nurse is reviewing the laboratory values of a patient newly admitted for congestive heart failure. Which of the following should the nurse report to the physician?

   A. Serum potassium 5.6 mEq/L

   B. Serum glucose 110 mg/dL

C. Serum creatinine 1.1 mg/dL

D. Platelet count 320,000

Intended Response: **A.** An elevation of serum potassium to 5.6 mEq/L places the patient at risk for potentially lethal arrhythmias and should be reported to the physician immediately. The remaining values are within normal limits.

9. A patient in acute congestive heart failure (CHF) is ordered to receive furosemide (Lasix) 80 mg IV daily. The patient's morning serum K^+ value is 3.8 mEq/L. In light of the serum K^+ value, which action should the nurse take?

   A. Phone the physician to question the medication order

   B. Administer the Lasix 80 mg IV as ordered

   C. Administer half of the ordered dose (40 mg)

   D. Withhold the Lasix and notify the physician

Intended Response: **B.** It is appropriate for the nurse to administer the diuretic as ordered because the patient's potassium level is within normal limits.

10. A nurse is caring for a patient in renal failure whose potassium value is 6.4 mEq/L. Which of the following actions would be most beneficial for the nurse to take?

   A. Maintain the patient's bed in high Fowler's position

   B. Apply oxygen at 2 L/min per nasal cannula

   C. Attach the patient to 3-lead continuous cardiac monitoring

   D. Place an artificial airway at bedside

Intended Response: **C.** Hyperkalemia can result in potentially lethal cardiac arrhythmias. Continuous ECG monitoring is indicated to monitor the patient's cardiac activity and direct treatment of arrhythmias should they develop. The remaining responses are interventions supporting ventilation and oxygenation, rather than cardiac function.

Acids and Bases

NANCY KORCHEK
MARRY L. WILLIAMS

Principle

Use a three-step method to identify acid–base imbalances and know the normal values of each.

Step 1—Determine arterial blood pH
Step 2—Determine CO_2 (carbon dioxide) level
Step 3—Determine HCO_3 (bicarbonate) level

Normal values: Arterial blood gas
pH 7.35–7.45
CO_2 35–45 mEq/L
HCO_3 25 mEq/L

Principle

When attempting to identify an acid–base imbalance, the nurse should first consider the "arterial blood pH." Arterial blood pH is the measure of acid–base balance in the human body. Normal arterial blood pH is 7.35–7.45.

Illustration of Principle

The pH is the cardinal indicator of acid–base balance in the human body. A decrease in pH from normal range indicates an acidotic state. An increase in pH from normal range indicates an alkalotic state. A pH that falls within normal range of 7.35 to 7.45 indicates that the acids and bases of the body are in balance or that excesses or deficits of acids and bases in the body are being compensated.

Normally, acid ions and base ions are retained and excreted by the body in a way that preserves a delicate balance between the two. This balance is indicated by an arterial blood pH value, which is normally between the extremes of 7.35 and 7.45. When an excess or deficit of chemicals and gases occurs in the body, the balance between acids and bases is disrupted, resulting in a change in the pH of arterial blood. For example, if an individual is unable to expire adequate amounts of CO_2, an excess accumulation of this gas occurs in arterial blood. Since carbonic acid is formed when CO_2 is combined with water, the acid nature of the blood increases.

Correspondingly, the arterial blood pH value drops, eventually falling below the low normal value of 7.35. This lowered blood pH, then, is an index of an acid–base imbalance. The body's compensatory mechanisms attempt to reestablish balance by altering retention or excretion of acids and bases as an automatic response to alteration in blood pH. Compensatory mechanisms are limited, however, and thus a change in the arterial blood pH from normal range presents an immediate concern for the nurse, because maintenance of pH within the narrow range of 7.35 to 7.45 is essential for life.

The human body has an incredible ability to maintain itself in equilibrium, or balance, in order to maintain optimal functioning. It is able to use its own resources, and its own compensatory mechanisms, in order to keep its systems operating at optimal levels of efficiency. Perhaps in no other area of bodily function is this maintenance of balance more evident than in the balance of acids and bases. Arterial blood pH is the ratio of bicarbonate to carbonic acid, rather than the actual values of the two components that determine pH. A ratio of 20:1 will give a pH of 7.40. It is important to keep in mind that ratio determines the pH. This concept is especially important when we discuss compensation.

MEMORY JOGS

*N*ormal arterial blood pH is 7.35–7.45

Acidosis is pH below 7.35 (accumulation of acids in the blood stream)

Alkalosis is pH above 7.45 (excess of base in the blood stream)

Compensatory mechanisms are available in the body to help maintain balance between acids and bases.

Principle

The second step in identifying acid–base imbalances is to consider the "CO_2" level of arterial blood. Normal CO_2 is 35–45 mEq/L.

Illustration of Principle

The arterial blood pH gives the nurse evidence that an acid–base imbalance is occurring. The CO_2 level will give information about which system is *causing* the imbalance, whether respiratory or metabolic.

If the arterial blood pH is abnormal, either acidotic (lower pH) or alkalotic (higher pH), look at the CO_2 next. If the CO_2 is normal, it implies that respiratory (CO_2) balance is at equilibrium, so look at bicarbonate (HCO_3) level next. But if the CO_2 level is abnormal, it indicates an imbalance.

If the CO_2 level is elevated (above 45 mEq/L), hypoventilation and thus retention of CO_2 is occurring, either as a primary reason or secondary to compensation.

If the CO_2 level is decreased (below 35 mEq/L) hyperventilation and thus loss of CO_2 is occurring, either as a primary reason or secondary to compensation.

The only way to determine whether CO_2, and thus the respiratory system, is the problem rather than a compensatory mechanism, is to look at the HCO_3 next. If CO_2 is abnormal and HCO_3 is normal, the respiratory system is the problem. If CO_2 is abnormal and HCO_3 is abnormal, one of them is compensating for the other.

Consider the following examples:

Example 1

pH: 7.30
CO_2: 50 mEq/L
HCO_3: 25 mEq/L

In this example, the pH value indicates an acidotic state, because the value is below the normal range for arterial blood pH (7.35–7.45). The CO_2 level is elevated above the normal range of 35 to 45, indicating an increased amount of CO_2 and thus an increased amount of acid. If HCO_3 is normal, an elevated CO_2 value indicates the patient is in *respiratory acidosis*. The respiratory system is causing the imbalance.

Example 2

pH: 7.31
CO_2: 32 mEq/L
HCO_3: 20 mEq/L

In this second example, the pH is decreased again, indicating acidosis. But the CO_2 level is decreased, reducing the amount of acid in the blood. The HCO_3 is also decreased—thus, the decreased CO_2 is compensating for the decreased pH. This patient, then, is likely in *metabolic acidosis* and is using deep, rapid respirations (Kussmaul) to "blow off" CO_2 in the body's compensatory effort to decrease arterial blood acidity. The metabolic system (GI tract) is causing the imbalance.

Principle

The final step in identifying acid–base imbalances is to consider the "HCO_3" level of arterial blood.

Illustration of Principle

Like the CO_2 value, the level of HCO_3 provides information about the cause of the acid–base imbalance. Likewise, its relationship to CO_2 levels will reflect the body's compensation for the imbalance. Consider the examples below:

Example 1
pH: 7.57
CO_2: 36 mEq/L
HCO_3: 29 mEq/L

In this example, the pH indicates an excess of base, an alkalotic state. The CO_2 is within normal limits. (The HCO_3 level is elevated, indicating an increase of HCO_3 in the serum, causing the alkalosis.) An abnormal HCO_3 with a normal CO_2 indicates that the problem is metabolic. The CO_2 level is within normal range, indicating that no compensation for this imbalance is occurring and that the respiratory system is not the problem. If compensation were occurring, the CO_2 level would be increasing to raise the acid level of blood to "buffer" the elevated base level. Remembering that pH is a ratio that allows you to know which way, up or down, the CO_2 would need to go in order to compensate. The patient is in *metabolic alkalosis*.

Whenever you think of compensation, think of ratio! You always want the ratio to be close together. In other words, if the CO_2 goes up, to keep the ratio together—to compensate—you must have the HCO_3 go up to correct things. When the ratio is close together, the pH will be normal. If one value, either CO_2 or HCO_3, goes up or down, the other value must go in the same direction to maintain the same ratio, and thus maintain equilibrium or normal blood pH values.

Example 2
pH 7.29
CO_2: 54 mEq/L
HCO_3: 29 mEq/L

In this second example, the pH indicates an acidotic state (below 7.35). The CO_2 level is increased, indicating greater retention of CO_2 in the body and hypoventilation. The HCO_3 level is elevated above the normal value of 25, indicating that the kidneys are attempting to compensate for the high acid levels in the body by releasing HCO_3 to "buffer" the acids and restore balance. The patient is in *respiratory acidosis*.

Principle

Conditions that involve "hypoventilation" lead to retention of CO_2 and potential "respiratory acidosis."

Illustration of Principle

The key to understanding respiratory acidosis is to focus on its symptomatic cause—hypoventilation. Although respiratory acidosis is associated with a variety of diseases, the hallmark feature of these diseases is a depression of respirations. Because hypoventilating clients have a decreased rate and depth of respirations, they are unable to release necessary amounts of CO_2 with expiration, thus increasing the CO_2 level of arterial blood. Carbonic *acid* forms when CO_2 mixes with water in serum, resulting in increased *acidity* of arterial blood. Increased acid levels, termed *acidosis*, cause a decrease in arterial blood pH. The evidence of respiratory acidosis, then, is a decrease of arterial blood pH below 7.35 with an accompanying increase in CO_2.

MEMORY JOGS

---

*R*espiratory Acidosis

pH: less than 7.35
CO_2: greater than 45 mEq/L
HCO_3: normal—25 mEq/L
This is respiratory acidosis without compensation. If compensation were occurring, HCO_3 levels would be greater than normal (25), and the kidneys would retain bicarbonate.

The symptoms of respiratory acidosis are directly related to its cause, which is hypoventilation. These symptoms include:

- Slow, shallow, weak respirations
- Declining level of consciousness, stupor
- Mental lethargy, confusion, disorientation
- Associated signs of impaired oxygenation, e.g., pallor, cyanosis

Diseases or conditions associated with hypoventilation and acidotic states include:

- Emphysema (retention of CO_2)
- Pneumonia (interference with alveolar gas exchange)

- Head trauma (damage to respiratory center of the brain that causes hypoventilation)
- Overdose (depression of respiratory center)
- Barbiturates
- Anesthetics
- Narcotics
- Respiratory or cardiac arrest (loss of O_2 and accumulation of CO_2)

Nursing Management

Nursing interventions for the patient with any acid–base imbalance should be focused first on addressing the underlying cause of the imbalance, and then on treating the related symptoms. In respiratory acidosis, the nurse needs to address first the underlying problem, hypoventilation, and thus hypoxemia, by providing sources of O_2 (cannula, mask, endotracheal intubation, or mechanical ventilation). Second, the nurse may be ordered to administer a sodium bicarbonate injection in an effort to increase the blood pH by increasing the bicarbonate ion (HCO_3) content of the blood. The nurse should monitor the patient's mental status and provide for safety needs as indicated. In order to ensure that these interventions are successful in reversing the acidotic condition, the nurse should consistently monitor serial arterial blood gas readings to identify changes in pH and CO_2 values that would mark patient progress. An increase in blood pH back to 7.35–7.45 and a decrease in CO_2 level back to 35–45 mEq/L would indicate reversal or correction of the acidotic condition.

MEMORY JOGS

*T*he first priority is to assess the cause, hypoventilation, and correct it.
The nurse should provide O_2 and support for ventilation, such as intubation, if needed. Sodium bicarbonate injection may be used to "buffer" the excess acid in the blood stream.

Principle

Conditions that involve "hyperventilation" lead to excessive loss of CO_2 and "respiratory alkalosis"

Illustration of Principle

The key to understanding respiratory alkalosis is to focus on its symptomatic cause—hyperventilation. Whereas respiratory acidosis is caused by retention of CO_2, respiratory alkalosis is caused by an excessive loss of CO_2 as a result of hyperventilation, and thus a low CO_2 level. Because a hyperventilating patient has an increased rate and depth of respirations, the patient begins to lose CO_2 by "blowing it off" with expiration. The excessive loss of CO_2 then causes a decrease in acid, disrupting the balance between acids and bases. This results in an increased arterial blood pH, indicating an alkalotic condition. The evidence of respiratory alkalosis, then, is an increase in arterial blood pH above 7.45 with an accompanying decrease in CO_2.

Respiratory Alkalosis
pH: greater than 7.45
CO_2: less than 35 mEq/L
HCO_3: normal—25 mEq/L
This is respiratory alkalosis without compensation. If compensation were occurring, HCO_3 levels would be less than normal because kidneys would excrete HCO_3.

MEMORY JOGS

The symptoms of respiratory alkalosis are related directly to its cause—hyperventilation—and are very similar to a common cause of hyperventilation, acute anxiety. These symptoms are:

· Rapid, deep, "blowing" respirations
· Acute excitation, trembling, nervousness
· Neuromuscular irritability
· Numbness and tingling of extremities

Diseases or conditions associated with hyperventilation and alkalotic states include:

· Asthma (acute bronchial constriction)
· Brain injury (stimulation of respiratory center)
· Overdose of
  Aspirin (attempt of body to eliminate ASA acids)
  Cocaine (stimulation of respiratory center)
· Acute anxiety ("fight or flight" response)

Additionally, women in active labor, who have been trained in Lamaze delivery techniques but who are losing control over their breathing patterns with an increased intensity of uterine contractions, may begin to hyperventilate, placing them at risk for the development of respiratory alkalosis as well.

Nursing Management

In order to correct the source of this imbalance, the nurse needs to take actions to increase the CO_2 level of the patient's arterial blood; in other words, the nurse must address the cause, which is hyperventilation. The nurse should attempt to identify any underlying issues or problems that may have precipitated the alkalotic episode, including fear, anxiety, or acute stress reaction with impaired coping. The nurse should use reassurance and supportive skills in an effort to reduce the patient's anxiety and irritability, which will in turn regulate the rate and rhythm of respirations. Ways to assist the patient in decreasing the rate and depth of respiration include:

- Coaching the patient's breathing pattern to slow, deep respirations (especially valuable in labor and delivery settings)
- Encouraging the patient to hold his or her breath for several seconds in between respirations
- Instructing the patient to breathe into a paper bag, allowing the patient to reinhale his or her own exhaled CO_2.

Antianxiety or sedative medication may be administered both to calm the patient and to depress the rate and depth of respirations, thus increasing the retention of CO_2. A decreasing pH with elevated CO_2 and return to normal respiratory rate and depth signal improvement of the alkalotic state.

MEMORY JOGS

*T*he first priority is to assess the cause—hyperventilation—and correct it. The nurse should provide reassurance and supportive skills to reduce anxiety, thus decreasing the rate and depth of respirations. Coaching breathing, breath holding, and paper bag breathing are helpful maneuvers. Antianxiety or sedative medications may be helpful.

Principle

"Metabolic acidosis" *is characterized by an* "increased loss of HCO_3," *or an increased retention of acid ions, resulting in a* "decreased arterial blood pH"

Illustration of Principle

Metabolic acidosis is associated with a variety of disease conditions without a hallmark characteristic or feature. Each, however, involves an imbalance of metabolism of food or fluid, commonly involving disorders of the gastrointestinal tract, making this acid–base imbalance easily discernible from respiratory acidosis. Clients with renal failure may develop this imbalance in response to the kidney's inability to excrete phosphate and sulfate acid ions.

Thus, in renal failure, inability of the body to metabolize and excrete fluids also causes an inability to excrete acid, resulting in an increased acid concentration of arterial blood. The lungs may attempt to compensate for the increasing levels of acid by increasing rate and depth of respiration in order to "blow off" CO_2. This type of respiratory pattern is termed "Kussmaul breathing" and is often associated with diabetic ketoacidosis, another example of metabolic acidosis (discussed in detail in Chapter 15, Hormonal Regulation).

The evidence of metabolic acidosis is a decrease in arterial blood pH below 7.35, with an accompanying decrease in HCO_3 below 25 mEq/L.

MEMORY JOGS

Metabolic Acidosis

pH: less than 7.35
CO_2: normal 35–45 mEq/L
HCO_3: less than 25 mEq/L
This is metabolic acidosis without compensation. If compensation were occurring, CO_2 levels would be less than normal (35) and respirations would increase to decrease CO_2.

The symptoms of metabolic acidosis are related to the drop in arterial blood pH and are typified by signs of central nervous system depression, including cardiac dysrhythmia, apathy and lethargy, disorientation, and eventually, coma. Other symptoms of acidosis are related to its underlying cause, such as an acetone odor to the breath in diabetic ketoacidosis, or oliguria or anuria in patients with renal failure.

Additional diseases or conditions associated with metabolic acidosis include:

- Severe or prolonged diarrhea (loss of bicarbonate ion in stool)
- Prolonged fasting (anorexia nervosa; anorexia associated with cancer chemotherapy)
- Diabetes mellitus (rapid metabolism of fats with accumulation of acid by-product in diabetic ketoacidosis [DKA])

Nursing Management

Because the causes of metabolic acidosis are so varied, the nurse must take steps to correct the underlying problem causing the acidosis *first*, and then provide for other supportive strategies to deal with the acidotic state. For example, the nurse caring for the client who is becoming acidotic as a result of prolonged diarrhea must *first* take measures to control the diarrhea, and *then* provide for reversal of the acidotic state by administration of sodium bicarbonate, if needed. The client in diabetic ketoacidosis must first receive an infusion of regular insulin to halt the rapid metabolism of fats, which produces ketone acid bodies. The nurse should also keep a close watch of the client's vital signs and level of consciousness, because central nervous system depression is a feature of metabolic acidosis. Continuous cardiac monitoring is an essential intervention, because cardiac dsyrhythmias are common in acidotic states.

The nurse can evaluate the patient's progress through the acidotic condition by monitoring serial arterial blood gas values, noting an increase in pH (back to 7.35–7.45) and an increase in HCO_3 levels (back to 35–45 mEq/L). The patient should show steady improvement in level of consciousness and alertness, but should still have safety precautions maintained during the recovery process.

Principle

"Metabolic alkalosis" *is characterized by a "decreased loss of HCO_3" or a decreased retention of acid, resulting in an "increased arterial blood pH"*

Illustration of Principle

Like metabolic acidosis, "metabolic alkalosis" is associated with a number of different disease conditions without a hallmark characteristic or feature. However, metabolic alkalotic conditions involve an imbalance of metabolism of foods or fluids commonly involving disorders of the gastrointestinal tract, making them easily discernible from "respiratory" alkalosis states. In metabolic alkalosis, there is an increase in the level of serum bicarbonate or a loss of acid, resulting in decreased levels of serum acid. This causes an increase in arterial blood pH accompanied by an increased serum HCO_3 level.

For example, if a client diagnosed with peptic ulcer overmedicates himself with antacid medications in a desperate effort to reduce abdominal discomfort, the client may develop an increase in serum bicarbonate levels, because antacids are highly alkaline. Likewise, if a client suffers a loss of acids from the body, such as one would with prolonged vomiting or gastric suction, the acid levels of the serum will decrease from loss of hydrochloric acid (HCl) from the stomach, resulting in an alkalotic state. The evidence of metabolic alkalosis, then, is an increase of arterial blood pH above 7.45, with an accompanying increase in HCO_3.

Metabolic Alkalosis

pH: greater than 7.45
CO_2: normal 35–45 mEq/L
HCO_3: greater than 25 mEq/L
This is metabolic alkalosis without compensation. If compensation were occurring, CO_2 levels would be greater than normal (45) and respirations would decrease to increase CO_2.

MEMORY JOGS

The patient experiencing metabolic alkalosis will demonstrate symptoms of central nervous system excitement, the exact opposite of the patient with metabolic acidosis. Symptoms include irritability, disorientation, muscular twitching, and seizures. The heart likewise will be overstimulated, resulting in dysrhythmia.

Nursing Management

First, the nurse should focus on correcting the underlying cause of the alkalotic condition so that acid–base balance may be restored. The nurse should be sure to monitor blood gas values in patients with upper gastrointestinal disturbances, so that an excess loss of acid ions does not go undetected, as it could in prolonged vomiting or improper gastric suction and irrigation. Likewise, the nurse should instruct patients with gastrointestinal problems, such as gastritis or peptic ulcer, to follow medication schedules carefully to prevent antacid overdose that could lead to alkalosis.

The nurse can determine a reversal of the metabolic alkalosis by serial arterial blood gas values that would indicate a decrease in pH (back to 7.35–7.45) and a decrease in HCO_3 values (back to 25 mEq/L).

Reasoning Exercises: *Acids and Bases*

1. Which of the following would place a patient at risk for developing respiratory acidosis?
   A. Frequent episodes of vomiting for 2 days
   B. Use of narcotic analgesia
   C. Rapid and deep "blowing" respirations
   D. Acute pain in the lower abdomen and pelvis

Intended Response: **B.** Narcotics, as central nervous system (CNS) depressants, can lower both the rate and depth of respiration, resulting in decreased oxygen intake and increased retention of carbon dioxide. Frequent vomiting could result in metabolic alkalosis, as acids are lost from the stomach. Rapid and deep blowing respirations will increase carbon dioxide loss, and are thus not associated with respiratory acidosis. The experience of acute pain increases the metabolic rate, which then typically increases rate and depth of respiration.

2. Which of the following assessment or diagnostic data would alert the nurse to the possibility of respiratory acidosis related to respiratory burns?
   A. Arterial blood pH of 7.36
   B. Singed nasal hairs
   C. Arterial blood CO_2 of 43 mEq/L
   D. Yellow/creamy colored respiratory secretions

Intended Response: **B.** Singed nasal hairs is a hallmark manifestation of respiratory burns, a significant cause of death in burn patients. Both arterial blood pH of 7.36 and arterial CO_2 value of 43 mEq/L are within normal limits. Yellow colored (purulent) respiratory secretions suggest respiratory tract infection.

3. Which of the following assessments would be the **earliest** indicator of respiratory acidosis?
   A. Restlessness
   B. Cool, clammy skin
   C. Mental confusion
   D. Decreased level of consciousness

Intended Response: **A.** As respiratory acidosis is associated with decreased oxygenation, restlessness and apprehension secondary to decreased oxygen supply to the brain are early indicators of this acid–base imbalance. The remaining responses are associated with respiratory acidosis, but occur as the imbalance develops with ever-decreasing oxygen saturation.

4. A patient is admitted to the emergency department with a diagnosis of angina pectoris (chest pain) and associated difficulty breathing. In an effort to **prevent** respiratory acidosis, which of the following physician orders should the nurse identify as the priority intervention?

   A. Collection of venous blood specimen for lab
   B. Administration of analgesia
   C. Initiation of IV fluids at keep vein open rate
   D. Administration of oxygen per nasal cannula

Intended Response: **B.** The experience of chest pain makes it difficult for a patient to fully respire, often resulting in hypoventilation with secondary retention of carbon dioxide. Administration of analgesia will reduce the sensation of pain, thus enhancing respiratory ease and depth.

5. A patient with a degenerative neuromuscular disease is being treated for *Haemophilus influenzae* (bacterial) pneumonia. On the third day of hospitalization, arterial blood gases (ABGs) reveal a pH of 7.33, CO_2 of 52 mEq/L, and pO_2 of 66. Which of the following nursing interventions would be appropriate?

   A. Document the results and continue to monitor the patient
   B. Encourage the patient to cough and deep breathe q 4 hours
   C. Instruct the patient to cover mouth and breathe nasally
   D. Administer oxygen per nasal cannula at 2–3 L/min

Intended Response: **D.** The patient's arterial blood gases suggest mild respiratory acidosis and hypoxemia, indicating the need for oxygen administration.

6. A patient with chronic obstructive pulmonary disease (COPD) is admitted with the following ABG values:

   pH 7.28; pCO_2 63 mEq/L; HCO_3 26 mEq/L; pO_2 76

Which of the following would indicate that the patient's acid–base imbalance is resolving?

A. pH increased

B. pCO_2 increased

C. HCO_3 decreased

D. pO_2 decreased

Intended Response: **A.** The patient's arterial blood pH indicates acidosis. Reversal of the acidotic state would be evidenced by an increase in pH.

7. A patient experiencing acute anxiety is hyperventilating, with a respiratory rate of 36 bpm. Which of the following nursing actions would be most beneficial to this patient?

   A. Maintaining the patient in a semi–Fowler's-to-sitting position

   B. Applying oxygen per nasal cannula at 2–3 L/min

   C. Encouraging the patient to cough and deep breathe at frequent intervals

   D. Administering prescribed sedative medication

Intended Response: **D.** Administration of sedating medication will suppress the respiratory center of the brain, resulting in a decreased respiratory rate and depth with decreased loss of carbon dioxide. Measures to enhance oxygenation A, B, and C are not indicated in this patient situation.

8. A patient in acute renal failure has metabolic acidosis. Which of the following serum lab values should the nurse **most** closely monitor related to the acidotic state?

   A. Hematocrit

   B. Potassium

   C. White blood count

   D. Calcium

Intended Response: **B.** As arterial blood pH decreases, serum potassium inversely increases, potentiating the serious cardiac dysrhythmias associated with this acid–base imbalance.

9. Which of the following clinical manifestations would indicate the body's effort toward compensation for metabolic acidosis?

   A. Rapid, blowing respirations

   B. Elevated temperature

C. Decreasing blood pressure

D. Polyuria

Intended Response: **A.** The lungs will attempt to compensate in metabolic acidotic states via rapid, blowing (Kussmaul) respirations to "blow off" carbon dioxide and thus lower serum acid levels.

10. The nurse notes that a diabetic patient is demonstrating rapid and deep "blowing" respirations. The nurse should take which of the following actions?

    A. Elevate the head of the bed to semi-Fowler's position

    B. Apply oxygen per nasal cannula at 2–3 L/min

    C. Administer a packet of sugar to the patient

    D. Request an order for stat arterial blood gases

Intended Response: **D.** The presence of rapid, blowing (Kussmaul) respirations in a diabetic patient indicates the body's efforts to "blow off" carbon dioxide in a metabolic acidotic state (DKA). Arterial blood gases should be drawn to quantify the seriousness of the imbalance and to monitor patient status during management. Measures to enhance oxygenation **A** and **B** are not indicated, as oxygenation of body tissues is not compromised in this patient situation. Because the patient is metabolizing stored fats (because glucose cannot be used for cellular energy) administration of glucose **C** is contraindicated.

Elimination

WAYNE NAGEL

Principle
Elimination has direct bearing on the body's ability to balance fluids and electrolytes

Illustration of Principle

Elimination is the process by which waste products are removed from the body. The principal systems include the gastrointestinal system and the urinary system. Alterations in gastrointestinal elimination, such as diarrhea or constipation, affect the body's balance of electrolytes and fluids. For example, diarrhea manifests as frequency of defecation, producing watery, loosely formed stools. During episodes of diarrhea, the organs associated with absorption are in a hypermotile state. Ingested foods pass quickly through the system, thereby decreasing the amount of time for nutrients and electrolytes to be absorbed. Since fluids and electrolytes essential to metabolic balance are primarily obtained from the foods and fluids that we ingest, alterations occur.

Constipation, a condition characterized by hard, dry stools and irregularity, results from hypomobility. Passage of ingested fluids and foods is slowed. Increased absorption of the nutrients occurs. Constipation can be a very uncomfortable condition for the client. Client knowledge deficits related to fiber intake is a frequent nursing finding.

*T*he key to assessing client regularity is determining whether the client's bowel patterns have changed.

Regularity can be defined as one bowel movement per day at the same time each day. Not everyone is "regular."

The urinary and renal system organs directly affect the composition and the volume of extracellular fluid. In addition to producing urine, these structures are involved with the excretion and absorption of water and electrolytes. Renal insufficiency potentially can produce fluid volume excess. This volume excess is related to an excess of sodium (Na). Renal nephron damage produces an inability to filter Na and to excrete water. Water is held in the extracellular compartments because Na is so osmotically active. This Na excess produces an excess of water and is observable in such conditions as hypertension, volume overload, and pulmonary edema. Excess fluid volume also increases the workload of the heart.

Potassium is another key electrolyte related to alterations in elimination. Potassium (K) excess is related to alterations in tubular secretory function. Rises in K related to altered excretion are responsible for a hyperkalemic state. Hyperkalemia can result from acute or chronic conditions affecting renal function, or from traumatic tissue injuries such as burns.

Hypokalemia can occur secondary to alterations in elimination when a hyperexcretory state exists. Rapid movement of fluid through the system minimizes the time in which K can be absorbed. Diuretics increase the elimination of fluids from the body; subsequently, K is lost with the increased urinary elimination. Client teaching regarding kalemic balance, including signs and symptoms and diets rich in K, is a significant nursing intervention.

*P*otassium has a very narrow normal range. Clients with conditions producing hypo- or hyperkalemic states should be monitored closely.

Alterations in renal tubular function affect magnesium (Mg) balance. Episodes of oliguria tend to increase Mg levels, and polyuric states that produce diuresis decrease Mg levels. The client who has been burned sustains Mg losses secondary to hypermobility of the gastrointestinal system.

Alterations in calcium–phosphate balance occur when vitamin D is not activated. Calcium (Ca) is absorbed from the intestines. The kidneys are responsible for activating exogenous vitamin D within the body. Renal disease decreases this response, allowing Ca to be lost. Hypermobility in the gastrointestinal system permits Ca to be lost in feces. Renal dysfunction inhibits the excretion of phosphates, resulting in elevated phosphate levels. The calcium–phosphate interaction is essential in maintaining healthy bone tissue.

Principle

The retention of metabolic wastes related to inadequate elimination affects multiple body systems

Illustration of Principle

The food and fluids that we ingest provide the body with the essentials to maintain structure, function, health, and balance. The body breaks down an ingested substance into substances that can be used. Substances that cannot be used are eliminated. By-products of metabolism become the wastes that are eliminated. Conditions causing inadequate elimination result in retention of these waste products. Renal and gastrointestinal dysfunctions result in the inadequate elimination of electrolytes and metabolic waste products. As the disease processes become increasingly severe, balance is more greatly affected, and the consequences to the body are more profound. The buildup of nitrogenous waste products, electrolytes, and other substances produces a toxic condition in the body.

Inadequate nutrition is frequently seen in clients experiencing retention of waste products. The by-products of ingested foods and fluids, as stated earlier, become these toxic substances when their ammonium exceeds what is required for balance. In a uremic toxic state, as the blood urea nitrogen level (BUN) elevates, a metabolic acidosis occurs. This condition occurs because the metabolic processes of the body are unable to produce buffers in sufficient quantity to keep up with the rising acidic state of the body.

As the metabolic acidosis worsens, the client becomes increasingly more anorexic. Protein substances do not taste good to the client with an elevated BUN. Foods high in K should be watched carefully because of the narrow range of normal limits of this electrolyte. Conditions such as renal failure may call for fluid restrictions; subsequently the client may feel very thirsty. Other associated conditions such as pain, elevated temperature, or immobility may decrease the client's desire for food.

> *P*rotein limitations or deficiencies can lead to muscle wasting. Small, frequent feedings are indicated in conditions in which intake intolerance is the identified problem.

MEMORY JOGS

Inadequate wound healing is frequently seen in clients experiencing retention of metabolic wastes. The buildup of intracellular waste products secondary to inadequate elimination of these substances results in the cells' inability to synthesize, differentiate, and multiply. Meticulous skin and wound care is essential to prevent complications. Buildup of metabolic wastes such as uric acid crystals on the skin is irritating and can produce integument breakdown. The client should be assessed frequently for signs and symptoms of skin breakdown. Clients who are bed bound or experiencing alterations in mobility are especially susceptible to skin breakdown.

Septicemia is a common complication in clients experiencing retained metabolic wastes. The toxic substances overwhelm the body. Because normal metabolism promotes the function of all body systems, alterations related to retained waste products place the client in a state of imbalance. The immune system suffers, in that it is unable to keep up with the increasing demands to protect the body from the aggressor pathogens. Pathogens then spill into circulating volume and are transported throughout the body. Multiple system injuries can ensue.

MEMORY JOGS

*M*eticulous care of invasive devices, intravenous lines, and catheters is important. These are direct portals of pathogenic entry into the body.

A buildup of metabolic waste products in the body can produce alterations in mental neurologic status. Waste products and their by-products can cross the blood-brain barrier. As this phenomenon occurs, the central nervous system is affected. Substances like ureas are osmotically active substances that attract abnormal amounts of body water into the central nervous system. The buildup of water produces swelling, which produces neuronal displacement or compression, which can produce disorientation, confusion, and seizures.

Activity intolerance is frequently seen as conditions become more chronic. The buildup of waste products, altered nutritional status, and lack of energy requirements and calories can and do impede a client's ability to participate in activities of daily living. Pain associated with the underlying pathological condition may produce malaise, and even fear of increasing discomfort. Anemias can occur, producing weakness and fatigue.

Sexual dysfunctions occur secondary to alterations in libido, potency, ovulation, and menstruation. These conditions result from the toxic effects of the circulating high levels of metabolic wastes that directly and indirectly interact negatively with the sexual function of the reproductive system.

*C*lients and families should be encouraged to discuss conditions affecting their sex lives and to seek counseling. Clients often feel that their sexual dysfunctions are unique to them.

MEMORY JOGS

Chronic conditions producing alterations in the ability to eliminate body wastes may be responsible for ineffective coping. A condition, for example, requiring ongoing dialysis certainly calls for significant lifestyle changes. These changes may produce feelings of powerlessness, may require financial adjustments that can be burdensome, and may limit one's physical stamina, thereby reducing quality of life. Support groups, community resources, individual counseling, and therapy are just some of the interventions available to promote effective coping. The buildup of metabolic wastes over a period of time may alter a client's ability to reason. This condition may require alternative long-term client placement.

Principle

Patterns of elimination are affected by psychosocial and physiological factors

Illustration of Principle

Alterations in patterns of elimination can be affected by functional disorders. Disorders such as tumors requiring bowel resection and resulting in colostomy may produce needs for dietary changes. The client who has to undergo hemodialysis secondary to kidney failure will be required to adhere to a dialysis regimen. These functional disorders may be temporary or permanent, but will require client compliance in order to maintain balance.

Clients may develop feelings of emotional stress, secondary to feeling different. This stress may decrease the client's ability to reintegrate into society, family, or a profession. Stress affects overall balance, because it increases the demands on the multiple systems to function in an optimal fashion. Hypermetabolic states can occur. These states increase the production of wastes, which increases the need for optimal elimination.

A client experiencing stress incontinence, for example, may be fearful of going shopping or going out to dinner because she may be embarrassed. Alterations in body image often produce a feeling of being "different." That sense of being out of the ordinary may produce withdrawal from social behaviors.

*D*iscussing the client's feelings with the client may relieve some discomfort. The goal is to promote client emotional comfort.

Reasoning Exercises: *Elimination*

1. Which of the following nursing diagnoses is most significant for a patient with renal insufficiency?
   A. Fluid Volume Excess
   B. Hyperthermia
   C. Fatigue
   D. Activity Intolerance

Intended Response: **A.** Because the patient with renal insufficiency cannot eliminate fluids, Fluid Volume Excess (FVE) is an expected, and often priority, nursing diagnosis. The kidneys do not directly affect temperature regulation **B,** and only with extreme fluid loss will temperature elevation appear secondary to dehydration. Although both Activity Intolerance **D** and Fatigue **C** are common features of renal insufficiency, neither is a specific enough diagnosis to be of greatest importance.

2. Which of the following changes in laboratory values is associated with renal insufficiency?
   A. Increased serum potassium
   B. Decreased serum creatinine
   C. Increased serum calcium
   D. Decreased serum BUN

Intended Response: **A.** Potassium as an electrolyte is excreted predominantly in urine. Because the patient with renal insufficiency has decreased urine production, serum potassium levels rise. Both serum creatinine **B** and serum BUN **D** increase as renal function decreases. Because the kidneys are responsible for activating exogenous vitamin D necessary for calcium absorption, persons with renal insufficiency demonstrate a decrease in serum calcium.

3. Which of the following interventions should the nurse include in a plan of care for a patient with fluid excess related to renal insufficiency?

   A. Push oral fluids

   B. Assess blood pressure q 8 hours

   C. Monitor strict intake and output

   D. Assess body weight weekly

Intended Response: **C.** Because the kidneys play such an essential role in fluid distribution and elimination, renal insufficiency commonly results in fluid volume excess. The nurse should monitor strict intake and output (preferably, *hourly*) and restrict oral fluid **A** to prevent a worsening of fluid volume excess. Because hypertension is a complication of fluid volume excess in renal insufficiency, blood pressure measurements must be more often than routine (once per shift). Because 1 kg of body weight = 1 L of fluid, body weight should be measured daily **D** to evaluate fluid volume status.

4. Which of the following clinical manifestations would correlate with anemia secondary to decreased production of erythropoietin in a patient with renal insufficiency?

   A. Abdominal cramping and diarrhea

   B. Weakness and fatigue

   C. Purpura and ecchymosis

   D. Edema and weight gain

Intended Response: **B.** Erythropoietin is an essential element in the production of oxygen-carrying red blood cells. A decrease in the kidneys' ability to manufacture erythropoietin results in chronic anemia, characterized by signs of decreased tissue oxygenation such as weakness and fatigue. Abdominal cramping and diarrhea **A** could be associated with hyperirritability of the lower gastrointestinal tract secondary to hyperkalemia (elevated serum potassium). Purpura and ecchymosis **C** are manifestations of decreased platelets (clotting cells). Edema and weight gain, although associated with renal insufficiency resulting from disturbances in sodium balance, are not indicators of decreased production of erythropoietin.

5. Which of the following is an expected effect of retention of metabolic wastes secondary to chronic renal insufficiency?

   A. Increased appetite

   B. Chronic hypotension

C. Sexual dysfunction

D. Persistent low grade fever

Intended Response: **C.** Toxic effects of circulating high levels of metabolic wastes affect the reproductive system, and thus, sexual function. Metabolic acidosis with renal failure causes increasing anorexia **A** in patients with impaired renal function. Hypertension **B** results from fluid volume excesses caused by decreased urinary output. Presence of a persistent low grade fever **D** is not expected in renal disease, and should alert the nurse to the probability of infection in this patient.

6. Which of the following nursing diagnoses is significant for a patient whose laboratory values indicate a marked decrease in serum calcium secondary to a renal failure?

A. Fatigue

B. High Risk for Injury

C. Altered Tissue Perfusion

D. High Risk for Infection

Intended Response: **B.** Patients with renal failure demonstrate a retention of phosphorus and a loss of calcium. Because calcium is essential to maintaining healthy bone tissue, loss of calcium renders the bones weak and fragile, placing the patient at risk for injury such as fracture.

7. Which of the following urine laboratory test values would provide the most valuable information to the nurse caring for a patient complaining of urinary frequency, urgency, and dysuria?

A. Ketones

B. Specific gravity

C. Occult blood

D. Culture

Intended Response: **D.** Because the patient's complaints strongly suggest the probability of a urinary tract infection, results of a culture of urine identifying the type and intensity of microorganism present would be most valuable in directing management of the patient. Although occult blood **C** may be present in urinary tract infection, this value is not specific to infection alone. Ketone bodies **A** result from rapid or excessive fat metabolism, and are not related to urinary tract infection. Specific gravity **B** changes with the fluid concentration of urine.

8. Which of the following findings would indicate to the nurse that continuous ambulatory peritoneal dialysis (CAPD) has been effective?

    A. Sodium decreasing, creatinine increasing

    B. BUN increasing, blood glucose increasing

    C. Blood glucose decreasing, potassium increasing

    D. BUN decreasing, creatinine decreasing

Intended Response: **D.** The primary purpose of CAPD treatment is to stimulate the kidney functions of fluid balance and waste removal and excretion. The decrease in BUN and creatinine levels evidence that these functions are being achieved by the CAPD treatments.

9. As a nurse is inserting a nasogastric tube for gastrointestinal suction, the patient suddenly begins to cough and gasp. Which of the following actions should the nurse take?

    A. Stop the insertion, allow the patient to rest, then continue inserting the tube

    B. Encourage the patient to take deep breaths through the mouth while the tube is being inserted

    C. Instruct the patient to take a few sips of water and swallow as the tube is being inserted

    D. Remove the inserted tube, allow the patient to rest, and then attempt to reinsert

Intended Response: **D.** The process of nasogastric tube insertion is not a pleasant one, and the nurse should anticipate that the patient will experience gagging sensations as the tube courses through the esophageal tract. However, symptoms of coughing and gasping indicate possible misplacement of the tube in the trachea or lung, and thus, the tube should be removed. The correct response is **D,** and following the tube removal, the patient should be allowed to rest briefly to fully oxygenate before the procedure is restarted.

10. Which of the following colors of gastrointestinal drainage would indicate the need for the nurse to perform a hemoccult test for gastrointestinal bleeding?

    A. Clear

    B. Pale yellow

C. Green

D. Dark brown

Intended Response: **D.** The presence of dark brown "coffee ground" coloration (response **D)** in gastric drainage indicates the need for a hemoccult test, which is used to determine the presence of blood in gastric drainage.

13 Infection and Inflammation

WAYNE NAGEL

Principle

The immune system differentiates between self and nonself

Illustration of Principle

This system protects the body against pathogenic organisms and other foreign bodies through a series of complex biochemical interactions. Humoral immune response produces antibodies to react with specific antigens that fight viral and bacterial infections. Through complex biochemical activity, this component of the immune system stimulates B-cells to produce invader-specific antibodies. Humoral response to the invading organism or virus may be immediate or may occur within 48 hours. Cellular immunity, also known as the cell-mediated response, produces T-lymphocytes that mobilize tissue macrophages. These macrophages then attack invading foreign bodies. The cellular immune system directly attacks the invading organism by producing appropriate numbers of white blood cells to identify, engulf, and destroy the invader. This system is also involved in what is commonly referred to as "resistance" to infection. Together, humoral and cellular immunity work as *self* in order to protect the body from the *nonself* pathogenic organisms and cancers.

*A*ntibodies are immunoglobins essential to the immune system. They are produced by lymphoid tissue in response to bacteria, viruses, or other antigenic substances. An antibody is specific to an antigen. *Antigens* are proteins that cause the formation of antibodies. Antigens react specifically with an antibody. The *antibody–antigen* reaction is the process by which specific B-cells recognize the invader or antigen, stimulate antibody production, and thereby protect the body from infection.

The immune response, therefore, becomes a defense function of the body that produces antibodies to destroy invading bacteria, viruses, and malignancies. The physiological weapons of self, therefore, become the antibody–antigen reaction. Immunity can be created by immunizing a client with vaccinations—for example, polio, tetanus, and rubella. Natural immunity, on the other hand, is a genetically inherited resistance to specific infectious organisms. Natural immunity is affected by components of health such as mental health, metabolism, diet, and environment, and is also affected by the strength of the invading organism. Balance is maintained when the self is able to effectively check the nonself (see Figure 13–1).

*V*accines are produced from attenuated or killed microorganisms and inoculated into clients to stimulate the immune system to induce active immunity. *Antibiotics, bacterials,* and *fungals* are synthesized chemically or produced from specific organisms. This group is effective in interfering with the production of the cell wall, protein synthesis, nucleic acid synthesis, or membrane synthesis. They also can and do inhibit critical biosynthetic pathways in the invading organism.

It is important, therefore, to summarize the physiology associated with the immune system. Referring back to our principle, *the immune system differentiates between self and nonself,* it is essential to understand that all components of the immune system work together. Through complex biochemical and physiological interactions, the immune system serves as the body's main defense against infections and cancers. As we later discuss inflammation, you will see the interplay in this system.

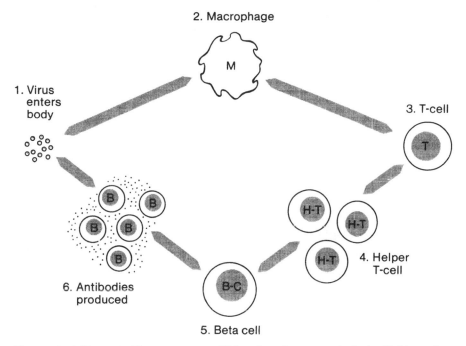

Figure 13-1. The normal immune system. (*1*) Invading *virus* enters the body. (*2*) *Macrophages* act as the alarm system. They identify the invading virus and biochemically notify the T-cells. (*3*) After being notified of the invader, the *T-cell* activates the immune system and begins producing helper T-cells. (*4*) *Helper T-cells* activate beta cells (B-cells). The B-cells begin producing antibodies. (*5*) In response to this direction, the *beta cells* increase in number, multiplying to meet the need for antibody production and fight the attacking virus. (*6*) The *antibodies,* warriors of the immune system, seek out and attack the invading virus. Once it is determined that the virus has been checked, *T-8 (suppressor cells)* are produced. These cells call off the attack, allowing the immune system to become balanced once again.

White blood cells (WBCs) are the main defense of the immune system in working to destroy invading organisms or cancer cells. Lymphocytes are a specific type of white blood cell and are considered the intelligence of the immune system. Lymphocytes possess the ability to recognize infectious agents and cancer cells; they direct the other white blood cells to destroy those agents. Humoral and cellular immunity work together, first to produce antibodies, and second to produce T-lymphocytes in order to combat infections and cancer cells through direct cellular contact. The T-lymphocytes consist of two subsets: T-4 helper cells and T-8 suppressor cells. For optimal balance of the function of the immune system, T-4 helper cells and T-8 suppressor cells must be present in sufficient quantities.

MEMORY JOGS

*C*onsider three terms relating to the immune system:
Immunomodulators: These substances act to alter the immune response. They are naturally present in the body or are pharmacologically reproduced.
Immunosuppression: This represents a significant interference with the ability of the immune system to respond to antigenic stimulation.
Immunoglobins: These are antigenically distinct antibodies that are present in the serum and external secretions of the body.

Clients experiencing immunologic deficits will exhibit signs and symptoms related to the etiology of the deficits. These etiologically specific deficits manifest in many different ways, depending upon which component of the immune system is being affected or inactivated. Pathogenic organisms, the nonself, produce unique and varied effects to which the immune system, the self, must respond. Because the immune system is made up of many components, certain diseases will require more activity from one component than another. Balance of this system requires that all components are able to function fully and optimally.

Consider the effect on the immune system when it is attacked by the AIDS virus (see Figure 13–2).

MEMORY JOGS

*A*IDS is a condition reflective of immunologic deficits. This condition is caused by the *human immunodeficiency virus* (*HIV*), which alters the balance between T-4 helper cells and T-8 suppressor cells. Skewing is in favor of the T-8 suppressor cells. This causes immune system suppression and increased susceptibility to infection.

Principle

The first barrier to infection is the epithelial layer covering the body, known as the skin

Illustration of Principle

Not only skin but also hair, mucous membranes, and secretions provide barriers to infection. The external and internal environments of a person are teeming with microorganisms. Internally, microorganisms are controlled by the overall good

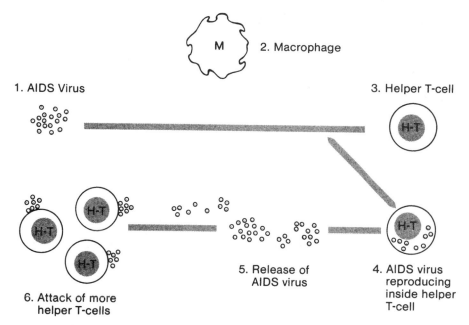

Figure 13-2. AIDS and the immune system. (1) When the AIDS virus enters the body, the macrophage is bypassed, and helper T-cells are attacked. The macrophage is ineffective as an alarm system, resulting in altered immunologic repsonse. (2) The helper T-cell is invaded by the AIDS virus. The AIDS virus remains in the helper T-cell but is inactive for a period of time. When the helper T-cell is attacked by another virus or bacteria, this stimulates the AIDS virus to begin reproducing itself. (3) The AIDS virus reproduces itself within the helper T-cell. The infected helper T-cell dies and the AIDS virus is released to infect other helper T-cells. (4) Newly released AIDS virus. (5 and 6) AIDS virus attacks other helper T-cells.

health of a person and a functional immune system. Exposure to microoganisms in the external environment is dependent upon several factors.

A break in the integrity of the skin or epithelial covering of the body is a major source of exposure to environmental microorganisms. Subsequent to this interruption, infections can and do develop. Such interruptions can occur in the urinary tract, gastrointestinal tract, and respiratory tract. Once a disruption occurs, microorganisms thriving in the external environment can enter the body. Microorganisms, bacteria, and viruses have the ability in some cases to escape the natural defenses of the host; because of this lack of detection, the invading organisms are able to generate infection and/or inflammatory responses.

Mechanisms of defense related to the integument differ from site to site. Characteristics of this phenomenon relate to the specialized functions of surface cells, including macrophages and cilia; flora that normally are present at the site and able to inhibit the colonization of pathogens; the skin and mucous membranes that act as a physical barrier to invading microorganisms; and secretions such as gastric acid, mucus, and saliva.

In general, the skin does not provide an optimal environment for microbial development. Epithelial cells are tightly compacted, thus providing a dense mechanical barrier. This barrier exists because of the multilayered structure that is created by the densely packed epithelial cells. The horny outer layer of the skin is being shed and replaced constantly. This phenomenon helps in the elimination of externally attacking pathogens. Moist areas of the body promote the growth of microorganisms. Most microorganisms require a nonacidic environment to promote their growth. The acidic pH of the skin repels this growth.

MEMORY JOGS

*T*he skin consists of two layers: the outer (epidermis) and the deeper (dermis).

The epidermis (outer layer) functions as a barrier to protect inner tissues from injury, chemicals, and organisms; as a receptor for a range of sensations (touch, pain, heat, and cold); and as a regulator of body temperature through radiation, conduction, and convection.

Impairment of skin integrity, either actual or potential, places the client at risk. Many factors can contribute to this state. It is important to consider that pathogenic organisms may contact the body in various ways, and disease does not always result. Contributing factors related to the disruption of skin integrity may include inadequate personal hygiene, which permits a medium for pathogens to grow and promotes excoriation of the skin. Inadequate nutrition does not permit optimal cellular growth and differentiation of this protective barrier. Other pathological conditions, such as impaired oxygen transport, related to anemia, cardiovascular disorders, metabolic conditions such as diabetes mellitus and cancer; or medications such as steroids, can and do contribute to skin disruption.

Other obvious conditions, such as penetrating traumatic injuries, burns, and surgical incisions, open the way for organisms to enter the human internal environment. Coupled with other compromising conditions such as shock, malnutrition, or previously existing pathology, the microorganisms can go on to reproduce and compromise human balance.

MEMORY JOGS

*D*ressings are mechanical barriers applied to the skin. Dressings absorb drainage, protect wounds from injury, control bleeding, serve as vehicle for mediation, and keep the wound clean. Types of dressings include pressure dressings, occlusive dressings, absorbent dressings, wet dressings, and antiseptic dressings.

Principle

The interactions among host defense mechanisms, microbial virulence, and environmental conditions are the determinants for development of infections

Illustration of Principle

Microorganisms enter the body in many ways. They can be ingested, as in the case of salmonella; inhaled, as in the case of mycobacteria in tuberculosis; or they may enter in other unknown ways, as in the case of cytomegalovirus. Natural resistance to infection relates to the overall health of the body in producing secretory or circulating immune globulins. Therefore, in addition to the physical barriers of skin and mucous membranes, there exists a series of chemical barriers.

Chemical barriers include all of the secretions or excretions of the stomach in the form of hydrochloric acid, digestive enzymes, bacteriostatic agents present in plasma, products released or activated by antigen–antibody reaction, and waxes and other fatty acids with bacteriostatic properties, such as cerumen.

Front line phagocyctic cells, which are part of the reticuloendothelial system, are filtering the circulating blood continuously. These cells are able to clear entering particles of bacteria from the bloodstream.

Principle

The process of infection can be interrupted at any point where the chain is broken. The most common interruption in the chain of infection is at the **mode of transmission**

Illustration of Principle

To keep in mind an understanding of this principle, the nurse must be aware that a series of events is necessary for an infection to occur. Required are a disease-producing agent, a reservoir, a mode of transmission, a portal of entry, and a susceptible host. Susceptibility is not well understood, but relationships exist among the virulence and number of organisms attacking the host, the immune system's ability to destroy invading organisms, and the overall health and nutritional status of the host. Susceptibility to disease is known to be influenced by factors such as psychosocial and lifestyle practices, the general environment that the host is exposed to, finances, recreation patterns, and stress.

As desirable as it is to use primary prevention by means of vaccination to prevent the transmission of infection, as with smallpox and polio, vaccination is not available for all pathogenic microorganisms. Thus, the essential goal of the nurse in the prevention of infection is interrupting the mode of transmission. This goal is best achieved by two measures: consistent, conscientious, and thorough hand washing; and the use of barrier protection such as gloves, mask, or gown.

To prevent transmission of infection, then, the nurse need only identify the mode of transmission of the infecting agent, and then apply barrier protection which will interrupt the mode. For example, if the agent is transmitted via a fecal route, the nurse should use enteric precautions, applying gloves as barrier protection whenever in contact with the patient's feces. Likewise, if the agent is transmitted via blood, the nurse should use blood-borne pathogen precautions, wearing barrier protection on any moist body surface (eyes, nose, mouth, and hands) which may come into contact with the blood or blood-contaminated secretions of a patient. The outbreak of HIV infection and an increasing incidence of hepatitis B alerted health care workers to the need to use blood-borne pathogen precautions routinely with all patients in all care settings. Thus, blood-borne pathogen precautions are frequently referred to as "Universal Precautions."

Nursing application in the form of promoting prevention through community education plays a major role in keeping infections in check. Nurses should assess clients' attitudes regarding infectious diseases, promote adequate personal and environmental hygiene practices, instruct clients regarding adequate nutrition and food handling, storage, and preparation practices, and assist clients in maintaining balance with regard to psychosocial and stress relationships.

MEMORY JOGS

*I**solation:* These practices are employed to prevent cross-contamination. Contamination can occur from an infected client to care providers or from care providers to the compromised client. The form of isolation employed should be specific to the needs of the client.

Important to keep in mind is that the isolation of clients places physical barriers between the client and the rest of the world. Barriers in the form of restricted access to the client's room and the use of gowns, gloves, and masks may lead to behaviors associated with withdrawal and sensory deprivation.

Hand washing: This practice continues to be one of the most effective mechanisms in the prevention of transmission of microorganisms. Inattention to this very important detail is unsafe nursing practice.

Principle

Inflammation works to limit the tissue damage, remove the injured cells, and repair the traumatized tissue

Illustration of Principle

Inflammation is a defensive response against cellular injury wherein the body attempts to restrict the injurious agent, neutralize the agent, and repair tissue that has been damaged by the harmful agent. Cellular damage can result from various causes. Regardless of the causative agent, the dynamics of the inflammatory response remain constant and are essential.

Damage that occurs in the body, of course, is dependent upon the invader and the condition of localized immune response. If the local reaction to the invader is weak or absent, the invading organism can enter the bloodstream and the lymphatic system. When the organism enters these systems, heat and pain are produced as signs of inflammation. Tissue damage occurs.

If the host has been exposed previously to the invading organism, antibodies may have been formed. This prior exposure provokes the immune system to respond more efficiently to rid the body of the invading organism. Immune system memory cells are responsible for this phenomenon. When the invading organism is new to the body, the inflammatory response is less efficient.

Inflammation is characterized by three stages: the vascular stage, the exudative stage, and the reparative stage. Look closely at the schematic of the inflammatory response (Figure 13–3), and you will see these stages. The end result of this response is to promote tissue healing and regeneration.

> *A* healthy body has the ability and capacity to protect and restore itself. In order to handle tissue trauma, the body is influenced by the extent of the damage and the individual's overall state of health. The body responds systematically to trauma in any of its parts and transports beneficial substances to the site of injury and harmful substances away from it. Circulating blood is the means of transport. Both open and closed wounds of soft tissue or bone can be invaded by pathogens, resulting in an inflammatory response. Normal healing is promoted when the wound is free of foreign substances such as bacteria. Wound healing occurs by first and second intention. Maladaptive responses to the invading organism include the symptoms associated with systemic inflammation, such as fever, chills, and myalgias.

MEMORY JOGS

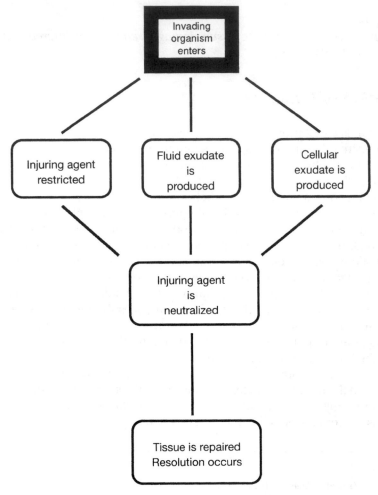

Figure 13-3. The inflammatory response.

Principle

Infection control guidelines are put into practice in an effort to prevent the transmission of pathogenic materials and microorganisms to our patients, to others around the patient, and to ourselves

Illustration of Principle

Infection control guidelines have been an essential component in the delivery of nursing care. The AIDS epidemic has heightened health-care workers' awareness of just what these guidelines are and should be. Now known as *Universal Precau-*

tions, they provide the familiarity and reliability of tested clinical practice. There is reassurance in knowing that these precautions will work in preventing the transmission of pathogenic microorganisms.

MEMORY JOGS

> **U**niversal Precautions
>
> Only effective if consistently applied
> Universal: Applies to everyone
> Precautions: Actions taken to promote safety and prevent harm

These guidelines have been formulated to prevent disease transmission. By adhering to these practices, the nurse promotes wellness by preventing harmful microorganisms and contaminants from causing illness. When appropriate, barrier protection is recommended. Barriers act as impermeable blockades to the harmful matter.

Specific Recommendations

Hand washing: Wash hands carefully with soap and water before, after, and in between patient contact. Well-lubricated skin is less likely to crack, preventing compromise of the first line of barrier defense.

Gloves: Use gloves when you expect to come in contact with blood, secretions, excretions, or other body fluids and tissue specimens. Gloves are not a substitute for hand washing and will not prevent a needle stick injury. Latex gloves have a tighter fitting cuff and provide greater sensitivity and dexterity.

Gowns: Wear one when coming in contact with blood or other body fluids. Gowns are most frequently indicated as barrier protection and should be the type with an impermeable layer. A cloth gown does not protect the wearer from contamination by fluids.

Masks and goggles: Use these devices when splashes from saliva, blood, or respiratory secretions are likely. Masks should be applied to patients with active pulmonary tuberculosis when they leave their rooms. It is recommended that nurses also wear a mask when working with the patient who is actively coughing and suspected of having a contagious pulmonary condition.

Additional Guidelines

- Never recap needles
- Use needle boxes made of puncture-proof material. Make them accessible where patient care is delivered.
- Clean spills with solutions that contain an antiviral agent or a bleach and water mixture.
- Laundry should be placed in an impermeable bag.
- Contaminated disposable waste items should be disinfected prior to disposal.

MEMORY JOGS

*B*ody Fluids

Blood, semen, vaginal secretions, and breast milk are linked most commonly to the transmission of HIV.

   Other pathogenic organisms can be transmitted by these body fluids, and by other fluids such as saliva, respiratory secretions, and cerebrospinal fluid.

Reasoning Exercises: *Infection and Inflammation*

1. Which of the following is an example of direct transmission of infection?
    A. Malaria infection transmitted by mosquito
    B. Gonorrhea infection transmitted by sexual intercourse
    C. Hepatitis A infection transmitted by contaminated food
    D. Influenza infection transmitted by shared handkerchief

    Intended Response: **B.** Transmission of infection can occur by either direct or indirect routes. Direct transmission involves human-to-human contact, such as sexual intercourse, or transfer by droplet nuclei, as in tuberculosis. Examples of indirect transmission include vector **A** and vehicle **C, D** transmission.

2. Which of the following culture results would be an example of an infection resulting from a disturbance of resident (normal) flora?
    A. *Staphylococcus* cultured in a wound following surgery
    B. *Escherichia coli* cultured in the urine

C. *Candida albicans* cultured in vaginal secretions following antibiotic therapy

D. Vancomycin resistant *Enterococcus* cultured in nasal passages

Intended Response: **C.** Not all bacteria in the body are pathogenic, or disease producing. Some bacteria, such as *E. coli,* reside in the body as normal flora. Disruption of the balance of normal flora, as occurs with the use of antibiotic therapy, can lead to imposed infection, such as *Candida* growth in the vaginal tract or *C. difficile* growth in the intestinal tract.

3. For which of the following purposes should a nurse wear gloves for administration of an intramuscular (IM) injection?

   A. To maintain sterility of the injectable medication and syringe

   B. To prevent contamination of the injection site

   C. To prevent blood-borne pathogen (BBP) exposure to the nurse

   D. To promote absorption of the injected medication

Intended Response: **C.** Administration of an intramuscular injection may involve contact with blood or bloody body fluids, thus placing the nurse at risk for transmission of blood-borne pathogens. Latex gloves will serve as barrier protection against potential transmission, but will not achieve any of the remaining responses.

4. Which of the following patients should the nurse consider at *highest* risk for the development of infection?

   A. An elderly woman who lives alone and seldom leaves her house

   B. A young adult woman taking corticosteroid medications for rheumatoid arthritis

   C. A teenaged boy closely monitoring his calorie intake to maintain his body weight class in high school wrestling

   D. An elderly man who drinks 1 or 2 glasses of wine with his evening meal

Intended Response: **B.** Individuals receiving treatment with immunosuppressive side effects (such as corticosteroids, anti-cancer chemotherapy, and anti-cancer radiation therapy) are at high risk for infection related to their immunosuppressed state.

5. The nurse examining a patient's decubitus ulcer notes a moderate amount of greenish-yellow, cloudy, and foul-smelling drainage from the wound. Which of the following laboratory tests would provide the most specific and useful information concerning the drainage?

A. White blood cell count

B. Wound culture

C. Red blood cell count

D. Sedimentation rate

Intended Response: **B.** The presence of greenish-yellow, foul-smelling drainage strongly suggests that an infectious process is occurring. A culture will identify which specific microorganisms are present and aid in determining which antiinfective therapy would be appropriate to eradicate that infection. The white blood cell (WBC) count and sedimentation rate, if elevated, would only indicate that an infectious process was occurring, but would not specify which microorganisms were present. Red blood cell (RBC) count is not affected by infectious processes.

6. An adult patient receiving cancer chemotherapy treatments as an outpatient is admitted to the hospital with a white blood cell (WBC) count of 700. In light of the patient's medical status, the admitting nurse would correctly place the patient in:

A. A semi-private room, with noninfected room partner

B. A semi-private room, with nonsmoking bed partner

C. A private room, with compromised host precautions

D. A private room, with enteric precautions

Intended Response: **C.** A white blood cell (WBC) count below normal limits (5,000–10,000) indicates a suppressed immune response, placing the patient at high risk for infection. In an effort to prevent infection, the nurse should place the immune-compromised patient in a compromised host precautions room aimed at protecting the patient from potential sources of infection.

7. The nurse notes oozing of serosanguineous drainage from a patient's abdominal surgical wound. When preparing to change the patient's wound dressing, which personal protective equipment for barrier protection should the nurse use?

A. Gloves

B. Face shield and gown

C. Face mask, gown, and gloves

D. Eye goggles, gown, and gloves

Intended Response: **A.** As only the nurse's hands will come in contact with the infectious drainage from the wound, only gloves are required to be worn as barrier protection against the transfer of microorganisms.

8. Which of the following represents a correct implementation of blood-borne pathogen precautions?

A. A needle used for an injection is recapped before disposal

B. Eye goggles are worn while providing a complete bed bath

C. Blood-contaminated materials are disposed of in a biohazard container

D. Alcohol is used to decontaminate blood-contaminated steel instruments

Intended Response: **C.** The goal of blood-borne pathogen precautions is to prevent or reduce potential exposure to blood or blood-contaminated fluids. Disposal of blood-contaminated materials in biohazard containers provides an extra degree of protection against accidental exposure. Needles should not be recapped, as this action significantly increases the risk of accidental needle stick injury. Eye goggles are necessary only in procedures bearing a risk of spray of body fluids, such as suctioning. Alcohol as a bacteriostatic agent will not eradicate HIV/HBV virus and should not be used as part of blood-borne pathogen precautions.

9. The nurse is caring for a patient in strict isolation. At which point should the nurse remove barrier protection?

A. At the bedside, immediately after completing work with the patient

B. Within the patient's room, just inside the doorway

C. Out of the patient's room, just outside the doorway

D. In the hallway, a significant distance from the patient's room

Intended Response: **B.** Regardless of the type of isolation, the nurse should always focus on limiting potential transmission of infection. Removing barrier protection away from the patient but within the patient's room prevents the exposure of others outside of the patient's room to microorganisms being isolated.

References

(1987). Recommendations for prevention of HIV transmission in health care settings. *MMWR* (suppl 2), 36, 1S–18S.

(1988). 1988 agent summary statement for human immunodeficiency virus and reports on laboratory acquired infection with human immunodeficiency virus. *MMWR* (suppl 4), 37, 1S–22S.

(1989). Guidelines for prevention of transmission of human immunodeficiency virus and hepatitis B virus to health care and public safety workers. *MMWR* (No. S-6), 38, 1–37.

(1991). Infection Control Guidelines for Health Care Workers. *AIDS Clinical Care* (2) 5,

Gerberding JL. (1986). University of California, San Francisco task force on AIDS, recommended infection control policies for patients with immunodeficiency virus infection: An update. *N Engl J Med*, 315, 1562–1564.

Gerberding JL, Sande MA. (1990). Infection-control guidelines: Health care workers. In: Cohen PT, Sande MA, and Volberding PA (eds.). *The AIDS Knowledge Base.* Waltham, MA: Massachusetts Medical Society, 1.0.2.1-15.

Grossman M. (1990). HIV and delivery room personnel. In: Cohen PT, Sande MA, and Volberding PA (eds.). *The AIDS Knowledge Base.* Waltham, MA: Massachusetts Medical Society, 10.2.4.

14 Movement, Sensation, and Cognition

MARIAN B. SIDES

Principle

The nervous system is a communication network that controls and coordinates activities throughout the body

Illustration of Principle

The nervous system plays a key role in humans' ability to interact meaningfully with their environment. Movement, sensation, and cognition are normal bodily processes that result from effective communication between the nervous system and the various parts of the body that it serves.

A key function of this system is to receive information from the environment, interpret it, and transmit electrical impulses to precise locations of the body for action. Thus, it controls and coordinates man's interactions and behaviors and is largely responsible for one's adjustments in life.

Principle

The flow of communication to various body parts depends upon the structural and functional integrity of the nervous system

Illustration of Principle

The nervous system conforms closely to the bony structure of the body. The skull and vertebral column contain the brain and the spinal cord, known collectively as the central nervous system. The cerebrospinal and autonomic nerves are located outside the bony structure and together form the peripheral nervous system.

Both the central nervous system and the peripheral nervous system have voluntary functions. The central nervous system is responsible for conscious behavior and includes all processes activated by the individual at will. The cerebrum is the largest part of the voluntary system (Figure 14–1).

Perception of this motor and sensory information is transmitted from the cerebrum through the cerebrospinal nerve fibers along the neuron pathway to its destination. Motor neurons, for example, cause muscles to contract. Sensory neurons bring forth an awareness of pain and temperature. These fibers or pathways from the brain cross over in the brain stem to communicate their messages to the opposite side of the body.

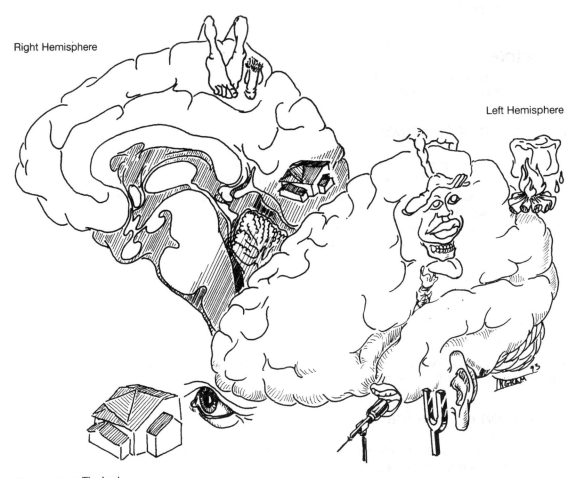

Right Hemisphere

Left Hemisphere

Figure 14-1. The brain.

Structural Integrity

A. Central nervous system
  1. Brain and spinal cord
  2. Inside bony structure
B. Peripheral nervous system
  1. Cerebrospinal and autonomic nervous system
  2. Outside bony structure

Functional Integrity

A. Voluntary
  1. Brain and spinal cord, cerebral nerves, and spinal nerves
  2. Control of cognition, movement, and sensation
B. Involuntary
  1. Autonomic nerves/sympathetic and parasympathetic nerves
  2. Control of visceral function

The involuntary or autonomic nervous system consists of a series of nerve fibers and ganglia that extend from each side of the vertebral column. They form two divisions that act in an apparently opposite but cooperative manner on the organs of the body. In concert, the sympathetic division accelerates, dilates, and stimulates bodily functions, especially in times of stress, while the parasympathetic system contracts, relaxes, or retards bodily functions in an effort to conserve energy.

The nervous system in these various configurations forms a communication network and provides a mechanism for the transmission of impulses to appropriate body parts. Internal balance and homeostasis depend upon the precision, synchronization, and patency of these systems.

Principle

A breakdown in the basic structure of the nervous system or in its communication network will result in neurological dysfunction

Illustration of Principle

The neuron is the most fundamental unit of the nervous system. It consists of a nerve cell that transmits impulses and stimuli to all parts of the body. Each cell has an energy-producing nucleus, a process called a dendrite that brings impulses to the cell, and an axon that sends impulses away from the cell. Several common neurological disorders can further demonstrate the phenomena related to the neurophysiology of the system and how they affect an individual's performance.

Hemorrhage or embolus formation causes cerebral vascular accidents (CVA), whereby motor and sensory pathways from the brain to corresponding body parts are blocked. Nerve cells have a continuous need for oxygen. When cerebral blood flow is interrupted on one side of the brain, for example, weakness and numbness may occur on the opposite side. A lack of oxygen to the posterior cerebrum will block vision, whereas ischemia to the anterior cerebral arteries may cause loss of memory and mood swings. Thus, movement, sensation, and cognition are affected.

MEMORY JOGS

*E*levated intracranial pressure kills

The brain is encased in a closed bony structure called the cranium. Brain tissue occupies about 78% of the cranial space, whereas blood occupies about 12%, and cerebrospinal fluid fills about 10%. These three fluid components exert a force called intracranial pressure, which is normally between 0–15 mmHg. Any change in the size, location, or amount of these contents will cause an increase in intracranial pressure. Causes of such change include head trauma—hematoma, contusion, and concussion—tremors, infection, and hemorrhage. As pressure in cerebral vessels increases, blood flow to the brain slows down. A decrease in circulation produces ischemia, an increase in metabolic waste products, hypoxia, and hypercapnia, accompanied by a decrease in level of consciousness. Classic changes in vital signs include widening pulse pressure, elevated blood pressure, and bradycardia. As cerebral edema increases, or a hematoma expands, cognition is altered. Cerebral circulation stops and brain death occurs.

Seizure activity can result from any dynamic that interferes with normal brain activity, such as head trauma, high fever, low blood sugar, drugs, and infection. This sudden outburst of electrical brain activity causes alteration in normal movement, sensation, and cognition.

Dementia is a degenerative syndrome caused by any disorder that permanently damages large association areas in the cerebral hemisphere. Huntington's disease is a rare hereditary disorder characterized by chronic, progressive chorea, psychological changes, and dementia. The most common cause of dementia is Alzheimer's disease, characterized by memory impairment, a progressive inability to recognize family and friends, and a loss of bodily functions.

Parkinson's disease is a degenerative disorder of basal ganglia cells. It is related to a deficiency in dopamine production, which is necessary for smooth, graceful movements. The absence of dopamine results in muscular rigidity, tremors, and an abnormal gait. Whereas Parkinson's disease is primarily a movement disorder, Alzheimer's disease is characterized by intellectual deterioration. A degenerative disease of cortical neurons, it eventually leads to motor deficits.

Inflammation of the peripheral or cranial nerves, with degeneration of the axons and myelin, as seen in Guillain-Barré syndrome, results in paralysis of affected body parts. This degeneration of peripheral nerves usually begins with weakness in the lower extremities, and may ascend to the respiratory muscles. Movement and sensation are affected. Cognition is not.

Amyotrophic lateral sclerosis (ALS) produces degeneration of the cell bodies of the lower motor neurons of the spinal cord and cranial nerves and results in muscle atrophy. Movement is affected, but cognition and sensation are not. On the other hand, spinal cord injury resulting from trauma can cause compression or severance of the spinal cord. Loss of function and sensation results.

Multiple sclerosis is a degenerative disease of the central nervous system that results in a breakdown of the myelin sheath in scattered areas of the brain and spinal cord. It causes interference in motor, sensory, and cognitive abilities, much like a lamp that has a frayed cord causes a short or interruption in the connection between the source of the electrical impulse and the light bulb itself.

These and other neurological disorders cause common disturbances in movement, sensation, and cognition resulting from structural or functional breakdown in the nervous system. The nurse's role in managing the patient care problems resulting from these neurophysiological deficits starts with recognizing clinical patterns as a basis for nursing care.

Principle
A common illness pattern characterizes most neurological problems and establishes the framework for management of care

Illustration of Principle

The exact etiology of many neurological problems is unknown. Regardless of cause, most neurological problems present a familiar clinical portrait or common illness pattern. They all have some variation in movement, sensation, and cognitive ability. These manifestations, along with specific individualized behavior, establish the framework for the management of care.

In preparing for boards, it is important that you try to grasp these fundamental concepts and common behavior patterns. It will be easier, then, to recognize the nursing care measures that are truly important in correcting these patterns. Likewise, you will not have to rely on the memorization of isolated facts and meaningless details.

Your nursing management begins with a neurological assessment. Since illness patterns of all common neurological disorders evolve around movement, sensation, and cognition, your assessment will focus on these functions.

MEMORY JOGS

*C*hecking the level of consciousness is the heart of the neurological assessment. It is the most reliable indicator of a life threat.

Regardless of the neurological disorder or its cause, a quick 90" assessment will help you sharpen your focus. Once you have established the level of consciousness, you will proceed to determine patency of airway, and presence of breathing and pulse. Analysis of these data will lead to problem definition or nursing diagnoses. Goals of care are directed at reducing life threats, maintaining body functions, preventing hazards of immobility, detecting changes in status, facilitating communication, establishing emotional stability, promoting rehabilitation, and returning to normalcy.

MEMORY JOGS

*N*ursing interventions in pursuit of these goals can be guided by the acronym SUPPORT:

    *S*pecialize
    *U*nderstand
    *P*rotect
    *P*revent
    *O*bserve
    *R*ehabilitate
    *T*each

Specialize. Although many commonalities exist in patients with neurological deficits, all patients will require specialized procedures and care measures determined by their individual needs. For example, the Guillain-Barré syndrome, characterized by progressive muscular weakness, is usually a medical emergency that can lead to respiratory failure and alterations in circulation. Astute airway management and support to other vital functions is critical to effective care. On the other hand, the patient with head trauma requires immediate life saving measures to reduce cerebral edema and restore oxygenation, circulation, and cognitive functioning.

Understand. These patients often face serious threats to self-esteem, autonomy, and independence. The CVA patient, for example, often loses control of normal bodily functions like walking and talking. The loss of movement control in the Parkinsonian patient or the forgetfulness of the Alzheimer's patient imposes a serious burden on self-concept. Adjustment to such degeneration is difficult and patients often reflect on their youth in an attempt to regain a healthy image (see Figure 14–2). The nurse should provide emotional support, be empathetic, be a good listener, and most of all, show respect.

Prevent. Patients with neurological disorders are at great risk for hazards of immobility. They often face regression to a previous illness state or further degeneration of their existing illness. An important goal of care is to prevent recurrence or worsening of deficits. The nurse must recognize signs of deterioration. To prevent a recurrence of a CVA, for example, the nurse must recognize danger signs and know how to deal effectively with them.

Protect. Safety is the fundamental goal of patient care. Safety measures span a broad range of activities. They include giving good skin care and maintaining proper positioning to prevent skin breakdown. For patients with movement deficits, the nurse will provide assistance in ambulation to prevent falls from unsteady gait. Other safety interventions include protecting the pathway of an airway to prevent respiratory failure, protecting the personal integrity of a patient who has suffered a loss of self-worth, and keeping a patient safe from personal harm during seizure activity.

Observe. Appropriate monitoring and observation are essential to detect changes in patient status. Patients with epidural hematoma can change rapidly, requiring immediate intervention. Changes in levels of consciousness may be subtle but critical evidence of life threats. Alteration in cognition and changes in vital signs, which accompany increased intracranial pressure, are also life threats. Accurate observation and decisive actions by the nurse may save a patient's life or prevent permanent injury.

Rehabilitate. Bringing a patient back to health can be a time-consuming and arduous task. In certain degenerative problems, as in ALS, rehabilitation is limited and primarily supportive. Conditions such as CVA and Guillain-Barré can have a good prognosis given extensive rehabilitative measures. Important objectives are to promote self-care and independence, and to assist the patient only in those activities he or she is unable to perform. These patients need encouragement and positive approval, as well as recognition, for even the smallest units of progress. An important nursing intervention is to provide opportunities for the patient to succeed, regain independence, and recognize progress.

Teach. Patient and family education are important for effective and optimal rehabilitation. Critical teaching areas include understanding of:

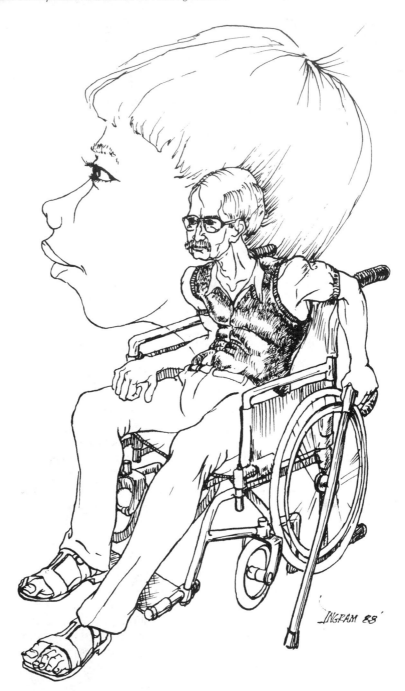

Figure 14-2. Reflection of the past.

1. Illness patterns and symptom manifestation
2. Diet and nutrition
3. Drugs, expected actions, and side effects
4. Hazards and benefits of rest and exercise
5. Health promotion and illness prevention

Each aspect of care should be evaluated on an ongoing basis to determine effectiveness in meeting patient care goals. The ultimate goal is to assist the patient and family in returning to the highest level of wellness, within the limitations of the illness and the patient's own abilities.

Reasoning Exercises: *Movement, Sensation, and Cognition*

1. A nurse is developing a plan of care for a patient experiencing "locked in " syndrome secondary to amyotrophic lateral sclerosis (ALS). Which of the following interventions would be most essential?

   A. Institute an alternative method for patient communication, such as eye blinks or eye movement
   B. Implement a regular schedule of turning and positioning
   C. Institute an alternative method for urinary elimination, such as an indwelling catheter
   D. Implement a regular schedule for bowel elimination

   Intended Response: **A.** Amyotrophic lateral sclerosis produces degeneration of the cell bodies of the lower motor neurons of the spinal cord and cranial nerves, resulting in muscle atrophy. Because cognition is not affected, the patient with ALS remains alert and aware, essentially trapped or "locked" in a body that no longer functions. For this reason, alternative methods for communication which will allow the patient to express cognitive processes and emotional needs are of great significance. Although remaining responses are appropriate for addressing the loss of motor control in this patient, only response **A** attends to the need for cognitive expression.

2. The nurse assessing a patient with Parkinson's disease would expect to note which of the following clinical manifestations?

   A. Unilateral flaccid paralysis of extremities
   B. Shuffling, propelling gait
   C. Facial twitching
   D. Rapid, repetitive speech

Intended Response: **B.** Parkinson's disease is caused by deficient production of dopamine, a neurotransmitter which affects motor function. Patients with Parkinson's disease demonstrate a decrease in desired purposeful movement (mask-like expression, and monotone speech) and an increase in undesired, nonpurposeful movement (resting tremors, and abnormal gait).

3. The nurse observing a patient with a closed head injury for signs of increased intracranial pressure should observe for which of these?
   A. Increasing pulse rate
   B. Decreasing urinary output
   C. Increasing systolic blood pressure
   D. Decreasing temperature

Intended Response: **C.** Increasing blood pressure is a hallmark manifestation of increased intracranial pressure. As pressure is exerted on the hypothalamus, regulation of vital signs is compromised, resulting in decreased pulse and respirations, and marked elevations of temperature. Change in urinary output **B** is not associated with increased intracranial pressure.

4. Which of the following clinical manifestations would be an early indication of increased intracranial pressure?
   A. Decreasing level of consciousness
   B. Nuchal rigidity
   C. Hyperreflexia
   D. Decerebrate posturing

Intended Response: **A.** All human cells require oxygen for life. As pressure increases within the closed compartment of the brain, compression of brain tissues results in damage and loss of function. A decrease in the level of consciousness is an early indicator that normal brain function is compromised by increased intracranial pressure. Nuchal rigidity (neck stiffness) is associated with inflammation related to infections such as meningitis. Loss of reflexive movement and posturing will occur as later signs of brain dysfunction secondary to increased pressure.

5. Which of the following would be a priority intervention for a patient with impaired judgment secondary to Alzheimer's disease?
   A. Provide frequent reality orientation
   B. Place the patient in a secluded, private room
   C. Provide frequent emotional support and reassurance
   D. Remove potential safety hazards

Intended Response: **D.** Judgment is the cognitive process that directs decisions regarding what is safe or unsafe, appropriate or inappropriate. As cognitive processes deteriorate in Alzheimer's disease, judgment will be impaired, placing the patient at risk for self injury. Reality orientation **A** would improve orientation and short-term memory. Emotional support **C** would serve to stabilize the disturbances in mood and affect associated with this disease. There is no indication to separate this patient from others; indeed, such isolation would likely exacerbate symptoms of Alzheimer's.

6. Which of the following is a priority need for a patient with HIV encephalopathy?
   A. Circulation
   B. Safety
   C. Elimination
   D. Love and belonging

Intended Response: **B.** The prefix "encephalo" refers to the brain or central nervous system; the suffix "pathy" means "disease of." HIV encephalopathy is a pathology of the brain caused by the invasion of human immunodeficiency virus, resulting in impaired cognition similar to what would be noted in Alzheimer's disease. Because cognitive processes are impaired, safety is of priority importance.

7. Which of the following interventions would be indicated to ensure the safety of a patient immediately after generalized seizure?
   A. Elevate the head of the bed
   B. Insert oral airway
   C. Apply soft cushioned restraints
   D. Insert a padded tongue blade

Intended Response: **B.** A generalized seizure is evidence of electrical chaos in the brain. Loss of systematic, synchronized firing of nerve impulses results in a loss of control over body movement, causing the jerking, spastic movement of seizure. Because the individual experiencing generalized seizure may lose the ability to clear his or her own airway, insertion of an oral airway to maintain patency is essential. The patient should be placed in a supine position **A** with the head turned to the side to prevent aspiration or choking. Restraints **C** could potentially cause fractures of the extremities, if another seizure were to follow. A padded tongue blade **D** is contraindicated, as it serves only to occlude the patient's airway and prevent proper ventilation.

8. Which of the following assessments of a patient in the period immediately after generalized seizure should cause the nurse the greatest concern?

   A. Blood pressure 180/110

   B. Pulse 120

   C. Pupils dilated, unreactive to light

   D. Respirations snoring and labored

Intended Response: D. Snoring and labored respirations would cause the nurse caring for the postictal patient the greatest concern because these indicate possible airway obstruction from the tongue, or accumulation of oral fluids in the mouth. The nurse noting labored respirations after seizure should immediately assess the patient's airway patency for possible obstruction.

Hormonal Regulation

NANCY KORCHEK

Principle

The primary role of the endocrine system is to maintain balance of various processes occurring in the human body

Illustration of Principle

The various glands that make up the endocrine system perform diverse tasks that influence a number of processes in the human body (Table 15–1). The thyroid gland, for example, releases hormones that directly affect metabolic processes in the body; the pituitary gland releases gonadotropin-stimulating hormones that influence reproductive cycles in the body. Even though the actions of the glands and the hormones produced in each gland differ, the primary role of each gland of the endocrine system is to maintain *balance* within the body. This balance, or homeostasis, is accomplished in the endocrine system essentially via the *feedback mechanism*, a communication network that signals glands to either release or inhibit hormone secretion. Through this feedback mechanism, the hormonal balance of the body can be ensured.

The following is a brief review of how the feedback mechanism works.

The *hypothalamus,* located in the brain, receives messages from the body's central nervous system, and it subsequently sends a message to the appropriate gland for either hormone release or inhibition. When hormone release has had its effect on the body's processes, feedback is sent to the gland and hypothalamus, so that balance may be maintained.

For Example

An individual who is exercising metabolizes carbohydrates more rapidly, and thus develops hypoglycemia.

195

Table 15-1. Hormones and their functions in selected human glands

Gland	Focus of Action	Deficit	Excess
ADRENAL CORTEX			
Hormones	Focus of Action	*Addison's disease*	*Cushing's disease*
Aldosterone	Promotes retention of Na$^+$ and H$_2$O, excretion of K$^+$ (by kidney)	↓ Na$^+$/H$_2$O excretion (dehydration, hypotension, ↓ CO, hypovolemic shock) ↑ K$^+$ retention (cardiac dysrhythmia, cardiac arrest)	↑ Na$^+$/H$_2$O excretion (weight gain, edema, "moon face," oliguria, hypertension) ↓ K$^+$ retention (thinning and wasting of extremity muscle, cardiac dysrhythmia, cardiac arrest)
Cortisol	Promotes gluconeogenesis to maintain serum glucose balance	↓ gluconeogenesis (hypoglycemia)	↑ gluconeogenesis (hyperglycemia, increased fat deposits)
Testosterone	Increase muscle mass and strength; bolsters physical endurance and stamina	↓ testosterone (muscle weakness, fatigue, decreased strength and stamina)	↑ testosterone (hirsutism, masculinization, acne, amenorrhea, infertility)
THYROID			
Hormones	Focus of Action	*Myxedema*	*Graves' Disease*
Thyroxine	Regulation of metabolic processes, including basal metabolic rate, body temperature, heart and respiratory rates, circulation, digestion	Hypometabolism (↓ BMR, hypoexcitability, lethargy and fatigue, mental lethargy and forgetfulness, depression, decreased body temperature, sensitivity to cold) CV changes (bradycardia, dysrhythmia, decreased extremity circulation, edema, bradypnea, SOB) GI changes (weight gain, constipation)	Hypermetabolism (↑ BMR, hyperexcitability, insomnia, sleep disturbance, loss of coordination, resting tremors, elevated body temperature, intolerance to heat, diaphoresis) CV changes (tachycardia, dysrhythmia, hyperpnea) GI changes (ravenous appetite, weight loss, diarrhea)
POSTERIOR PITUITARY			
Hormones	Focus of Action	*Diabetes insipidus*	*Syndrome of Inappropriate ADH (SIADH)*
Vasopressin (Antidiuretic hormone, ADH)	Promotes retention of H$_2$O by the kidneys	Fluid imbalance: *Dehydration* (thirst, dry mucous membranes, dry hot skin, sunken eyeballs, doughy abdomen) *Polyuria* (4–10 L/day output, dilute urine, low specific gravity) Electrolyte imbalance (hypernatremia, hypokalemia) CV changes (tachycardia, dysrhythmia, hypotension)	Fluid imbalance: *Overdehydration* (weight gain) *Oliguria* (minimal output, concentrated urine, high specific gravity) Electrolyte imbalance (hyponatremia, hyperkalemia) CV changes (tachycardia, dysrhythmia, hypertension)

The central nervous system sends a message to the hypothalamus that the individual is hypoglycemic.

The hypothalamus sends a message about the hypoglycemia to the pituitary gland, stimulating the pituitary to release growth hormone. The release of growth hormone increases the glucose level of the blood.

Once the glucose level begins to rise because of the release of growth hormone, a feedback message is sent to the pituitary and hypothalamus to inhibit further release of growth hormone. Thus, a balance of glucose metabolism is maintained via the function of the feedback mechanism of the endocrine system.

In this example, the reader can see how the communication of bodily messages via the feedback mechanism of the endocrine system serves to maintain balance or homeostasis of bodily processes. An excellent illustration of this communication network and the results of failure in the communication network is provided in the following discussion of the endocrine disease, diabetes mellitus.

Principle

Insulin is required by the body for the metabolism of carbohydrates, fat, and protein

Illustration of Principle

Although we tend to think of diabetes mellitus as a disease characterized by an incomplete metabolism of carbohydrates, it actually involves the metabolism of fats and proteins as well. In the nondiabetic, insulin serves nutrient metabolism in a number of ways, including assisting glucose to enter fat and muscle cells to be used as energy; stimulating the production of fat cells; inhibiting the release of stored fat cells into the bloodstream; and stimulating the liver to make and store unused simple carbohydrates in the form of glycogen, a complex carbohydrate.

Therefore, in the absence of insulin, normal metabolic processes cannot be maintained. Since the diabetic patient's pancreas does not manufacture and release insulin, the energy needs of the body cells cannot be met by carbohydrate metabolism. Because insulin is not available to control the rate of fat metabolism, the diabetic patient is prone to rapid destruction of fat cells in order to provide for cellular energy needs. This rapid metabolism causes the release of free acid bodies (ketones) into the serum, precipitating an acidotic state in the body called *diabetic ketoacidosis* (an acidosis caused by accumulation of ketone acid bodies in the serum), a serious complication of *hyperglycemia* and lack of insulin.

It is evident, then, that the principal management of the insulin-dependent, or Type I, diabetic patient is the administration of insulin. Because insulin is primarily a protein, it would be metabolized too quickly by the salivary enzymes of the mouth, and thus must be administered by injection, typically into subcutaneous (fatty) tissues of the body. The goal of insulin administration is to provide this essential hormone in order to balance the glucose levels in serum, promote glucose metabolism for cellular energy, and encourage glucose storage in the forms of glycogen and fat for future energy needs.

MEMORY JOGS

*I*n the absence of insulin, the diabetic patient metabolizes body fat rapidly for energy. This releases acidic by-products that accumulate in the serum, causing *acidosis*.

Principle

Glucagon is a hormone of the pancreas that serves to increase serum glucose levels

Illustration of Principle

In the nondiabetic, the alpha cells of the islets of Langerhans of the pancreas manufacture the hormone *glucagon*, whose primary action is to *increase* blood glucose levels when those levels drop below generally accepted normal parameters (60–100 mg/100 mL). Thus, insulin and glucagon work "hand-in-hand" to maintain *balance* of serum glucose, which in turn supports the metabolism energy requirements of the cells. In the diabetic patient, however, the pancreas does not manufacture insulin, creating a disturbance in the "hand-in-hand" balance between insulin and glucagon.

Thus, just as the diabetic patient will require injections of insulin to lower the blood glucose level, he or she may also require intermittent injections of glucagon to counteract abnormally low blood glucose levels that have caused symptoms of *hypoglycemia*.

*T*he pancreas manufactures two hormones that affect glucose serum levels. Insulin lowers blood glucose; glucagon raises blood glucose. Balance between insulin and glucose is essential.

MEMORY JOGS

Principle

Insulin, in the nondiabetic individual, is released on a prn basis

Illustration of Principle

This basic principle highlights a major difference between the nondiabetic individual and his or her diabetic counterpart. Normally, insulin is released from the beta cells of the islets of Langerhans of the pancreas on an as-needed or prn basis as foodstuffs are ingested, or as glucose levels of serum rise. The process of timely insulin release is controlled by the feedback mechanism of the endocrine system, with its secretory and inhibitory properties. Because the insulin-dependent diabetic's pancreas is *not* functioning properly, the feedback mechanism of the endocrine system that guides insulin secretion and inhibition is nonfunctional, resulting in a lack of control over glucose levels and metabolism.

Because the insulin-dependent diabetic does not manufacture insulin in his or her own pancreas, he or she must receive needed insulin by injection. Insulin injections, whether administered subcutaneously or for more rapid absorption by IV route, cannot simulate the prn release of insulin of the nondiabetic pancreas. Rather, the peaks and diminutions of insulin levels in the diabetic are dependent upon the *type* of insulin administered, with regular or crystalline insulin having a much more rapid peak than Isophane Insulin (NPH), for example.

*E*ach type of insulin the diabetic uses in the management of the disease has a different "peak" action. Whereas regular insulin acts on blood glucose levels and peaks rapidly, the longer-acting NPH insulin peaks at a much later time after injection. Thus, glucose levels of a diabetic patient may vary throughout the course of a day, depending upon the type of insulin being administered.

MEMORY JOGS

Nursing Management

Because of this fact, patients receiving insulin injections must be monitored consistently to ensure adequate and appropriate "coverage" by the administered insulin for the body's metabolic needs. As metabolic needs of the body change, such as with exercise or fever, insulin requirements of the body also change, calling for adjustment of insulin type and dose. It is impossible, then, for the diabetic patient to determine a preset insulin requirement and maintain that same coverage level throughout life. An important nursing intervention with the diabetic patient, then, is to provide teaching about what processes may alter metabolic needs and thus insulin coverage requirements, so that the diabetic patient learns to be flexible and sensible about providing insulin injections in relation to body need.

A time-honored method of helping the diabetic patient to recognize changes in insulin coverage requirements is routine testing of urine samples for the presence of glucose and acetone bodies. If the patient is "spilling" glucose or acetone into his or her urine, it is recognized that blood levels of glucose or acetone are elevated, and additional insulin coverage is needed.

Advanced technology has allowed nurses and diabetics alike to use much more accurate methods of evaluating glucose levels and insulin needs, with blood glucose chemstrips and blood glucometers. Urine testing is used less and less often. Regardless of the method used, the nurse should be aware that ongoing evaluation of blood glucose and acetone levels is essential in the management of the diabetic patient.

MEMORY JOGS

*I*t is essential that the diabetic patient monitor blood glucose values in conjunction with insulin therapy. Since injected insulin cannot enter into the bloodstream on an "as needed" or prn basis, the patient and nurse should anticipate fluctuations in glucose levels and corresponding insulin requirements.

Principle

The goal in the management of the insulin-dependent (Type I) diabetic is to achieve balance among three critical factors: insulin, diet, and activity or rest

Illustration of Principle

Once the suspected diabetic patient has been differentially diagnosed by means of classic signs and symptoms of hyperglycemia (polyphagia, polydipsia, and polyuria) coupled with diagnostic results of a glucose tolerance test, the goal of management is to achieve balance among three critical factors: insulin, diet, and activity or rest.

The glucose tolerance test involves the administration of a set concentration of glucose with sequential blood glucose value analysis. If the patient is a Type I diabetic, glucose levels of the blood will not decrease with sequential blood samples, indicating a lack of insulin production. With this information in mind, nurses and physicians must work together to find the correct plan of management for the patient, focusing on the following points:

- Type, amount, and frequency of insulin administration
- Dietary requirements for calories, carbohydrates, proteins, and fats
- Metabolic needs of the body and changes occurring with altered patterns of rest and activity

Insulin

Each type of insulin has a different effect on blood glucose because of varying peak action. Patients are often maintained on an intermediate-acting insulin (such as NPH) or a long-acting insulin (such as Ultralente) in order to get adequate around-the-clock coverage of serum glucose values. Regular insulin, with its rapid, peak action, would be indicated for an acutely elevated blood glucose value and should not be used in routine diabetic management.

Unit amounts of insulin are gauged according to serum glucose values as well, until an ideal dosage is identified for the individual patient. Dosage and frequency of insulin injections, then, may vary quite a bit from day to day until the patient's insulin needs are ascertained. If, for example, a morning injection of NPH Humulin insulin, 40 units, causes the patient to experience hypoglycemic reactions, the dosage may be lowered, or the injections may be altered in frequency.

*I*nsulin needs of each diabetic patient are highly individualized. The type of insulin and the frequency of administration will depend on a number of factors, including age, metabolic rate, caloric intake, and activity level. Periodic adjustment of insulin coverage should be expected.

MEMORY JOGS

Diet

Although the diabetic patient has difficulty with carbohydrate metabolism, carbohydrates are essential for energy production, and thus are included in the diabetic diet. In fact, the American Diabetic Association (ADA) diet comprises food exchange selections, to match a prescribed caloric intake, that are approximately 60% carbohydrates. The nurse should explain to the diabetic patient that, although carbohydrates make up over half of the total caloric allotment, they must be *complex* forms of carbohydrates, such as breads and fruits. The diabetic patient must avoid simple forms of sugar, such as candies or sweetened carbonated beverages, because simple sugars cause rather rapid and unpredictable elevations of blood glucose.

The diabetic patient can readily maintain optimal nutrition as well as diabetic management by adhering to the prescribed food exchanges in each category of nutrient (carbohydrates, fats, and proteins). Only when the diabetic patient is experiencing acute hypoglycemia should simple forms of sugar (e.g., table sugar, candies) be taken in small amounts. The patient should be advised of the importance of eating regularly scheduled meals to maintain optimal balance of glucose/insulin levels, and should be cautioned to avoid skipping meals or overeating at one meal, making caloric and nutrient distribution unequal for the day.

MEMORY JOGS

*T*he diabetic patient is allowed a substantial amount of carbohydrates in his or her diet. The diabetic should avoid simple carbohydrates, such as candies or carbonated beverages, though, since these will cause rapid fluctuations in blood glucose.

Activity and Rest

Activity levels will affect diabetic management and required insulin administration because activity requires energy, which is acquired through glucose metabolism by the cells. Regular activity or exercise plans are desirable for the diabetic patient, since these will increase circulation and may even reduce requirements for insulin. Because the diabetic patient is prone to the development of atherosclerotic deposits in his or her arteries, caused by deposits of unmetabolized glucose and other solids, exercise is indicated and should be encouraged to stimulate improved circulation. However, the diabetic should plan exercise and activity under the guidance of a physician, because increased activity levels may bring about a hypoglycemic episode, if proper insulin and diet management have not been maintained prior to exercise. The nurse should instruct the patient to follow closely the physician's prescription for activity and rest and to report any unusual signs or symptoms during or following activity and exercise that might indicate a precipitous change in blood glucose values.

Principle

An imbalance of glucose, above or below normal serum glucose parameters, results in the development of hyperglycemic or hypoglycemic states, with associated symptoms and signs

Illustration of Principle

Because the Type I diabetic patient does not manufacture insulin, balance of serum glucose levels is often difficult to maintain. When a diabetic patient receives too much insulin per injection, or takes the usual dosage of insulin but does not take in adequate food supply, serum glucose levels will fall, because pancreatic control of insulin production and release is not functional. Similarly, if the diabetic patient takes the usual dosage of insulin but experiences changes in body metabolism, as would occur after vigorous exercise, carbohydrates will be metabolized too rapidly, and blood glucose will decrease. As serum glucose levels fall below the normal or accepted parameters of 60–100 mg/100 mL, the patient will show evidence of a *hypoglycemic* (hypo—little; glycemic—serum glucose) state, manifested by characteristic symptoms, including:

- Headache
- Slurred speech
- Disorientation
- Nervousness
- Tremor
- Convulsion
- Loss of consciousness

The hypoglycemic state should be treated as an emergency, with prompt and expedient action. It is critical that the nurse readily identify symptoms of hypoglycemia and respond, in conjunction with the physician, with appropriate administration of some form of rapidly metabolized glucose—by means of IV administration of glucose solution if the patient is unresponsive, or by oral administration of simple sugars, as in orange juice, candy, or table sugar, if the patient is able to swallow without difficulty.

*T*he symptoms of hypoglycemia are primarily central nervous system (CNS) changes. Hypoglycemia can rapidly result in loss of consciousness and must be treated as a medical emergency. When unsure of the diabetic patient's status, it is wisest to treat the condition as hypoglycemia until diagnostic values can confirm hypoglycemia *versus* hyperglycemia.

Following the administration of some form of glucose, the patient should show rapid improvement in CNS functioning, and blood glucose values should begin to elevate toward normal parameters. When the opposite phenomenon occurs, and the diabetic patient receives too little insulin per injection, or when metabolic needs of the body are changed, causing an increased *need* for insulin, serum glucose levels will rise, resulting in a *hyperglycemic* state. Because circulating insulin levels are not adequate to allow glucose to enter into body cells to be metabolized and used as an energy source, the glucose remains in the serum, causing blood glucose levels to rise, and leading to characteristic symptoms. The nurse should assess the patient for indications of hyperglycemia, including elevated blood glucose, polyuria, polydipsia (excessive thirst), and polyphagia.

The nurse may determine a "spilling" of glucose into the patient's urine from urine glucose testing. If the hyperglycemia goes unchecked, the patient may begin to evidence signs of ketoacidosis, an acid–base imbalance that occurs when glucose cannot be metabolized for energy by the cells, and fats are metabolized at a rapid and uncontrolled rate, releasing fatty acids into the bloodstream. Symptoms of diabetic ketoacidosis (DKA) are those of a metabolic acidosis and are accompanied by signs of acute dehydration: warm, dry, flushed skin; soft, sunken eyeballs; poor skin turgor; increased body temperature, pulse, and respirations; and decreasing blood pressure. In response to the compensatory efforts of the body, the nurse will note an acetone odor to the patient's breath, sometimes described as fruity or sweet.

Arterial blood gases will reveal a decrease in pH, because of the accumulation of fatty acids in the serum, with an accompanying drop in HCO_3 values, signifying a metabolic acidosis. The CO_2 may be decreased in a compensatory effort as the ketoacidotic patient begins to breathe rapidly and deeply in an effort to "blow off" CO_2 to reduce acidic content to arterial blood. Thus, the presence of the Kussmaul respirations described above indicates the body's drive toward compensation.

The hyperglycemic or ketoacidotic patient requires immediate administration of a rapid-acting form of insulin in order to correct the elevated blood glucose values and halt the subsequent rapid metabolism of fats that leads to ketoacidosis. The nurse should plan for administration of regular (crystalline) insulin to the patient. Arterial blood gases should be assessed for evidence of metabolic acidosis. Administration of sodium bicarbonate may be necessary to reverse or "buffer" the excess acid bodies in the serum. Vital signs and urine output should be measured so that a fluid and electrolyte imbalance secondary to polyuria does not progress unchecked. Because insulin is required to allow potassium (K) into cells, hyperglycemic states may result in hyperkalemia with an associated increase in cardiac irritability. Thus, the patient's apical pulse and cardiac rhythm should be monitored for evidence of tachycardia and dysrhythmia.

The nurse will evaluate the progress of the patient through the hyperglycemic episode as serum glucose levels begin to diminish back to normal or to more acceptable levels. The patient will become more responsive and mentally alert and will no longer evidence excessive thirst or polyuria. If the patient's hyperglycemic state advances into ketoacidosis, the nurse should note a decrease in both glucose and ketone levels following administration of insulin. Arterial blood gases would evidence an increasing blood pH and a corresponding increase in HCO_3, demonstrating reversal of the metabolic acidosis. The patient's respiratory pattern should return to normal with cessation of Kussmaul respirations. Vital signs should return to normal ranges, and evidence of dehydration should begin to reverse.

The nurse should continue to monitor the patient's cardiac function carefully, because the administration of insulin will force serum K into the cells, with a resultant drop in serum levels precipitating hypokalemia. Serum glucose levels should be continuously monitored after the hyperglycemic or ketoacidotic episode to ensure that insulin treatment has not caused a precipitous *fall* in blood glucose that could result in a hypoglycemic reaction. For this reason, patients recovering from hyperglycemic reactions may be given intermittent orange juice to ensure adequate glucose values following insulin therapy.

Reasoning Exercises: *Hormones, Diabetes Mellitus*

1. Which of the following subjective data would correlate most closely with a diagnosis of posterior pituitary insufficiency?

    A. Visual disturbances

    B. Weight gain

    C. Muscle twitching and cramping

    D. Polydypsia

Intended Response: **D.** Insufficient production of antidiuretic hormone in the posterior pituitary (diabetes insipidus) causes polyuria, resulting in symptoms of fluid volume deficit such as excessive thirst. As potassium is over-excreted in polyuria, hypokalemia may result, causing muscle weakness. Weight loss due to excessive fluid loss is common. Visual disturbances are not associated with this hormonal disturbance.

2. Which of the following assessment criteria should the nurse use to determine whether medication prescribed for a patient's posterior pituitary insufficiency is causing the intended effect?
   A. Decreasing blood pressure
   B. Increasing level of consciousness
   C. Decreasing apical pulse
   D. Increasing urinary output

Intended Response: C. Pulse rates should decrease and stabilize as fluid volume deficit is corrected with medication therapy (Vasopressin) for posterior pituitary insufficiency. As normal fluid balance is re-established, blood pressure A will correspondingly increase as the previously excessive urinary output D decreases. Changes in level of consciousness are not associated with this hormonal disturbance.

3. Which of the following would be an expected finding in a patient with syndrome of inappropriate antidiuretic hormone (SIADH)?
   A. Hypokalemia
   B. Hypercalcemia
   C. Hyponatremia
   D. Hyperglycemia

Intended Response: C. Because antidiuretic hormone is overproduced in SIADH, fluid volume excess develops with corresponding dilutional hyponatremia. Oliguria associated with this hormonal disturbance causes hyperkalemia. Neither change in glucose nor in calcium is associated with this hormonal disturbance.

4. Which of the following would a nurse appropriately include in a plan of care for a patient with syndrome of inappropriate antidiuretic hormone (SIADH)?
   A. Seizure precautions
   B. Comprised host isolation
   C. Bleeding precautions
   D. Contact isolation

Intended Response: A. SIADH is characterized by fluid volume excess and secondary hyponatremia, an electrolyte disturbance which may result in seizure activity. This hormonal disturbance is not associated with infection **D,** immune response **B,** or abnormalities of clotting **C.**

5. A patient with Cushing's disease has the following laboratory values. Which should the nurse report to the patient's physician immediately?
   A. Glucose = 132 mg/dL
   B. Na$^+$ = 148 mEq/L
   C. BUN = 12 mg/dL
   D. K$^+$ = 3.0 mEq/L

Intended Response: **D.** Overproduction of aldosterone in Cushing's disease causes retention of both sodium and water, with corresponding excretion of potassium. As hypokalemia can lead to dysrhythmias, the potassium value should be reported immediately to the physician. The glucose **A** value is elevated due to excess production of cortisol. Although both glucose and sodium values are abnormal, they are not as great a concern as the serum K$^+$ value. The BUN value is within normal limits.

6. The nurse is preparing a teaching plan for a patient newly diagnosed with insulin-dependent diabetes mellitus (IDDM). The nurse should instruct the patient that requirement for insulin is decreased by which of the following factors?
   A. Physical activity
   B. Fever
   C. Emotional stress
   D. Infection

Intended Response: **A.** Exercise, by increasing metabolic rate, increases utilization of glucose by the cells for fuel, thus reducing insulin requirement. All remaining responses increase the need for insulin, as each causes blood glucose to elevate.

7. Which of the following clinical manifestations would correlate to a stat blood glucose value of 360?
   A. Cool, moist skin
   B. Nervousness and irritability
   C. Thirst
   D. Headache and uncoordinated movements

Intended Response: **C.** A blood glucose value of 360 indicates hyperglycemia, evidenced by excesses of thirst and urination. The remaining responses are all associated with hypoglycemia, a below normal blood glucose.

8. The nurse caring for a patient in diabetic ketoacidosis (DKA) should **most** closely monitor which of the following laboratory values?

    A. Hematocrit

    B. Potassium

    C. Blood urea nitrogen

    D. Sodium

Intended Response: **B.** As insulin is required to move potassium into the cells, the patient in DKA has a significant risk for hyperkalemia, which could result in potentially lethal arrhythmias. Close monitoring of serum K^+ levels is indicated both before and during treatment for ketoacidosis. Serum sodium, hematocrit, and BUN may increase in DKA, evidencing fluid volume deficit; however, none of these are as critical to assess as serum potassium.

9. Which of the following types of insulin should be indicated for a patient with a glucose value of 620 and a serum acetone value of 32?

    A. Regular

    B. NPH

    C. Navalin 70/30

    D. Lente

Intended Response: **A.** Serum acetone is normally zero, as fats are not normally metabolized at such a rapid rate as to release acetone bodies into serum. The lab values indicating both hyperglycemia and ketosis (fat breakdown) indicate the need for a rapid-acting insulin which may be administered intravenously. The remaining types of insulin are not rapid-acting enough and cannot be administered intravenously.

10. Acute hypoglycemia reaction in a conscious patient is best reversed by prompt administration of which of the following?

    A. 2 or 3 teaspoons (packets) of sugar in a cup of orange juice

    B. A cup of apple juice followed by skim milk

    C. 4 or more saltine crackers with butter or jelly

    D. IV administration of 10% dextrose injection

Intended Response: **B.** Hypoglycemia in a conscious patient can be promptly and readily reversed with administration of a simple glucose (apple juice) followed by a more complex form of glucose (skim milk) to stabilize blood glucose values. Response A is an excessive amount of glucose and is thus not indicated. Response **C** is a complex carbohydrate which will not increase blood glucose values promptly enough. IV administration of dextrose **D** would be an appropriate intervention if the patient were not conscious.

16

Cell Division

BARBARA ETLING MURPHY

Principle

The cell is the basic structural and functional unit of the human body

Illustration of Principle

A cell is the smallest intact component of a living organism. It is life in its simplest form, a nucleus floating in cytoplasm, encased in a membrane. Yet the cell is not a simple structure. Each individual cell in a living organism is a complex unit of information, activity, and function.

The nucleus of the cell acts as its control center. It is the "brains" of the operation, directing all of the cell's activities. The nucleus also contains the cell's genetic information. Chromatin material, made up of deoxyribonucleic acid (DNA) and protein, develops into threadlike structures known as chromosomes. Segments of the DNA strands, the genes, contain coded information that ultimately determines the individual characteristics of the organism (e.g., eye color, and hair texture). In humans, all this information is organized into 23 pairs of chromosomes. Each individual cell nucleus is actually a blueprint of the entire organism.

---

*T*he nucleus is the cell's control center.
It directs and coordinates all intracellular activities.
It influences how the cell interacts with the extracellular environment.
It contains the cell's genetic information.

MEMORY JOGS

In order to survive and function, the cell must have some means of meeting its own metabolic needs. It must be able to nourish itself. It must be able to synthesize the materials it needs to perform its various functions. It must have some means of transporting these materials throughout the cell. Finally, it must have access to a power source capable of keeping all these mechanisms running. These activities occur in the cytoplasm of the cell. The cytoplasm lies between the nucleus and the cell membrane. It houses a number of different structures, known as organelles, that perform the actual work of the cell. Organelles are distinct, self-contained systems, working together to maintain balance within the cell.

MEMORY JOGS

*U*nder the direction of the nucleus, the organelles in the cytoplasm perform the actual "work" of the cell.

The nucleus and the cytoplasm of the cell are held together by the cell membrane, which serves to protect the cell from the outside environment. The membrane itself is composed primarily of lipid and protein and contains openings or "pores" that allow the internal mechanisms of the cell to communicate with the outside environment. However, the cell membrane does much more than just separate the cell from the outside world. Under the direction of the nucleus, it performs a number of critical functions that are essential to the survival and proper functioning of the cell.

The cell membrane participates in certain chemical reactions occurring within the cell. Digestive enzymes, located in the membrane, initiate the processes by which necessary nutrients are made available for use by the cell. The cell membrane also acts as a site for the activation of adenosine triphosphate (ATP), the cell's fuel, into a form of energy the cell can use to carry out its various chemical reactions. However, one of the cell membrane's most significant functions involves its control over the passage of materials into and out of the cell. This mechanism is essential for maintaining balance within the cell. The ease with which this is accomplished depends on how permeable the cell membrane is. Most cell membranes are considered semipermeable, which means that certain substances, like water, can pass freely into and out of the cell, whereas other substances cannot. Some of the factors that influence membrane permeability include the following:

The molecular size of the substance attempting to enter the cell, in relation to the size of the pores in the membrane.

The composition of the substance attempting to enter the cell. The cell membrane has a high lipid content, so lipid-soluble substances have an easier time passing through the membrane than nonlipid soluble substances.

The electrical charge carried by the substance attempting to enter the cell, as compared with that carried by the cell membrane. Two like charges repel each other and make passage through the membrane difficult.

The presence of active transport mechanisms within the cell membrane. Using energy, these "carriers" transport substances into the cell that might otherwise not be able to enter.

If this system were perfect, the cell membrane would be permeable to the substances that the cell needs for growth and reproduction and impermeable to the substances that could harm it. Unfortunately, the system is not that specific. Because of these properties of cell membrane permeability, appropriately prescribed medication is able to reach its target tissues and perform its functions appropriately. However, when medication is taken by a pregnant woman, these cell properties also allow drugs to cross the placental membranes, and may potentially result in damage to the developing fetus.

> *T*he cell membrane separates the intracellular environment from the extracellular environment and controls the passage of substances into and out of the cell.

MEMORY JOGS

The cells of living organisms all go through similar processes in performing their individual functions. They take in and process nutrients, they eliminate wastes, and most of them reproduce. A single-cell organism, like the protozoa, is just that—a single cell. This one cell must independently perform all of the activities necessary to ensure its survival. It is by necessity a relatively simple organism. As the number of cells in an organism increases, they become less able to perform all functions independently. Therefore, the various cells tend to specialize in whatever function they are best suited for, counting on their fellow cells to fill in the gaps. For example, nerve cells are capable of absorbing nutrients, but are primarily involved in transmitting impulses back and forth between the brain and other parts of the body. These cells depend on the cells in the intestinal mucosa to process nutrients for use by the entire body. The end result is an effective division of labor. Groups of specialized cells function interdependently to meet the needs of the organism as a whole.

> *M*ulticellular organisms, like human beings, are made up of groups of specialized cells, functioning interdependently to meet the needs of the organism as a whole.

MEMORY JOGS

Human cells come in a variety of shapes and sizes, depending upon the kind of work they do. Muscle cells are long, so that they can shorten and create a force when they contract. Red blood cells are round and flat to provide an increased surface area over which O_2 and CO_2 can cross. Nerve cells are long and spiderlike because they cover extensive areas, connecting all the body's tissues with the brain and spinal cord. In health, the functions of these and all of the other cells in the human body are coordinated so that balance is maintained within the organism. However, if part of this system fails, the balance is disrupted. The impact that this has on the individual human being depends on what cells are involved and to what extent.

Principle

In order to function appropriately, cells must grow and divide in an orderly, systematic manner

Illustration of Principle

Human life begins as a single cell, the product of the union between a female egg and a male sperm. Each of these parent cells offers their offspring 23 chromosomes, one-half the full human complement of 46. The mechanism by which this occurs is known as meiosis. The human sex cells, the ova and the spermatozoa, are the only cells in the human body capable of this type of cell division. The result of their union is a new life, a single cell with a full complement of 46 chromosomes, in a unique combination of the best and the worst characteristics each individual parent cell has to offer.

MEMORY JOGS

> *M*eiosis is a form of cell division in which the full human complement of 46 chromosomes is halved. The ova and the spermatozoa are the only human cells capable of this type of cell division.

This single cell, the zygote, spends its first few days of life dividing and increasing in number. It accomplishes this through a mechanism known as mitosis. This process allows the cell to make exact, genetic duplicates of itself. It is a continuous process that involves dissolution of the nuclear membrane and division of the 46 chromosomes into two identical sets, which migrate to opposite ends of the cell. The cell membrane constricts, dividing the cytoplasm in half. Finally, the nuclei reorganize around their respective chromosomes, and the division is complete.

MEMORY JOGS

*M*itosis is a mechanism of cell division in which the cells of living organisms are able to make exact, genetic duplicates of themselves.

Once the zygote reaches the uterus, it has developed into a mass composed of several hundred cells. It then begins a process of differentiation. The physical properties and functions of the cells change as they begin to develop into the different structures in the body. Initially, this process involves a separation between the developing embryo and the placenta. Eventually, the cells will differentiate into the germ cell layers from which all body tissues and structures develop. If all goes well, that one single cell will develop into a complex system of specialized tissues and organs—the human body.

When problems occur at this point in development, they usually arise from one of two possible origins, either a genetic defect in the zygote or a failure of the zygote to differentiate appropriately.

When a zygote inherits a defect from either or both parent cells, the eventual outcome and the impact it has on the developing offspring depend on the nature of the defect. For example, cystic fibrosis is a chronic metabolic disease that results in defective exocrine gland function. Although cystic fibrosis patients are usually of normal intelligence, they suffer from a variety of respiratory and digestive complications and may only survive into early adulthood. This disease can be traced to a single defective gene, directly transmitted from parent to offspring. Down syndrome, or trisomy 21, occurs when a zygote inherits an extra twenty-first chromosome from either of the parent cells. The syndrome includes a number of physical abnormalities, mental retardation, and occasionally heart and intestinal defects. However, with appropriate care, these individuals can live near-normal life spans. Not all genetic defects have as significant an impact on their victims as these two disorders have. However, it is important to understand that any genetic defect is an inherent part of the individual's entire cellular structure, and no technology currently available can correct these defects once they have occurred. Therefore, intervention is aimed at supporting the individual and family and counseling them as to their chances of having more similarly affected offspring.

MEMORY JOGS

*G*enetic defects originate somewhere in the female egg cell or in the male sperm cell, or in both. A defect is inherent in the newly formed organism from the time it is a single-cell zygote.

Hydatidiform mole is an example of what occurs when a zygote fails to differentiate appropriately. Instead of developing into the specialized tissues and structures that become a fetus, trophoblastic cells proliferate wildly into a cluster of fluid-filled, grapelike structures. Although this mass is composed of gestational tissue, it will never develop into a human being. Treatment involves evacuation of the tissue and support of the family who have experienced the loss. Since hydatidiform mole has also been associated with subsequent malignancy, follow-up of these women is extremely important.

Most cells do not live forever, but their life spans vary. Certain blood cells may only live a few hours or days, whereas nerve cells may live as long as the human being does. In order for a living organism to survive, its cells must be able to grow and reproduce. This mechanism allows the body to replace dead cells with cells that are identical in structure and function, thereby preserving the integrity of the tissue and the balance within the entire organism. Cell reproduction also allows the body to grow and develop as the infant grows to adulthood.

The rate of cell growth and reproduction varies among cell types and is genetically regulated. Skin and blood cells reproduce rapidly, because their average life spans are short. If there happens to be a deficiency of these cells in the body, they will reproduce even more rapidly until an appropriate balance is regained. It is for this reason that a surgical wound heals in a relatively short period of time. Skin cells, damaged by the scalpel, are quickly replaced by newly generated tissue. Similarly, a healthy individual can tolerate donating a unit of blood without compromising on his or her circulatory status, because replacement blood cells are produced rapidly by the bone marrow. Nerve cells, on the other hand, do not reproduce at all, which is why no amount of time or effort can fix a spinal cord once it has been transected.

**MEMORY
JOGS**

*T*he rate of cell growth and reproduction is regulated genetically in the nucleus of the cell and varies among cell types.

With the exception of highly differentiated cells, like the nerve cells, a deficiency in the number of any kind of cell in the body triggers an increase in the rate of that particular cell's reproduction. The impact this has on the entire system depends on what cells are involved and how many. For example, if an individual cuts himself and loses 100 cc of blood, he has fewer red blood cells available to deliver O_2 to all the tissues in his body. However, since 100 cc is a relatively small percentage of her total blood volume, this blood loss should have little effect on her overall health. In an attempt to achieve a balance, his body will reproduce red blood cells until his normal red blood cell count is regained. However, if this individual happens to cut an artery and loses most of his total blood volume, the consequences are considerably more significant. If blood isn't circulating, O_2 is not being delivered to the tissues, which can lead to significant tissue damage and death. Because the body can't possibly reproduce enough red blood cells quickly enough to reverse the situation, this individual will need outside intervention in order to survive. The goal of treatment is to help her regain balance by augmenting her body's own efforts. This will involve controlling the bleeding, replacing the fluids, and providing supportive therapy.

> *I*n an attempt to maintain balance within the organism, a deficiency in the number of almost any kind of cell in the human body will trigger an increase in the rate of that particular cell's reproduction.

MEMORY JOGS

Principle

Cell growth and reproduction require O_2 and nutrients

Illustration of Principle

It is an indisputable fact that human beings must eat and breathe in order to survive. Since the human body is actually a complex organization of specialized cells, it follows that each individual cell must also eat and breathe in order to survive. Nutrients are acquired through digestion of foodstuffs in the gut and transported to the various tissues by means of the circulatory system. Oxygen is acquired through respiratory activity in the lungs and is also transported to the various tissues by means of the circulatory system. Once these products are available at the cellular level, the cells assimilate them through either active or passive processes.

> *J*ust as human beings must eat and breathe in order to survive and thrive, each individual cell in the human body must be able to acquire nutrients and O_2 to perform its specific function.

MEMORY JOGS

Passive processes occur as a result of concentration gradients and pressure differences. They are referred to as passive because no energy is required for these processes to take place. The cell uses several passive mechanisms to acquire necessary nutrients.

Osmosis is the passage of water across a membrane, from an area of higher water concentration to one of lower water concentration. Water concentration is determined by how much material, or solute, is present on either side of the membrane. The greater the concentration of solute, the lower the concentration of water. In an attempt to establish a balance of water and solute on both sides of the membrane, water is drawn through the membrane to the side with the higher concentration of solute. If there is a greater concentration of solute inside the cell, water will enter, causing the cell to swell. If there is a greater concentration of solute outside the cell, water will leave, causing the cell to shrink. The ability of the human body to deal with either of these extremes depends on how many cells are affected, for how long, and to what extent.

For example, many commercially prepared infant formulas come in condensed forms that require dilution before they can be fed to an infant. An error in the appropriate dilution of this formula could result in a preparation that is either too concentrated or not concentrated enough. A single feeding of this preparation probably won't affect a healthy newborn significantly. However, if this error persists over a period of time, it may have very serious consequences. Highly concentrated formula in an infant's gut will draw water out of his bloodstream and tissues, resulting in diarrhea and dehydration. A formula that is too dilute will provide the infant with inadequate nutrients per volume of fluid, resulting in cellular malnutrition. If these conditions are not corrected, they may result in serious fluid and electrolyte imbalances and even death. The implications for nursing's role in parent education are obvious.

Diffusion refers to the mechanism by which substances move from an area of higher concentration to one of lower concentration in an attempt to distribute themselves evenly. A membrane is not required for this process to occur. For example, in the lungs, the air drawn into the alveoli during inspiration has a relatively high concentration of O_2. The blood vessels surrounding the alveoli have a low concentration of O_2. Therefore, O_2 will diffuse into the bloodstream from the alveoli and will be carried away for delivery to the various body tissues. Conversely, blood returning to the lungs from the rest of the body is loaded with CO_2, the waste product of respiration. Since the concentration of CO_2 is higher in the blood than it is in the alveoli, it will diffuse into the alveoli and be expelled through expiration.

Filtration occurs when substances are forced across a membrane because the pressure on one side of the membrane is higher than the pressure on the other side of the membrane. This process only works when the substance attempting to cross the membrane is small enough to pass through. The passage of waste products from the bloodstream into the kidneys, under the influence of the body's blood pressure, is an example of how this mechanism operates in the human body.

*T*he cell acquires some of the materials necessary for its survival through passive processes that depend on concentration and pressure gradients instead of energy. They include

· Osmosis

· Diffusion

· Filtration

When the materials necessary for the growth and reproduction of a cell are unable to enter passively, the cell facilitates their entry by using active processes. They are referred to as active because they require an energy expenditure on the part of the cell.

Active transport is the principal mechanism by which the cell acquires essential components such as amino acids, electrolytes, glucose, and vitamins. Because of their size, composition, and electrical charge, these substances otherwise would not be able to pass through the cell membrane. This process requires a coordinated effort by certain cellular components, including the carrier molecule, specific enzymes that assist the substance in attaching to and detaching from the carrier molecule, and an energy source. With this mechanism intact, substances entering the cell can overcome the passive barriers of both concentration and pressure gradients.

Pinocytosis is an active process by which the cell acquires very large molecular substances such as proteins. These large particles attach to indentations in the outer surface of the cell. The cell membrane folds around the molecule, allowing it to sink in toward the inner aspect of the cell. As the cell membrane closes around it, the particle finds itself floating in an intracellular compartment, to then be dealt with by the appropriate structures within the cell.

The cell also uses an active mechanism to dispose of the waste products of cellular metabolism. This process is known as phagocytosis. Organelles, known as phagocytes, digest the cellular debris, which is then transported out of the cell by various active and passive mechanisms. Phagocytosis is also one of the mechanisms by which the cell attempts to rid itself of bacteria and other foreign substances.

*C*ertain materials necessary for the cell's growth and development, which cannot enter the cell passively, are acquired through active processes that require an energy expenditure. These include

· Active transport

· Pinocytosis

· Phagocytosis

When an individual is healthy, intracellular and extracellular environments are balanced. This means that sufficient amounts of O_2 and appropriate nutrients are available to the cells, and the cells are capable of using them. When one or more components of this system fail, the balance is disrupted, which may result in cellular damage or death. As always, the impact that this has on the health of the individual depends on what cells are affected and to what extent.

In considering the concepts of cellular oxygenation and nutrition in humans, it is tempting to view them in black and white. If an individual is adequately nourished and oxygenated, he or she survives and thrives; if not, he or she dies. However, in reality, there is an enormous gray zone between these two extremes. Problems with cellular oxygenation and nutrition usually arise from one of the three following sources:

1. An inadequate supply of O_2 and nutrients available for use by the body
2. An ineffective mechanism for transporting O_2 and nutrients to the various tissues of the body
3. An inability of the individual cells to use O_2 and nutrients appropriately

If O_2 and nutrients are not available to a living organism, its cells cannot survive. For example, the individual who is in the process of drowning is anoxic. He has been cut off from his supply of O_2. His body will continue to function only as long as the O_2 remaining in his system lasts. Similarly, the individual who has no food to eat will eventually starve. Less dramatic examples include the individual with COPD, whose O_2 intake is limited by the condition of the lungs, and the infant with failure-to-thrive, whose nutritional intake is limited by various physiological and psychological factors. These individuals may have enough O_2 and nutrients to sustain vital functioning, but probably do not have enough of a reserve to maintain a normal activity level or to grow and develop. No matter what the cause, the goal of treatment is the same. Adequate oxygenation or nutrition must be restored, or when that is not possible, attempts must be made to help the individual make the best possible use of what he or she has.

The ineffective transport of O_2 and nutrients to the tissues of the body can also emerge as either an acute or a chronic condition. For example, the trauma victim who is hemorrhaging has a defect in his O_2 transport system. His lungs are capable of supplying adequate amounts of O_2, but he has no means of delivering it to the tissues. As the blood pours out of his body, it takes the O_2 with it. Similarly, the individual with a bowel obstruction may have access to an adequate supply of appropriate nutrients but is unable to deliver them to the intestines where they would ordinarily be processed for use by the body. Unless these conditions are remedied in a timely fashion, these individuals will die.

A child with cyanotic heart disease illustrates how a chronic deficiency in O_2 transport affects a living organism. Because of a defect in the circulatory system, the body is unable to deliver adequate O_2 to all its tissues. Subsequently, O_2 is shunted to the vital organs at the expense of the rest of the body. This results in a stunting of the child's physical and developmental growth.

Regardless of the cause, intervention is aimed at correcting the defect in O_2 nutrient transport, whether this involves suturing an arterial laceration or surgically correcting a congenital heart defect. When this is not possible, treatment focuses on supporting the individual and potentiating whatever function is intact.

---

*A*dequate cellular oxygenation and nutrition depend on three factors:

1. An adequate supply of O_2 and appropriate nutrients
2. An effective transport mechanism to deliver these materials to the bodily tissues
3. The ability of each individual cell to use these materials appropriately

---

MEMORY JOGS

Assuming that adequate amounts of O_2 and nutrients are available and that they have been appropriately transported to the various tissues in the body, cell growth and reproduction will continue only if the individual cells are capable of using these materials appropriately. Consider the individual who has suffered tissue necrosis secondary to a temporarily inadequate blood supply, which has been corrected. In spite of the fact that adequate amounts of O_2 and nutrients are available and have been delivered directly to the tissues, the cells can't use them because they are already dead. Treatment is therefore aimed at removing the dead tissue and promoting the growth and development of surrounding tissue, with the hope that the healthy cells can make up for those cells that were destroyed. Although this mechanism works effectively for many tissues in the body, certain cells cannot be replaced once they are destroyed (e.g., nerve cells). The impact this has on the individual will depend on what tissues are involved, over what period of time, and to what extent.

Principle

When cells grow and reproduce too rapidly, they are unable to provide for their own nutrition

Illustration of Principle

Cell growth and reproduction in the healthy human body are organized and controlled. Each individual cell, within the context of its own particular function, life span, and rate of reproduction, participates in the dynamic processes required to assure a balanced state of health. When cells grow and reproduce rapidly, they can't always nourish themselves adequately, because most of their energy and effort are involved in cell division. They therefore must rely on other cellular systems to provide this nourishment for them.

**MEMORY
JOGS**

> *W*hen cells grow and reproduce rapidly, they frequently are unable to nourish themselves adequately and must rely on other cellular systems to provide this nourishment for them.

Very rapid cell division in the human body can be of either a physiological or a pathophysiological origin. For example, the developing fetus is undergoing cell growth and reproduction at a rate that is unparalleled at any other point in human life. The fetus depends on the pregnant woman to supply the O_2 and nutrients necessary to support this growth. This is accomplished by way of the placenta, which is the functional unit for cellular growth and metabolism in the developing fetus. Subsequently, all of the cellular systems in the pregnant woman readjust to accommodate the growing fetus. However, when rapid cell division is the result of a pathologic condition, like cancer, adaptive mechanisms are not in place. Cancer is cell division out of control. These cells seize the available O_2 and nutrients at the expense of the body's healthy cells.

Subprinciple

The placenta is the functional unit for cellular growth and metabolism in the developing fetus

Normal cell growth and reproduction in the developing fetus is explosive. In approximately 40 weeks, a single-cell organism evolves into a trillion-cell, highly differentiated, living, breathing human being. Adequate nutrition and oxygenation are of paramount importance if this phenomenon is to occur. However, these fetal cells are so busy growing into a baby that they don't have the time or the means to acquire these necessary materials independently. This is a job for the placenta.

Placental development begins in the third week of life, at the site of embryo implantation. It is divided into two parts, a maternal segment and a fetal segment. The maternal side of the placenta has a red, fleshy appearance. It comprises a tissue layer known as the *decidua basalis* and its corresponding circulation. The fetal side of the placenta comprises a tissue layer known as the chorion and its corresponding circulation. An adherent, amniotic membrane covers the fetal side of the placenta, giving it a shiny, gray appearance and making it easy to distinguish from the maternal side. Within the placenta, these two separate tissue layers interlock by means of a series of fetal chorionic villi that project into intervillous spaces formed by the maternal decidua, similar to the way the teeth of a zipper fit together. Fetal and maternal circulatory systems are separated by a chorionic membrane layer, which is only a few cells thick. Under normal situations, nutrients and gases can pass through this membrane without allowing the two separate blood supplies to mingle.

By the fourth week of life, the placenta has completely taken over the responsibility for metabolic exchange between the fetus and mother. The maternal circulatory system delivers O_2 and nutrients to the placenta by means of the maternal arterioles. This blood spurts into the intervillous spaces, under the influence of the maternal blood pressure. Through various active and passive mechanisms, O_2 and nutrients cross the chorionic membrane and enter the fetal circulation, where they are delivered to the fetus by means of a single umbilical vein. Carbon dioxide and other fetal waste products return to the placenta in reverse fashion by means of two umbilical arteries, where they are delivered to the maternal circulation for disposal.

MEMORY JOGS

*T*he placenta is the functional unit for cellular growth and metabolism in the developing fetus.

It supplies the fetus with O_2 and nutrients.

It disposes of the waste products of cellular metabolism.

It produces hormones essential to the continued growth and development of the fetus.

In addition to the mechanisms previously discussed, the placenta participates in a number of other metabolic activities, including endocrine and immunologic functions. The placenta produces hormones (i.e., progesterone, estrogen, human chorionic gonadotropin [HCG], and human placental lactogen [HPL]) that are essential for maintaining fetal well-being and promoting appropriate fetal growth and development. It is also thought that certain hormones produced in the placenta interfere with cellular immunity during pregnancy. This may be the reason why the maternal immune system does not seem to recognize the fetus as foreign and attempt to reject it.

When the maternal-placental-fetal unit is intact and functioning appropriately, it would seem reasonable to assume that the fetus has an excellent chance of growing and developing normally. Indeed, appropriate fetal growth and development are dependent on this maternal-fetal relationship. However, this fact alone cannot guarantee a good fetal outcome. In fact, the very nature of this relationship may put the fetus at significant risk in situations in which teratogenic substances are involved. The placenta's major function is to provide the fetus with O_2 and essential nutrients, but it is not particularly selective about what substances are allowed to pass to the fetus. Countless drugs, chemicals, viruses, and bacterias have been proven to cross the placental membranes to enter fetal circulation, often with tragic results. Prenatal counseling and appropriate education play a significant role in minimizing these hazards.

> *P*lacental membranes are not particularly selective about the substances they allow to pass from the maternal circulation into the fetal circulation. Substances that do not adversely affect the mother may have teratogenic effects on the developing fetus.

When the maternal-placental-fetal unit is not intact, both the developing fetus and the mother may be in jeopardy. The disrupting factors may be either acute or chronic. The effect this has on both mother and fetus depends on the extent of the problem, how long it persists, and at what point in fetal development it occurs. For example, placental abruption is the premature separation of the placenta from the uterine wall, which disrupts the supply of O_2 and nutrients to the fetus. If the separation is minimal, the rest of the placenta usually can accommodate fetal needs adequately. However, if the abruption involves the entire placenta, the mother hemorrhages into the uterus, and the fetus' lifeline is cut.

An example of a more chronic form of placental compromise is the uteroplacental insufficiency that frequently accompanies pregnancy-induced hypertension. In addition to the classic symptoms of hypertension, edema, and proteinuria, patients with pregnancy-induced hypertension experience generalized vasoconstriction and hypovolemia. This results in a decreased blood supply to the placenta, with a subsequent compromise in fetal oxygenation and nutrition. These infants are frequently growth retarded and may have a difficult time tolerating the stress of normal labor. Management of the patient with pregnancy-induced hypertension is aimed at improving uteroplacental blood flow by means of physical rest, stress reduction, and medication, while monitoring the condition and growth of the developing fetus. The final "cure" for pregnancy-induced hypertension is delivery of the infant. The route of delivery (i.e., vaginal versus cesarean section) will depend on whether there is enough placental reserve to support the fetus adequately during the stress of labor.

> *D*isruption in the function of the placenta interferes with the delivery of O_2 and nutrients to the fetus. A deficiency in essential nutrients may result in intrauterine growth retardation.

Subprinciple
Cancer is cell division out of control

Cell division in the healthy human body is organized and controlled, so that the various cell types will grow and reproduce at an appropriate rate. Cancer is a disease that attacks the nucleus of the cell, causing genetic mutations that destroy these control mechanisms. The result is a rapid, uncontrolled reproduction of mutated cancer cells.

An occasional mutated cell is not unusual in an organism composed of trillions of cells. Under ordinary circumstances, it has no effect on the human body. The immune system views it as abnormal and eliminates it. How and why these isolated cells develop into cancer is not well understood. However, certain predisposing factors have been identified, including radiation exposure, chemical carcinogen exposure, chronic tissue inflammation, and various hereditary factors.

Once cancer cells have established a foothold in the human body, their nuclei are no longer able to control the growth process, and they reproduce rapidly and aggressively. They also tend to separate from each other and travel throughout the body by way of the circulatory and lymphatic systems. This tendency results in metastasis of the cancer to additional sites in the body.

Like any other cell in the human body, cancer cells require O_2 and nutrients to survive. They compete with the body's normal cells for these materials. Because their growth and reproduction are so rapid, they consume the available nutrients at the expense of the rest of the body's tissues. Eventually, the body's healthy cells starve to death.

MEMORY JOGS

*M*alignant cells compete with healthy cells for available nutrients. Because malignant cells reproduce so rapidly, they consume these nutrients at the expense of the rest of the body's tissues.

The goal of treatment in cancer patients is to stop the growth and reproduction of these mutant cells and eliminate them from the body. Surgical excision, in combination with chemotherapy and radiation therapy, is commonly employed to achieve this goal. In general, chemotherapy and radiation therapy attempt to interfere with the metabolism and reproduction of the malignant cells. However, since these malignant cells mutated from healthy cells and are still quite similar in form and function, it is frequently impossible to kill the cancer cells without wiping out a significant number of healthy cells as well. Killing the patient in order to kill the cancer is not an acceptable treatment outcome. Subsequently, chemotherapy and radiation doses are tailored to kill as many cancer cells as possible, while holding healthy cell destruction to a minimum. Cancer patients require substantial physical and emotional support to help them deal with the stresses of both the disease and the treatment.

MEMORY JOGS

> *T*he effective treatment of cancer with chemotherapy and radiation therapy is inhibited by the fact that in order to kill malignant cells, healthy cells are also destroyed.

Reasoning Exercises: *Cell Division*

Patty Daniels is a 25-year-old white female, pregnant with her first child. She is being seen in the obstetric clinic for her first prenatal visit.

1. Patty tells the nurse, "I drank a glass of wine at a party before I found out that I was pregnant. I'm worried that I might have hurt the baby." Based on an understanding of alcohol use in pregnancy, which of the following responses is the most appropriate?
   A. "We don't really know how much alcohol is too much during pregnancy. Don't drink anymore and try not to worry about it."
   B. "As long as your drinking is moderate, I wouldn't worry about it. There were plenty of healthy babies born to drinking mothers before they ever discovered fetal alcohol syndrome."
   C. "An occasional drink shouldn't hurt the baby. Research has shown that the risk to the fetus increases as the amount and frequency of alcohol consumption increase."
   D. "I can understand why you're so upset, but an occasional drink shouldn't hurt the baby."

Intended Response: **C.** This patient needs two things from the nurse: information about alcohol use in pregnancy and reassurance about the potential risk to her own baby. Alcohol is a known teratogenic substance, but it is unclear how much alcohol it takes, and at what point in development, to adversely affect the fetus. Research has shown that the incidence of fetal alcohol syndrome and related disorders increases as the amount and frequency of alcohol consumption increase. An occasional drink should not harm the fetus. **C** is the correct response because it is the only answer that offers reassurance and accurate information without catastrophizing the situation.

2. The nurse explains to Patty that good prenatal nutrition is essential for the healthy growth and development of her baby. Which of the following nutritional factors has the most significant impact on the eventual outcome of her pregnancy?

    A. The severity of first trimester nausea or vomiting and its interference with adequate nutritional intake

    B. The ready availability of the essential minerals (e.g., calcium and iron) necessary for proper tissue and organ formation

    C. The availability of appropriate nutrients at critical points in fetal development

    D. The percentage of protein intake, compared with the intake of other nutrient groups

Intended Response: **C.** Growth and development in a fetus occur as a result of an increase in both the number of cells (i.e., cell division) and cell size. This requires an adequate supply of appropriate nutrients, available to the fetus when needed. When dietary deficiencies interfere with cell growth, it is possible to reverse the process by eliminating the deficiency. However, if dietary deficiencies interfere with cell division, they may result in permanent defects that will have a permanent effect on the fetus.

Situation Update

Patty is now at 41 weeks' gestation. A nonstress test performed in her physician's office was nonreactive. She has been admitted to the labor and delivery unit to undergo a contraction stress test.

3. The contraction stress test (CST) is used frequently in the management of postdate pregnancies. The main reason that a CST is performed is which of the following?

    A. To determine whether the fetus is ready to be delivered

    B. To determine whether the placenta is adequately oxygenating the fetus

    C. To determine whether the fetus can tolerate normal labor, prior to elective induction

    D. To determine whether the uterus will be able to contract efficiently enough to establish an adequate labor pattern

Intended Response: **B.** The CST identifies the fetus at risk for intrauterine asphyxia, by monitoring the fetal heart rate in response to uterine contractions. Labor is normally an asphyxiating condition. If the fetal-placental unit is healthy, there is enough O_2 reserve to support the fetus during the stress of the contraction. In postdate pregnancies, the placenta begins to degenerate so that there is less O_2 reserve available.

4. During the CST, the baseline fetal heart rate was 130 to 140 beats/min. Which of the following findings gives the best indication that Patty's fetus may not be able to tolerate labor?

   A. A series of late decelerations, with a drop in fetal heart rate to 116 beats/min

   B. A single variable deceleration, with a drop in fetal heart rate to 90 beats/min

   C. A series of early decelerations, with a drop in fetal heart rate to 116 beats/min

   D. A single late deceleration, with a drop in fetal heart rate to 90 beats/min

Intended Response: **A.** Early decelerations result from fetal head compression and do not indicate fetal distress. Variable decelerations result from umbilical cord compression and may or may not indicate distress. A single, isolated variable deceleration is probably not ominous. Late decelerations result from uteroplacental insufficiency and indicate fetal distress. A persistent run of late decelerations is more ominous than a single, isolated one.

5. Based on the results of the contraction stress test, the decision is made to deliver Patty's baby by cesarean section. Which of the following observations at birth indicate that the infant may have experienced intrauterine stress–asphyxia at some point earlier in the pregnancy?

   A. 1 min Apgar = 5; 5 min Apgar = 8

   B. Thick, bright green meconium present in the amniotic fluid

   C. Vigorous stimulation required to initiate respiration

   D. Yellowish-brown, stained amniotic fluid; infant's skin stained similarly

Intended Response: **D.** Meconium-stained amniotic fluid is a classic sign of fetal asphyxia or distress. Fresh meconium is bright green in color, but it turns a yellowish-brown color as it ages. The correct response is **D,** because yellowish-brown, stained amniotic fluid and infant skin indicate that the fetus passed meconium at some point earlier in the pregnancy.

6. Which of the following is commonly associated with malignancy, regardless of cell type?

   A. Generalized lymphadenopathy

B. Weight loss

C. Abnormal bleeding or discharge

D. Cardiac dysrhythmias

Intended Response: **B.** Malignant cells compete with healthy cells for available nutrients. Because malignant cells multiply more rapidly than normal cells, malignant cells consume nutrients at the expense of the rest of the body's tissues, resulting in weight loss. Generalized lymphadenopathy **A** could suggest a malignancy of the lymphatic system, such as Hodgkin disease. Abnormal bleeding or discharge **C**, though noted in some cancers, such as endometrial or breast, is not characteristic of all malignancies. Cardiac dysrhythmias **D** are typically not associated with malignant processes.

7. The nurse is developing a plan of care for a patient who is to begin receiving anticancer chemotherapy. Which of these potential side effects should the nurse evaluate as being of greatest concern?

   A. Scalp alopecia

   B. Transient nausea and vomiting

   C. Oral stomatitis

   D. Fatigue and dyspnea

Intended Response: **D.** Anticancer chemotherapy has the unfortunate action of destroying normal cells as well as malignant ones, causing a number of side effects. The side effect of greatest concern is bone marrow suppression, involving depression of red blood cell production (anemia), platelet production (bleeding tendencies), and white blood cell production (susceptibility to infection). Red blood cell suppression would be evidenced by signs of decreased oxygen transport to tissues, including fatigue and dyspnea.

8. Which of the following interventions aimed at maintaining nutritional status should be included in a plan of care for a patient who is to begin receiving anticancer chemotherapy?

   A. Administer antiemetic medication prior to chemotherapy

   B. Limit oral intake of fluids

   C. Administer antipyretic medication following chemotherapy

   D. Limit caloric intake to 1800 calories daily

Intended Response: **A.** As nausea and vomiting are expected side effects of nearly all anticancer chemotherapeutic agents, medications to prevent or alleviate nausea and vomiting should be administered before the initiation of chemotherapy drugs. Oral intake of fluids **B** and high caloric intake **D** should be encouraged as much as the patient may tolerate to counteract fluid and nutritional imbalances related to anorexia. The administration of antipyretic (fever-reducing) medication would have no effect on nutritional status.

9. Which of these assessment data would indicate a chemotherapy-related fluid and electrolyte disturbance?

   A. Urine output averages 900 mL per shift

   B. Serum K⁺ level is 3.6

   C. Blood pressure ranges from 120/64 to 132/70

   D. Serum BUN is 34 with creatinine of 1.0

Intended Response: **D.** An elevated blood urea nitrogen (BUN) coupled with a creatinine level within normal range suggests fluid deficit (dehydration). Responses **A, B,** and **C** are all within normal parameters, suggesting no fluid and electrolyte disturbance.

10. The nurse notes that the platelet count of a patient who is receiving anticancer chemotherapy has dropped to $58,000/mm^3$. Which of the following nursing diagnoses should be added to the patient's plan of care?

    A. Fatigue

    B. High Risk for Injury

    C. Altered Tissue Perfusion

    D. High Risk for Infection

Intended Response: **B.** The patient's platelet count is well below low normal values, indicating a risk for injury related to impaired clotting. Fatigue **A** would be associated with a decrease in oxygen-carrying red blood cells or hemoglobin. Altered tissue perfusion **C** is associated with conditions impairing arterial blood flow. High risk for infection **D** would be associated with a decrease in white blood cell production.

11. A patient is receiving external beam radiation therapy for treatment of a lung carcinoma. Which of the following interventions regarding care of irradiated skin should the nurse plan?

    A. Wash chest area with tepid water and mild soap

    B. Lubricate chest area with topical emollients

    C. Apply antiinfective ointments to chest area

    D. Cover chest area with a dry gauze dressing secured with tape

Intended Response: **A.** Like chemotherapy, radiation therapy damages and destroys normal, healthy cells as well as malignant cells. Thus, persons receiving external beam radiation may develop damage to skin tissues similar to sunburn damage caused by exposure to ultraviolet rays. Damaged tissue should be washed with water only or water and mild soap. Neither lotions **B** or ointments **C** should be applied. Skin should be left open to air to enhance healing. Tape should be avoided to prevent adhesive tears on damaged skin surfaces.

17

Mobility

MARIAN B. SIDES

Principle

The human body functions best when it can move about freely in its environment

Illustration of Principle

Mobility is a quality of the human body that enables males and females to move about freely and interact with the world around them. This freedom to move about ranges from no movement (comatose) to excessive movement (hyperactivity). Optimal mobility occurs when the body strikes a comfortable balance between these two extremes.

The ability to move freely and purposefully in the environment enables one to satisfy basic human needs, move away from danger, and move toward pleasant events. When the body is able to maintain balance through movement, nursing intervention is minimal. As immobility increases and autonomy decreases, the nurse plays a more active role in providing care.

Principle

A decrease in the quantity and quality of mobility reduces self-control and threatens self-image

Illustration of Principle

The freedom to control motor activity is very important to one's self-image. Self-worth is directly related to independence and autonomy. For example, the patient with upper extremity burns may not be able to perform the basic activities of daily living. Although this limitation is focused and temporary, the need to rely on others is threatening. The patient who has debilitating rheumatoid arthritis and is bedridden feels an even greater threat to independence and self-worth because this limitation is generalized and progressive. In planning care for this type of patient, the nurse must be sensitive to the psychological impact of these limitations and promote independent functioning whenever possible.

Principle

The extent and duration of immobilization determine the kind of intervention required

Illustration of Principle

Mobility takes on characteristic features related to extent and duration when illness occurs. These features help shape and give direction to nursing intervention. For example, the patient who has a hip spica cast or a Stryker frame requires greater assistance for a longer period of time than the patient who has a cast following a surgical reduction of a limb fracture. The nurse must be sensitive to the extent and duration of immobility that limits the individual's freedom to function independently.

The manner in which the immobilization is imposed upon the patient is also important in determining appropriate nursing response. For example, the patient who is recovering from a myocardial infarction may be ordered to limit activity to conserve energy. Patient compliance in this case requires self-discipline and an understanding of the relationship between activity and recovery. The patient must be willing to cooperate and follow protocol. After all, the patient knows that he or she *can* move about but *must* not.

The patient in traction for a fractured femur is immobilized by the mechanical treatment protocol (traction) as well as the functional disability (fracture). In this case the patient knows he or she can't move about *now* but will be able to later.

The patient with lower extremity amputations is limited primarily by his or her own functional disability rather than by some external medical protocol. This patient has permanent restrictions on mobility. He or she is not mobile now and will not be later.

Each of the above limitations creates a different set of circumstances to which the patient must adjust. It is important to understand the threat imposed by each type of immobility. The nurse must carefully assess the patient's understanding of his or her limitations and the way in which the patient is coping, and then must provide the necessary interventions, including safe physical care, emotional support, and adequate health teaching.

MEMORY JOGS

---

*I*n establishing your plan of care, ask yourself these questions:

1. How long *has* the patient been immobilized?

2. How long *will* the patient be immobilized?

    To what extent is the patient immobilized?

4. How is the patient coping with this limitation?

Principle

A decrease in mobility increases the risk for complications in major body processes

Illustration of Principle

Situational immobilization of a body part, such as with a cast on the arm or a brace on the knee, imposes little threat to normal body functions. However, patients who are subjected to prolonged and extensive immobilization are at risk for many complications and hazards related to immobility. The impact of immobility on major body processes and the selected nursing management of deviations from normalcy are discussed in the following sections.

Musculoskeletal Processes

The bones and muscles of the body provide a structural framework that enables it to perform purposeful and independent activities. In turn, the constant motion of the body keeps the musculoskeletal processes in good working order and helps maintain structural integrity. When movement is curtailed, rapid and progressive deterioration in bony structure and muscle mass occurs. Prolonged immobilization is accompanied by an increase in the loss of calcium from the bones. The incidence of fractures may increase in bones unable to support body weight. Debilitating changes in joint structure result from immobilization of body parts. These changes are manifested in a loss of flexibility in the joints and a gradual decrease in range of motion. The joints eventually become stiffer, and contractures result.

MEMORY JOGS

> *I*mmobilization causes a deterioration in musculoskeletal strength and a loss of joint mobility.

The initial step in managing the actual or potential health hazards caused by immobility is to make an accurate assessment of your patient's mobility status. The nurse must know the processes causing immobilization, limits imposed by the medical treatment regimen, and the health status prior to immobilization. These assessment data are a necessary baseline for establishment of your patient care goals.

The intervention behaviors of the nurse are directed at supporting the normal functions of the body and maintaining the strength, endurance, and flexibility of the musculoskeletal system. All nursing actions are directed at providing a safe environment and preventing injury and complications.

Exercise

A planned exercise program should be executed to maintain and recover muscle strength and joint mobility. The amount and type of exercise needed will depend upon the patient's physical limitations and medical restrictions. Range-of-motion exercises, transfer activities, and ambulation will help maintain joint mobility and reduce loss of calcium from the bone.

The nurse should encourage the patient to perform independently all activities that are permitted by his or her limitations in order to achieve an optional level of mobility. In other words, the nurse should not perform activities that the patient can do alone.

Diet

The nurse should monitor the patient's dietary intake of calcium when mobility is curtailed. A healthy diet, including an increase in foods rich in calcium, is important to produce adequate calcium levels and to reduce skeletal muscle loss. Calcium supplements should be taken cautiously because overingestion may lead to hypercalcemia. A well balanced diet will counter muscle weakness and fatigue and maintain bone integrity.

Positioning

Good body alignment is essential to optimal musculoskeletal functioning and joint mobility. It is also essential to prevent complications. The nurse should be highly sensitive to the need for proper positioning and appropriate body supports, and the need to change position as frequently as necessary.

Comfort

Changes in musculoskeletal processes are often accompanied by joint pain, inflammation, edema, or surgical discomfort. The nurse should respond to alternatives in comfort by taking appropriate measures for pain control, particularly before exercise and activity. These measures may include administering pain medication, changing positions, providing support to extremities and body parts, or making heat or cold applications.

Your patient's progress must be monitored and evaluated in an ongoing manner to determine the effectiveness of your interventions. The initial assessment data are used to determine the extent to which your goals are achieved.

> *H*ow well does your patient perform range-of-motion exercises in comparison with his or her initial performance? What changes in muscular strength, endurance, and joint mobility indicate that you were successful in your nursing interventions?

MEMORY JOGS

The success of your exercise program, for example, can be evaluated by observing skeletal strength and muscle tone by means of normal activities of daily living. Success also may be evaluated by observing how long a patient can perform a particular task before becoming fatigued. The patient is frequently a good evaluator of progress.

Respiratory Processes

Normal ventilation is necessary to keep the lungs expanded and to prevent respiratory infection in the immobilized patient.

A decrease in physical activity reduces the stimuli for breathing and decreases the movement of air in and out of the lungs. When a person is supine, respiratory secretions collect in the lungs and create ideal media for bacterial growth. Atelectasis or collapse of alveoli can result from a decrease in ventilation.

MEMORY
JOGS

*T*he patient who is immobilized is at risk for development of respiratory infection and collapse of the alveoli.

The first responsibility of the nurse in caring for the immobilized patient is to conduct a thorough assessment of the quality of his or her breathing. The goal of nursing care is to reduce pulmonary secretions and increase pulmonary ventilation. Interventions aimed at this goal will prevent infection and alveolar collapse. These interventions include deep breathing and coughing exercises, frequent change in position, and room humidification. Suctioning and hyperventilation may be necessary to assist the patient who is unable to perform these exercises.

MEMORY
JOGS

*W*hat are the key indicators that adequate ventilation is being accomplished? What is the respiratory pattern? What are the blood-gas values? How do the lungs sound? How does your patient look?

Circulatory Processes

The heart must work harder when the body is in a supine position to redistribute blood from the legs to other parts of the systemic circulation. As noted earlier, muscular strength decreases with immobilization, thus further reducing the effectiveness of the peripheral pumping action and increasing the stress on the heart. Likewise, the pumping action that occurs in the blood vessels in the extremities markedly slows when the body is moving. Venous thrombosis can begin to form almost immediately after immobilization in patients whose health is compromised. Individuals at risk include the elderly, persons with cardiovascular problems, the obese, and those who are severely ill.

MEMORY
JOGS

*P*hysical immobilization reduces the pumping action of the heart and slows the emptying of vessels. The longer the immobilization, the greater the risk of venous thrombosis.

The nurse should monitor carefully the cardiovascular status of all patients who are immobilized. The primary goal is to maintain circulatory status and prevent complications. Mobilization of the extremities with range-of-motion exercises should be performed as indicated. Vital signs should be monitored, and the nurse should assess the patient for clinical signs of venous thrombosis. Common signs are edema in the extremities, pain, tenderness, and erythema. Intolerance of postural changes may be accompanied by a decrease in blood pressure, an increase in pulse rate, dizziness, and blurred vision. A sudden change from supine to upright position should be avoided. The nurse should assist patients in sitting up for the first time after surgery and after long periods of immobilization to avoid hypostatic problems.

Pulmonary emboli can occur in patients who are immobilized with cardiovascular problems or other conditions that compromise the pumping action of the heart. Dyspnea is the most common obvious symptom. The nurse must constantly evaluate the patient's tolerance of immobility and response to efforts to increase mobility.

---

*A*sk yourself these questions: Are vital signs within your patient's normal limits? Can he or she change position from supine to upright without difficulty? Are the feet swollen? Is there pain or tenderness in the calves? Are there any other signs of poor blood flow? How does your patient feel?

MEMORY JOGS

Immobilization contributes to problems in elimination. Alterations in gastrointestinal and urinary functions are discussed in Chapter 12. Problems related to neurological processes are also precipitated by immobility. These issues are addressed in Chapter 14.

Patients who are immobilized are at great risk for skin breakdown. Ischemic change in the skin and muscles results from prolonged pressure on body parts and bony prominences. A turning schedule or pattern of movement should be established. Meticulous skin care and a well-balanced diet are essential preventive measures.

The ultimate goal of nursing intervention is to assist the patient in returning to an optimal level of wellness and to minimize the untoward effects imposed by the restriction on movement (see Figure 17–1). Pathological changes in each body system should be anticipated. Efforts should be directed at maintaining functional capacity and preventing deterioration of body processes.

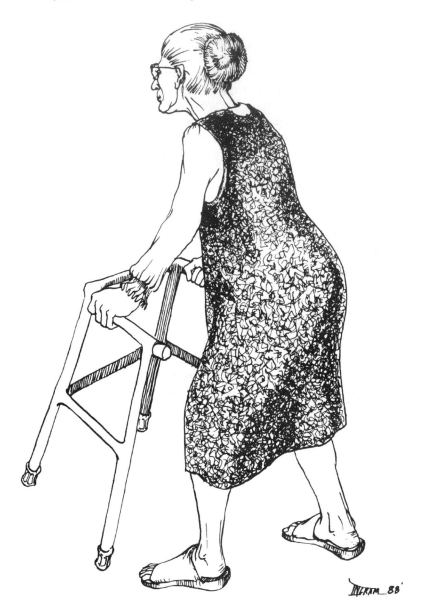

Figure 17-1. Maximizing potential for movement.

*F*or each of the physiological processes identified under hazards of immobility, ask yourself these questions: What can I do for this individual that will make the most difference in his or her health status? What can I do to prevent pneumonia, constipation, decubiti formation, thrombi formation, and muscular weakness? If these problems have already developed, then what can I do to correct them and help the patient to regain normalcy or accept the limitations?

Most interventions that support the normal functioning of body processes can be performed independently by the nurse. If these opportunities are recognized and acted upon in a timely manner, the nurse can expedite the patient's return to wellness. Astute decision-making and nursing judgment must be carefully exercised in selecting intervention measures so that actions are appropriate and relevant to each situation. For example, skin massage may be appropriate to prevent skin breakdown and promote circulation, but leg massage may be contraindicated for patients who are on prolonged bed rest. Nursing intervention, therefore, must clearly and sensibly relate to the underlying patient care problems.

Maintain functional capacity

Optimize return to normalcy

Build ego strength

Individualize care

Listen to your patient

Intervene only when necessary

Teach good therapeutic care

Yes, I can do it, attitude

Reasoning Exercises: *Mobility*

1. Which of the following nursing diagnoses would be of priority for a patient diagnosed with decalcification of bone secondary to prolonged immobilization?

A. High Risk for Injury

B. Body Image Disturbance

C. High Risk for Infection

D. Altered Nutrition: Less than Body Requirements

Intended Response: **A.** Decalcification of bone renders bony processes more porous, and thus more fragile, placing the patient at significant risk for pathologic fracture. Although demineralization can result in structural deformity, Body Image Disturbance **B** is not the priority concern. Because decalcification is related to prolonged bed rest, improved nutritional intake **D** alone will not prevent further demineralization. Infection **C** is not associated with bone decalcification.

2. Which of the following is the primary purpose of range-of-motion (ROM) exercises?

A. Increase muscle strength

B. Enhance cardiovascular tone and fitness

C. Maintain joint mobility

D. Improve venous circulation to extremities

Intended Response: **C.** Prolonged bed rest may result in joint stiffness and ultimately, joint contracture. Range-of-motion exercises allow for either active or passive movements of body joints to maintain joint mobility.

3. The nurse is caring for an elderly patient at risk for decubitus ulcer development secondary to bed rest. Which of the following interventions would be most effective in ulcer prevention?

A. Turn and position the patient q 2 hours

B. Apply soft protective padding to bony prominences

C. Encourage oral fluid intake

D. Apply emollient lotions to areas of dry skin

Intended Response: **A.** All human cells require oxygen for life. Skin tissue cells that are deprived of a steady and adequate supply of oxygen due to interruption in circulation lose viability, resulting in decubitus ulcers. Relief of pressure via regular turning and positioning schedules is the ideal method of decubitus ulcer prevention.

4. A nurse is preparing to transfer a patient from bed to wheelchair (w/c). As the patient rises from supine to sitting position, he complains of (c/o) feeling "lightheaded and dizzy." Which of the following actions should the nurse take next?

A. Lift the patient quickly into the wheelchair

B. Ask the patient to dangle at bedside while leaving the room for a few seconds to get assistance

C. Have the patient sit at the side of the bed for a few minutes while supporting his back and shoulders

D. Return the patient to supine position and apply a safety vest

Intended Response: **C.** The patient's complaints are indicative of orthostatic hypotension, a sudden decrease in blood pressure caused by change of position from supine to sitting, which is common in immobilized patients. Because this phenomenon is typically transient, the nurse should wait a few minutes for blood pressure to stabilize while supporting the patient's back and shoulders to prevent falling or injury. Dangling a patient experiencing orthostatic hypotension is appropriate, but leaving the patient alone at bedside **B** or attempting to transfer him quickly **A** places him at significant risk for injury. A safety vest **D** is not necessary or indicated in this situation.

5. Which of the following clinical manifestations would alert the nurse that an immobilized patient has developed a lower extremity thrombus?

A. Lightheadedness and dizziness

B. Cramping pain in the calf

C. Extremity weakness and numbness

D. Aching pain in the joints

Intended Response: **B.** The presence of a thrombus (blood clot) in an extremity vein results in inflammation, including cramping pain, tenderness, swelling, and redness.

6. An immobilized patient has an increased risk of developing a thrombus. Which of the following would be most beneficial in helping to prevent thrombus development?

A. Elastic stockings

B. Semi-Fowler's position

C. Oxygen therapy

D. Heel protectors

Intended Response: **A.** Elastic stockings (TED hose) support venous structures, which thus increases blood flow through the veins, reducing the likelihood of clot formation. None of the remaining responses will have a preventative effect.

7. Which of the following clinical manifestations would alert the nurse that an immobilized patient has developed a pulmonary embolus?

    A. Sudden onset of dyspnea and restlessness

    B. Complaints of fatigue and muscle weakness

    C. Insidious onset of confusion and disorientation

    D. Complaints of headache and visual changes

Intended Response: **A.** Because a pulmonary embolus interferes with normal oxygenation processes, symptoms are those of hypoxemia, including dyspnea and restlessness. The remaining responses are not pertinent to this hazard of immobility.

8. A nurse is planning interventions to prevent the development of pneumonia in a patient who will be immobilized following open reduction of a fractured femur. Which of the following interventions should the nurse include in the patient's postoperative care plan?

    A. Administer oxygen therapy as needed

    B. Restrict oral fluid intake

    C. Turn, cough, and deep breathe q 2 hours

    D. Provide respiratory suction q 1 hour

Intended Response: **C.** It is essential to mobilize respiratory secretions in order to prevent the development of pneumonia. Turning, coughing, and deep breathing can help achieve this outcome. Oxygen therapy has no preventative effect for the accumulation of fluids in the lung fields. Oral fluid intake should be increased as tolerated to keep respiratory secretions liquefied, and thus easier to expectorate. Suction should be provided only as necessary to maintain an unobstructed airway.

Communication

NANCY KORCHEK

Principle

Humans are social beings who are in constant communication with others in their environments

Illustration of Principle

Males and females, in general, are entities who both seek and receive pleasure from socialization with others—through speech, action, expression—even through tools of communication such as painting, poetry, or song. Both are constantly engaged in processes of communication, even when not consciously aware of it. For example, an individual who removes himself or herself from the crowd at a large party and remains in a quiet corner of the room sipping a drink is not actively speaking with others at the party, but *is* communicating! The separation from the group communicates a message of "I wish to be alone for awhile" or "I don't feel comfortable in this large group." Humans, then, communicate in a variety of ways, both verbal and nonverbal. A smile shared with a familiar face, a handshake with an old friend, or an embrace with a beloved family member communicates a message as effectively and clearly as the spoken word.

Illness presents an *increased* need for the individual to communicate, because illness causes new situations with new needs, problems, and concerns. At the same time, however, illness may alter the individual's ability to communicate effectively, thus requiring health care givers to implement measures that facilitate the patient's expression and communication. For example, a patient who has undergone surgery for tracheostomy has a definite *increased* need to communicate with his health care provider; at the same time, he has a *decreased* ability to communicate by virtue of his surgical experience.

245

Nurses, then, must become critically aware of their essential roles as communicators—of receivers and transmitters of thoughts, feelings, desires, and fears. The establishment of effective helping relationships depends heavily on the nurse's ability and willingness to be an open listener and communicator, ready to hear the patient's communicated messages and accept the value of those messages to the patient.

Principle

Verbal communication involves the relaying of ideas, thoughts, emotions, and drives through the content, speed, volume, pitch, and pattern of speech

Illustration of Principle

The process of communication between human beings involves more than just the transmission and receipt of a spoken message; *how* the message is sent, and thus, received, influences communication as much as *what* is being said. Because nursing is a service involving constant interaction with individuals, both requiring and providing health care, understanding the elements of the communication process is critical to the provision of holistic and comprehensive nursing care.

The elements of verbal communication are as follows:

Speech Content

Content comprises what is being said or discussed, the topic of the conversation, and the message idea. The nurse, in order to fully appreciate speech content, must practice being an attentive *listener,* so that the message that is intended can be fully appreciated or accepted. The nurse should take note that the spoken message is congruent with other elements of verbal communication, such as pitch or volume. For example, if the patient verbally denies any pain or discomfort and states, "I'm fine, really," but at the same time is clenching his teeth and has an unusual pitch in his voice, the nurse may need to reevaluate the patient's denial of pain.

In conversations with patients and staff, the nurse should use astute listening skills to keep focused on the speech content, rather than on the attempt to formulate responses. No pat answer to a spoken message exists; if unsure about what to respond to a message, the nurse should simply repeat what has been said to encourage the patient or other individual to express himself or herself more fully.

Consider this example:

Patient: "I've been in the hospital for over two weeks now. I don't think I'll ever get better."

The nurse caring for this client may be unsure of the true meaning of the patient's statement and may feel ill at ease with providing a sense of reassurance that may not be warranted. The best response is one that *encourages the patient to express himself or herself more fully,* so that the nurse can gather more information and thus understand the patient's statements.

An example of an effective response might then be, "You seem concerned about getting better."

Speech Pitch or Tone

Speech pitch is the intonation or pitch in the voice with which a verbal message is communicated. Clearly, all of us can appreciate that a certain tone or pitch in voice definitely can change the meaning of a spoken message. A complimentary message such as "Your new hairstyle is so different!" quickly can be changed to a negative, disapproving message with a tone of sarcasm added to the verbal message. Tone or pitch, then, reflects an attitude, opinion, or emotion about the speech content that cannot be ignored if one is to fully comprehend and appreciate the communicated message. Nurses should not only concentrate on picking up the tone of the messages received from patients but must also focus on avoiding sending messages with tones of disapproval, doubt, shock, or disgust back to patients and others.

Consider this example:

Nurse 1:   "Do you really think the biopsy will show a malignancy?"

Nurse 2:   "Do you _really_ think the biopsy will show a malignancy?"

With the addition of the underlined word "really" in the second message, a new tone is established in the nurse's statement to the patient, one that may indicate doubt or disapproval to the receiver of that message.

Speed and Volume of Speech

Speed and volume are listed in unison, because they tend to work together in speech. When an individual is feeling very saddened, is experiencing grief or loss, has undergone a difficult period of adjustment or of failure, or is embarrassed about what is being said, the volume and speed with which that individual speaks tend to decrease. Few students, for example, would announce loudly to their colleagues, "Look! I've failed an important exam!" That difficult message would much more likely be communicated in a slow, hesitating manner, and in a soft or low volume. Likewise, when an individual is feeling intense emotion such as anger or fright, or experiencing joy, elation, or significant accomplishment, he or she is most likely to communicate with increased volume and speed. Consider a group of fans at a football game cheering on their team with especially loud volume, or a married couple engaged in a heated argument that has escalated from quiet, slower speech to a feverish pitch of loud interchanges between the two.

Thus, the nurse must be attuned to changes in volume, speech, and pitch to pick up unspoken messages that patients or colleagues may be expressing. Likewise, the nurse would do well to alter his or her own volume and speech to better coincide with the person with whom he or she is communicating. In the example of a patient speaking in a soft voice to the nurse and saying, "I think that I may have made a mess in the bed," the nurse should note the softness of the volume and comprehend that the patient is not only expressing a need for assistance—but is also expressing a sense of possible embarrassment over losing control of elimination.

Speech Pattern

Speech pattern involves the rhythm with which we speak, and words that are interspaced in communicated messages that alter that rhythm. Common interspaced words that affect speech patterns include "uh," "er," "you know," and "like." Changes in speech pattern, like changes in pitch, volume, and speed, may indicate a feeling, tone, or emotion that the patient is expressing. For example, persons who are unused to public speaking and feel ill at ease in front of a group or audience tend to stammer a bit with their words and will use the words "uh" and "er" a great deal in their speech. This change in speech pattern highlights the speaker's sense of anxiety and discomfort in public speaking. Consider these examples. What feeling tone might be expressed?

A 15-year-old male patient explains his purpose for seeking medical attention to the admitting clinic nurse.

> Patient: "I think ... uh ... that I ... you know ... I ... uh ... have ... like I might have V.D."

Here the speech pattern clearly indicates the patient's discomfort over his medical problem and may also indicate his anxiety over discussing it openly with the nurse.

An 18-year-old college freshman tells her classmate how she fared on her first class examination.

> Student: "Well, I mean, I did okay, I guess, I mean, I didn't flunk, or anything like that, you know, I mean, you know, it was an okay grade, you know, I guess I did all right."

An astute listener could pick up, in this situation, that the student is avoiding the discussion of her test score with her classmate by never really answering the classmate directly; by using multiple speech patterns, she is expressing her own insecurity about her test performance.

When the nurse becomes aware of changes in speech pattern, the nurse should focus on listening attentively and allowing the patient added time to complete his or her thoughts and formulate those thoughts into messages. Avoid hurrying the patient or attempting to complete the patient's sentences, because these actions will likely impair the communication process.

Patient: "I need my . . . uh . . . you know . . . that thing . . . that blue thing . . . uh . . . "

Nurse: "You need your bedpan? Your blanket? Your towel? What do you need? Your robe?"

In the above example, the nurse frustrates the communication with the patient by attempting to finish the patient's sentence and hurry his or her thoughts. It would be more appropriate to encourage the patient to think for a few seconds and to identify what is needed, than to interrupt his speech and risk blocking communication.

Principle

Messages may be communicated without the use of words, by nonverbal communication. Nonverbal communication involves the postures, movements, expressions, mannerisms, and gestures of the human body that relay messages and meanings

Illustration of Principle

Nonverbal communication, sometimes referred to as "body language," is an unspoken expression of thoughts, feelings, and drives that is as useful a tool in the communication process as verbal or spoken messages. Consider the behavior of an expectant father in a waiting room. The nurse might note pacing, hand wringing, or an inability to sit in a chair for more than a few minutes. The individual may flip through various magazines without really reading or comprehending even a single paragraph. He may drink one cup of coffee after another or smoke excessively. All of these behaviors reflect his mental and emotional states, and are thus valuable tools of communication. Consider also the behavior of young children when they see a department store Santa Claus, the facial expressions of a young bride and groom as they exchange marital vows at the altar, or the body postures of a row of students sitting through a long and tedious lecture on an un-interesting topic. It is obvious that nonverbal communication can be a useful tool of human expression.

The nurse must learn to be a keen observer of nonverbal cues that convey a message in order to completely comprehend and appreciate a patient's conveyed message. Focusing on *all* aspects of a patient's communication style will help the nurse to better understand the patient and anticipate his or her needs.

Golden Rules of Effective Communication

1. Always choose responses that allow or encourage the patient to express him-self or herself more fully.

   Because human beings have an inherent need to express themselves, and because illness often increases that basic need, responses by the nurse that facilitate greater expression for the patient are often the most satisfactory in a helping relationship. Reflecting or restating what the patient has said pre-viously helps the patient to focus and clarify the ideas or feelings he or she is trying to express. The nurse may also encourage expression directly. Such re-sponses might include these examples:

   "Tell me more of what you have been feeling."
   "Go on."
   "Can you share more of that experience with me?"

   It is evident that the above responses communicate to the patient the nurse's interest, concern, and openness to the patient's ideas and feelings.

2. Listen for the "feeling tone" of the patient's communicated message.

   Remember that feelings and emotions often are not stated directly, but rather, are expressed by the intonation, speed, or volume of the speech. The nurse ought to be attentive for such signals in the communication process that will assist her in better understanding the real message being conveyed to her by the patient. Consider the example. What feeling tone is being ex-pressed?

   "I just can't go on like this! Sometimes I think I can't do *anything* right!"

   Here the patient is clearly expressing feelings of frustration, helplessness, and even hopelessness. The nurse could facilitate further expression of these feelings by responding in the following manner:

   "You seem frustrated. Can you tell me a bit more about your situation?"

By focusing on the feeling tone of what has been said by the patient, the nurse helps draw the patient's feeling out in the open, to be better understood and thus more effectively managed.

3. Encourage hope in the patient, but avoid providing false reassurances.
It is well documented that all patients need and benefit from a sense of hope—no matter how critically, chronically, or terminally ill. However, the nurse must be careful not to provide the patient with a false sense of comfort or reassurance, because this may cause the patient to experience increased anxieties when the reality of the situation does not reflect the reassurance provided. Thus, the nurse must exercise caution when expressing personal beliefs about the patient's situation, prognosis, or outcome.
Examples of falsely reassuring responses include the following:

"I'm sure everything will turn out okay with your surgery."
"I know you've done everything you could."
"Your physician is very experienced with this disease. I'm confident you'll be well in no time."

No human being can ever safely predict the future or fully understand the present, and responses to patients such as those listed above attempt to achieve those unreachable goals. Such responses may, in fact, backfire in the future, when the falsely reassured patient does not experience in reality what the nurse blithely promises.

4. Avoid responses that catastrophize the patient's situation.
Patients facing illness, surgery, or medical interventions may view their situations with reservations based upon fear, anxiety, or lack of understanding. Nurses may easily escalate the patient's sense of discomfort by catastrophizing, that is, creating an even worse scenario than the patient has visualized.
Consider this example:

Patient: "I didn't know what to do! I couldn't get my breath, and I felt like I was choking!"

Nurse: "You must have been terrified! What a frightening experience you've had!"

Even though it is appropriate for the nurse to reflect to the patient that she appreciates the patient's sense of fear in the above situation, she makes the patient's situation sound much worse than the patient perceives it, or than it was in reality. Telling the patient that he or she "must have been terrified" is an example of catastrophizing, and the nurse here, rather than supporting the patient, may cause the patient to have even greater concern, worry, or fear about the situation encountered.

5. When unsure about what the patient is saying, either verbally or nonverbally, clarify!

    Effective communication is dependent upon the perception and understanding, or comprehension, of the relayed message. If the nurse is unsure about what is being said, or if she questions her comprehension of the patient's true meaning in the message, it is appropriate and necessary to ask for clarification. This rule may also apply if the patient's speech is impaired and difficult to understand; if the patient uses colloquialisms or slang; or if the patient speaks in dialect. Asking for clarification of what has been conveyed expresses to the patient the nurse's interest in him or her, and the nurse's need to fully appreciate the thoughts and feelings being expressed. Consider this example:

    Patient: "Nurse, I need to pass water. Get me that bottle, would you?"

    The patient is using a different term for urination than the nurse might be familiar with by stating "I need to pass water." Likewise, he refers to the urinal as a "bottle." The nurse, if unsure of the patient's meaning, should clarify his statements so that effective and helpful communication may take place.

6. Avoid negating feelings that are being expressed.

    Patients, as stated previously, will have unique perceptions of their illnesses, treatment, care, and progress that may or may not be rooted in fact. The nurse should use responses to patients that will aid them in clarifying and expressing their feelings, and avoid responses that negate or diminish the patient's feelings or concerns. Nurses are most prone to use statements that diminish patient's feelings when the patients are expressing negative emotions, because the caring nurse does not wish the patient to endure psychic unrest or pain. However, the patient needs to express negative emotions just as much as positive ones, and negating or diminishing thus does not serve the patient in a helping way.
    Consider this example:

    Patient: "I hate being in the hospital! I don't like being so dependent on others."

    Nurse: "It's not really that bad, is it?"

    In this situation, the nurse intended to reduce some of the patient's negative perceptions of hospitalization, but in responding, instead negated the patient's perception, and thus feelings, as being unwarranted and exaggerated. This response would likely frustrate the patient and may well block any further communication of the patient's true feelings.
    A more effective response by the nurse in this situation would be

    Nurse: "It sounds as though you're having a difficult time being hospitalized."

With this response, the nurse calls for further clarification of the issues and concerns of this patient, and likewise expresses her interest in the patient's state of well being.

7. Avoid confronting the patient until the situation is fully known and understood.

   When a patient's behavior is inappropriate and requires limitations or restrictions, such as acting-out behavior in the psychiatric setting, confronting the patient may be necessary. The nurse confronting the patient should identify calmly and concisely the inappropriate behavior that the patient has engaged in; how that behavior has influenced the patient, others, or the environment; and finally, what steps should be taken to alter the situation and decrease or halt the behavior labeled inappropriate. The nurse must be cautious with the use of confrontation, however, and should be sure to examine all the facts of the situation before making a decision to confront. The use of direct confrontation with patients may escalate their feelings of self-doubt or insecurity, because this exchange between patient and nurse is, by nature, often anxiety-provoking.

8. Extend "communication courtesy" to patients.

   Simple measures of communication courtesy can go a long way to enhance the communication process between individuals. If the patient senses that the nurse is truly interested and attentive, he or she is obviously much more likely to feel comfortable in expressing thoughts. Therefore, to create an atmosphere more conducive to communication, the nurse should observe some basic rules of communication courtesy:

Don't interrupt when the patient is speaking.

Don't rush the patient to complete a message, or attempt to complete sentences for him or her.

Maintain good eye contact with the patient.

Maintain a comfortable distance from the patient.

Use touch with the patient as appropriate.

These measures will help the nurse to facilitate communication with patients, and thus, foster helping relationships.

Reasoning Exercises: *Communication*

1. An adolescent girl is admitted for evaluation of lower abdominal pain. She tells the nurse, "I wish my friends would come to visit me. I

don't like being here alone." Which of the following would be the most appropriate response of the nurse?

A. "You must be terribly lonely. When do you expect your friends?"

B. "I'm sure your friends will come to see you soon."

C. "It's a little too early for visiting hours. You'll have to wait until this afternoon."

D. "It's hard to be alone. Would you like me to stay with you awhile?"

Intended Response: **D.** This response acknowledges the patient's feelings and offers support. Response **A** tends to catastrophize the patient's situation by saying "you must be very lonely." Response **B** provides false reassurance, because the nurse has no real way of knowing if in fact friends will come to visit. Finally, **C** is incorrect because it provides only a factual response and does not attend to the feeling tone of the patient's remarks.

2. A nurse is planning to teach a 4-day postoperative patient about care of his incision, in preparation for discharge. Which of these assessments of the patient should cause the nurse to postpone the teaching session?

A. "I'm anxious to go home to my family. I'm looking forward to a good home-cooked meal!"

B. "It's still a little sore where they did my surgery, but I manage pretty well."

C. "I'm feeling nauseated now. I think that antibiotic is making me feel sick to my stomach."

D. "I didn't realize this incision would be so big. Do you think I'll have a scar?"

Intended Response: **C.** This patient has an increased need for communication with a health care provider by virtue of his surgical experience. However, the patient's present nausea will prevent him from focusing completely on the important information being communicated. The nurse should postpone the interaction with the patient until he is feeling more physically able to share in the communication process.

3. A patient scheduled for lumpectomy asks the nurse, "Will I have a lot of pain with this type of surgery?" Which of the following would be the most appropriate response of the nurse?

A. "You seem worried about your upcoming surgery."

B. "Your physician will order medications to control any pain you experience following your surgery."

    C. "All patients react differently to surgery—it's impossible to tell what pain you might experience after the procedure."

    D. "The nurses will make sure that you don't have any pain following your surgery."

Intended Response: B. Response B provides the most accurate information about pain and pain management following surgery. Response A focuses on the patient's concerns and possible fears but supplies no information about postoperative pain management. Response C is incorrect, because postoperative pain is predictable and expected. Response D may offer the patient false reassurance, because it isn't always possible to eliminate a postoperative patient's pain completely. Much as we nurses would like our patients to be pain-free, this goal is clearly unrealistic.

4. A nurse caring for a child hospitalized because of parental abuse says to the unit supervisor, "I don't think I can do this . . . I find myself feeling so angry at those parents! We'll care for this child, and then he will go back to those same parents who beat him! What's the point?" Which of the following initial responses by the unit supervisor would be most appropriate?

    A. "We have a number of child abuse cases here. It might be best for you to request a transfer to a different unit."

    B. "I know this is a very difficult situation, but we must care for our patients."

    C. "Let's make a time for us to sit and talk. It may help you to share what you're feeling."

    D. "You've cared for abused patients before without being so upset. Is something else bothering you?"

Intended Response: C. The goal of the initial intervention with a nurse experiencing difficulty in coping with the stress of caregiving should be to establish an avenue for support. Response C acknowledges the nurse's need for emotional support and opens up lines of communication for further exploration of feelings.

5. A nurse checks on a patient awaiting surgery the following morning and finds her alone quietly weeping. Which of the following would be the most appropriate initial response of the nurse?

    A. Leave the room quietly and close the patient's door.

    B. Apologize for disturbing the patient and return to the room later.

    C. Sit with the patient silently and use therapeutic touch.

    D. Ask the patient if there is a family member the patient would like to be with.

Intended Response: **C.** Sitting with the patient and using touch therapeutically conveys the nurse's interest in and concern for the patient, which will help to reduce the patient's preoperative fears and anxieties. Responses **A** and **B** convey a message of avoidance of the patient and offer no support to the patient. Response **D** is ineffective because the nurse is not offering himself or herself, but rather a family member to support the patient.

Personal Integrity

ANN FILIPSKI

Principle

A sense of self begins to develop early in life and is dependent upon nurturance and external validation

Illustration of Principle

Each person begins life in unique circumstances. With an innate set of individual characteristics determined by genetic material and the influences and events within the prenatal and birth environment, each human being begins the complex and lifelong task of continued growth and development. Despite individual differences in physical experiences, makeup, and life circumstances, there is a logical and orderly progression to human development that has been observed by personality theorists like Freud, Erikson, and Sullivan.

> *T*heories of human personality recognize a progression through "stages" of development that are dependent upon the physical maturation of the individual and the response of the surrounding environment.

MEMORY JOGS

Because of the relative immaturity of their physiological and psychological apparatus, all infants and young children must rely upon the external environment and those within it to meet their needs. Just as the maturing body's physical

257

survival and growth are dependent upon the provision of food and shelter, the maturing self or "emotional body" must be provided with nurturance and external validation.

Early psychological needs are met in many seemingly simple ways. Physical contact with the world can produce varied sensations for the infant, some pleasant and some not so pleasant. Witness the different responses by most children to a cold, wet diaper versus being held and rocked by a familiar adult. Being protected from environmental threats or disruptions in a comfortable state, and consistent contacts with caring others, lead to a sense of the world and those within it as safe, reliable, and pleasing. Further, contacts and interactions with the larger world and other beings provide the developing individual with many opportunities to both validate experience and learn more about oneself.

Ideally, over time, the individual can gain an awareness of his or her physical being (or body image), a sense of identity (both real and desired), a means of developing and preserving self-esteem (coping mechanisms), and the ability to examine oneself and one's behavior (self-awareness). The foundation for this multifaceted, dynamic sense of self is firmly rooted in the individual's early experiences, but it continues to mature and be subject to alteration throughout life.

MEMORY JOGS

*T*he aspects of the person to be integrated into the "self" include body image, identity, self-esteem, and self-awareness.

Contacts with patients in many varied settings and states of health place the nurse in a unique position to assess for potential or actual alterations in sense of self, formulate appropriate nursing diagnoses, and intervene in a manner designed to facilitate further growth and development. These efforts must be guided by an awareness of the "normal" process of human development. Further, the nurse must recognize that even when the patient's physical being is the priority or focus of attention, *no* nursing contact or intervention is without potential impact upon the patient's self.

MEMORY JOGS

*E*ach nursing action has an impact upon the patient's self and potential for fostering integration of the personality.

Principle

The self is the vehicle in which one functions in the larger world

Illustration of Principle

The self of any individual is dynamic and multifaceted. Aspects of the self are made known or communicated to others through behavior. One's observed conduct is often used as a tool in understanding or gaining knowledge about that person. We recognize that behavior has meaning, and because humans are complex, an action is influenced by a multiplicity of factors.

Internal influences upon behavior include the individual's perceptions, thoughts, feelings, and actions. External influences include such things as the environment and setting, cultural norms, and the expectations of others. Thus, any attempt to understand an individual's behavior must consider both the self (or unique attributes of the person) and the context of the larger external environment.

> *B*ehavior is complex, meaningful, and multidetermined.

MEMORY JOGS

Most observers tend to evaluate others' behavior strictly from their own perspectives. The nurse, however, is responsible for expanding this narrow focus. An awareness of both the internal and external influences upon the patient's behavior must be included in the use of nursing process.

Any given behavior may be the result of unique or altered internal influences. For example, patients with sensory impairments may have altered perceptions about a given situation. Those who are intellectually limited because of handicaps or physical immaturity will likely respond differently to varied patient education efforts. An impulsive patient may handle frustrating situations in characteristic and often counterproductive ways. With knowledge of the unique internal influences upon a patient's behavior, the nurse is better prepared to intervene therapeutically.

The nurse must also be aware of many external influences upon patient behavior. For example, the setting may well influence an individual response to the statement "Undress, please." Or the behavioral response to being served rare roast beef may vary depending on whether one is a vegetarian, a Hindu, or a cattle rancher in the Midwest. Finally, the expectations of others may also influence how one behaves. The patient giving his or her own insulin injection for the first time may respond very differently to "I'll help if you need me," versus "I don't know if you can manage."

Sensory stimuli > perceptions
Perceptions (interpreted and labeled) > thoughts
Thoughts and evoked memories > feelings
Feelings experienced and acted upon > behavior

Armed with the knowledge of patient behavior and the various influences upon it, the nurse can direct interventions toward the individual and/or the environment. The overriding goal is always to foster the patient's ability to function as effectively as possible.

Principle

Each individual must develop means of maintaining the integrity of the self in altered circumstances

Illustration of Principle

All living organisms must be able to adapt to changing circumstances in life. Thus, in human beings both physiological and psychological means are available to help maintain "normal" homeostatic balance.

For example, exposed to infectious agents within the environment, a human being has certain protective mechanisms that automatically assist in maintaining a healthy body. Certain physical and chemical barriers, the inflammatory process, and the immune system all act to sustain physical integrity. Similarly, in interaction with the external environment, the human being has *psychological* mechanisms available to help sustain emotional health. Mechanisms such as denial, repression, sublimation, and compensation are used to safeguard the self. They help to preserve self-esteem while allowing for some modification in one's sense of identity and desired self-image when faced with environmental limitations or the demand for change. Like the physiological mechanisms mentioned earlier, these defense mechanisms are also somewhat "automatic." Frequently used in normal everyday life, they may be called upon to maintain the integrity of the self long before the individual is even aware of any personal threat. They are vital to emotional health and the ability to sustain the self.

> *D*uring normal maturation, the individual develops a collection of defense mechanisms or coping skills that aid in maintaining the health of the self.

MEMORY JOGS

Successful adaptation for the individual in a physical sense means that the protective mechanisms have maintained an acceptable level of homeostasis and bodily integrity. The state of health may be disrupted, however, if the bodily threat is so severe as to be overwhelming, the protective mechanisms are themselves deficient or impaired, or the prolonged use of the normal mechanisms leads to exhaustion and further vulnerability to insult.

Psychologically, successful adaptation allows the individual to preserve personal integrity without causing undue distress for the self or others. If the defense mechanisms are inadequate in number or quality, the external assaults or environmental stresses are too severe, or the use of the defenses themselves jeopardizes the individual or others, then emotional health is disrupted.

> *S*uccessful adaptation allows the individual to meet the demands of the environment without causing undue distress or disruption for the self or others.

MEMORY JOGS

The focus of nursing attention is always related to the variables of patient, environment, and health. Thus, in any situation, the nurse will be seeking to maximize the state of the patient's self.

This may be accomplished through the use of any or all of the following interventions:

- Assisting the patient in recognizing and responding to changing environmental circumstances
- Supporting the patient's use of effective, adaptive coping or defense mechanisms
- Identifying alterations in health or deficits in the patient's ability to act autonomously or maintain personal integrity, and means to remedy these
- Lending the assistance of the self of the nurse to the patient's efforts to acquire new or more effective defense mechanisms and continue psychological growth and development

Principle
Threat to the individual results in fear or anxiety

Illustration of Principle

The experiences of fear and anxiety are universal. Both responses serve protective functions in that they alert the individual to potential threats and disruptions in one's normal, steady state. *Fear* is generally considered object-specific. This means that a readily identifiable threat exists (often to one's physical well-being) in the environment. As a result, the individual experiences distress (fear) and responds with a "flight, fight, or fright" reaction. Both the threat and the subsequent response would be understood or viewed as predictable by most individuals. For example, if while crossing the street one were suddenly to see a speeding car approach, both fear for one's safety and attempts to run from the path of the vehicle would be common reactions.

MEMORY JOGS

> *F*ear is a response to the presence of an immediate environmental threat to the individual's survival or physical well-being.

In contrast, *anxiety* is a more subjective experience. The anxious person feels uncertain and ill at ease or may even experience an acute sense of panic and impending doom. Often with anxiety, the individual may be uncertain or unclear about the source of his or her distress. Even if identified, the "threat" is often highly individualized and may be unrealistic. The experience is generally precipitated by an assault to one's sense of self or other aspects of one's personal integrity.

MEMORY JOGS

> *A*nxiety is a sense of vague uneasiness and discomfort experienced in response to the presence of subjectively determined threats to the self.

Principle

Anxiety elicits the use of defense mechanisms and coping strategies in attempts to preserve the integrity of the self

Illustration of Principle

The experience of anxiety serves to alert the individual faced with actual or potential threats. Although some patients may be able to describe or label their internal, subjective experience as "anxiety," more often the nurse infers its presence

Levels of Anxiety	*Manifestations*
Mild—common event in everyday life. Use of defense mechanisms prevents significant impairment in ability to function.	Physiological ↑Pulse and respirations Mild GI symptoms—*i.e.,* "butterflies" Dry mouth ↑ Diaphoresis—*i.e.,* "sweaty palms" ↑ Muscle tension
	Emotional Some sense of tension—"nervous" Mild lability—giggling or nervous laughter, more easily irritated or tearful
	Cognitive Able to focus attention ↑ Awareness of environment
Moderate—present when faced with excessive or repeated demands for change or threats to the self. May see exaggeration of normal defensive operations or some impairment in ability to function.	Physiological Tachycardia and tachypnea Nausea, anorexia, constipation, or diarrhea Excessive perspiration Restlessness, excessive motor activity, painful muscle tension Urinary frequency or retention
	(continued)

Levels of Anxiety	*Manifestations*
	Emotional
	Labile mood—irritability, anger, hostility or tearfulness, withdrawal, apathy
	Cognitive
	↓ Concentration and attention
	↑ Distractibility
	↑ Preoccupied
	↓ Recall
	↑ May see distortions in perceptions or judgment and decision-making
Severe or Panic State—present when the threat to the self is overwhelming; defensive operations have been inadequate, disruptive, or failed. *Marked* impairment in ability to function results.	Physiological
	Autonomic nervous system symptoms remain and may become the focus of patient's attention or concern. Frank somatic symptoms such as fainting, chest pains, shortness of breath may be reported or observed. Marked psychomotor agitation or assaultive behavior may be seen. Hypervigilance
	Emotional
	Unstable mood and poor affective regulation or control
	Terror, rage, or aggression
	Inappropriate affect
	Cognitive
	Poor reality testing
	Internally focused and preoccupied
	Difficulties with attention
	Impaired judgment
	Faulty decision-making

from observation of the patient. Anxiety produces physiological, emotional, and cognitive manifestations in all individuals, and these manifestations are closely related to the severity of the distress experienced. Further, these same manifestations may produce behavioral change.

The use of defense mechanisms to safeguard the self is generally an adaptive mechanism. Their use allows the individual to function effectively in the face of new or unusual circumstances. Sometimes, however, the mechanisms are inadequate, and the anxiety no longer serves merely as a signal of potential threat. It may become so pronounced as to impair functioning and lead to disruption in the experience of the self.

> *T*he presence of anxiety can be inferred from observation of patient behavior.

MEMORY JOGS

The role of the nurse with the anxious patient is as varied as the manifestations and severity of anxiety. Thus, the importance of accurate assessment is clear, as is the need to select interventions that will be effective and appropriate to the level of anxiety.

In general, patients need assistance in containing the manifestations of anxiety and in preserving the self, particularly with increasing levels of distress or impairment. As anxiety increases, nursing interventions use verbal or cognitive modes of a less sophisticated nature. And conversely, with less disruption at mild levels of anxiety, it is more appropriate to assist the patient in identifying the presence of anxiety and its manifestations, gaining insight into its causes, and developing means to manage it more effectively or adapt to changes.

> *F*actors to be considered in determining nursing interventions for patients experiencing anxiety include the level of current distress, the nature of defense mechanisms, and the integrity of the self.

MEMORY JOGS

Reasoning Exercises: *Personal Integrity*

A woman is admitted to a psychiatric hospital with a diagnosis of obsessive-compulsive reaction. She spends hours carrying out a routine of washing her hands and cleaning the toilet facilities and the sink. She is careful to wash all food and dishes before she eats.

1. The patient's obsessive-compulsive behavior is characterized by an overuse of which of the following?

   A. Sublimation

   B. Conversation

   C. Undoing

   D. Suppression

Intended Response: **C.** The obsessive-compulsive patient attempts to "undo" the underlying feelings that caused the obsession and may act out the associated compulsive behaviors.

2. A patient says to the nurse, "I have so much cleaning to do. Germs, you know, they're everywhere." Which of the following explanations of the patient's compulsive washing is most accurate?

   A. It serves to keep the patient distracted from her real fears.

   B. It serves to decrease anxiety by eliminating the obsession.

   C. It helps the patient to control or modify her obsession.

   D. It represents a symbolic method through which the patient can face her fear.

Intended Response: **C.** Although the patient explains her compulsive washing rituals by claiming that she is concerned about germs, the reality is that the patient is attempting to control her underlying obsession by conducting her compulsive rituals. Although the compulsive behavior may reduce her anxiety, the obsession will not be eliminated.

3. One realistic goal for the patient is that she will:

   A. Express insight into obsessive thoughts

   B. Accept limits on ritualistic behaviors

   C. Initiate new forms of activity

   D. Stop ritualistic and repetitive behaviors

Intended Response: **B.** The acceptable goal for the obsessive-compulsive patient is that she will accept some limitation on the compulsive behavior. It is unrealistic that the patient will surrender her compulsive rituals altogether, as the rituals serve to decrease anxiety.

4. On the third day of the patient's hospitalization, the nurse notes that she is repeatedly late to group sessions and activities. Which of the following comments by the nurse to the patient would be most appropriate?

A. "You must realize that these washing behaviors are unnecessary."

B. "I will have to limit you to one session of washing per day."

C. "You'll need to start earlier so you can complete your washing in time to go to group session."

D. "You will only get better if you go to your sessions. You'll have to control your washing routines."

Intended Response: C. As stated in the above rationale, a realistic goal for the patient is to accept limitation on the ritual. The patient must learn to adjust such rituals in order to accept other responsibilities, such as attendance at therapy sessions. Use of a rational approach **A, D** is ineffective, as ritualistic behavior is rooted in the patient's experience with anxiety. Limitations of rituals must be realistic and nonpunitive **B.**

5. Which of the following statements indicates a realistic short-term measure of improvement in the patient?

   A. "Wow, I never realized how ridiculous I was acting!"

   B. "I'll do whatever you think is best, nurse."

   C. "I wish I knew why I feel so anxious and scared all the time."

   D. "I should be able to get my cleaning done more quickly tomorrow."

Intended Response: C. The patient is evidencing an initial insight into the true source of her obsessive-compulsive behavior—anxiety.

6. A young adult male is brought to the emergency room by the police, who describe him as "uncooperative" and "suspicious." Although the patient will provide no information to the admitting physician, his family is contacted using identification information in his wallet. Additional history is obtained from the patient's family and past medical records. He has been diagnosed as suffering from schizophrenia, paranoid type. Emotional arrest in such patients is most likely to have occurred during what stage of development?

   A. Autonomy versus shame and doubt

   B. Intimacy versus isolation

   C. Generativity versus stagnation

   D. Trust versus mistrust

Intended Response: D. The nature of this disorder's symptoms and the defenses used to protect the self suggest that very early emotional trauma has left the patient with difficulty in establishing trusting relationships with others.

7. The patient tells the nurse, "You know I'm the last Czar of Russia don't you? The KGB and CIA are both looking for him!" The nurse must recognize that these statements likely reflect all of the following *except*:

   A. Delusional beliefs

   B. Use of defense mechanisms

   C. Impaired self-concept

   D. Sense of entitlement

Intended Response: **D.** Delusions of persecution or grandeur are common features in this subtype of schizophrenia. Both reflect attempts to defend against underlying feelings of isolation and low self-esteem. Thus, the patient provides himself with the delusional explanation that his differentness is *special* in some way. It allows the fear and anxiety to be externalized to an environmental source.

8. The patient is admitted to inpatient psychiatric services. He remains aloof and distant, seeming to avoid contacts with other patients or unit staff. In order to establish a relationship, it will be most helpful if the nurse

   A. Approaches him directly and converses about topics like unit events or daily activities

   B. Encourages him to participate in cooperative activities with other patients

   C. Provides warm and supportive contact, allowing him to select the focus of conversation

   D. Asks him to discuss his obvious discomfort in the presence of others, to gain insight

Intended Response: **A.** The remaining responses are likely to be interpreted as threatening by the patient and would thus serve to *increase* his anxiety. With increased anxiety, his abilities to test reality are likely to decrease, leading to further impairment in functioning.

9. A 48-year-old woman is transferred from medical ICU following management of a suicide attempt. Her provisional diagnosis upon admission to the psychiatric unit is acute depressive episode. In conducting a thorough assessment of the patient, the nurse notes all of these problems. Which should be the priority for intervention?

   A. Lack of interest in personal hygiene and appearance

   B. Loss of appetite

   C. Narrowed perception and impaired problem-solving

   D. Disturbance in sleep pattern

Intended Response: **D.** As physiological needs are more basic to wellness than psychosocial needs, a disturbed sleep pattern is the problem of priority **D.** Altered sleep patterns may lead to deprivation of REM sleep, potentiating disturbances in thought and behavior. Additionally, if sleep/activity patterns and corresponding basal metabolic rates are not stabilized, nutritional needs cannot be met effectively.

10. Which of these approaches by the patient's primary nurse would be most therapeutic?
    A. Firm and restrictive
    B. Cautious and withdrawn
    C. Friendly and accepting
    D. Supportive and nonjudgmental

Intended Response: **D.** A supportive and nonjudgmental approach to a patient with depression offers that patient potential for self-acceptance and improvement in self-esteem and worth.

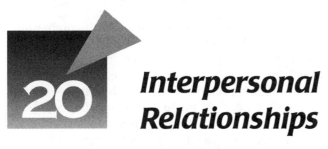

20 Interpersonal Relationships

ANN FILIPSKI

Principle

Humans are social beings, ever in interaction with others in the environment

Illustration of Principle

From the moment of birth until death, humans are in contact with the environment and those within it. Initially, the physical and emotional needs of an infant, a dependent being, must be met by others. These contacts provide the means for the developing infant's continued survival and growth. Additionally, although early interactions may seem unidirectional (the caretaker gives, the infant receives), they rapidly become *progressively more reciprocal* in nature. For example, the caretaker gives warmth and reassurance; the infant experiences pleasure and smiles. The caretaker feels capable and gratified; the infant comes to know "I am pleasing." Thus, a pattern is established, and the developing self of the child comes to have certain expectations of, needs for, and capacities to affect other humans.

> *H*uman interaction is reciprocal in nature.

MEMORY JOGS

Over time and with repeated interactions, humans develop relationships. The nature of a relationship is influenced by the present and past events and experiences of each individual involved. Thus, no two relationships are ever exactly alike.

271

Relationships also vary in degrees of depth. Our contacts with another may be brief or limited in scope; even though they may be repeated, little personal exposure results, and such a relationship would likely be considered superficial or social in nature. In contrast, with increasing levels of personal exposure or shared experience, a friendship may result. In this case, it is also likely that the relationship meets a larger number of needs for each individual or is more mutually gratifying. Intimate or deep relationships are those in which extensive exposure of aspects of the "self" of each person occurs. Further, the quality or quantity of shared experience also continues to increase.

MEMORY JOGS

> *R*elationships vary in degrees of depth. There is often an inverse relationship between depth of interaction and the number of relationships of that type a given individual has.

The obvious means of sharing past and present experiences or revealing aspects of the self is through *communication.* This tool is essential in establishing and maintaining a relationship.

Principle
Behavior occurs in the interpersonal context

Illustration of Principle

Behavior, or how one "acts," communicates much about an individual to the larger world. It reveals much about one's psychological or *inner world*—how one perceives, thinks, feels, or actualizes intentions. In addition to these internal influences upon the individual, behavior is also shaped by *external* factors. These external influences are all related to aspects of the social or interpersonal environment. How one interprets cues in a given setting or environment, experiences others' expectations, or interprets what one's culture dictates, all influence behavior and the responses of others to a given behavior.

MEMORY JOGS

> *T*here is a constant dynamic interplay between one's social or relationship experiences and one's inner emotional state.

Principle

Interpersonal relations are governed by the needs of the individuals involved, their respective interactional skills, and the social context in which they occur

Illustration of Principle

Our individual needs and wants influence our relationships with others. Because of our early infantile experiences, in which others met our physical and emotional needs, this pattern of relationships may feel comfortable, and at times we may wish to have it continue. However, with further growth and development, and the capacity to gratify many of our own needs, autonomy is also experienced as pleasurable. Thus, from early childhood into old age, a constant individual balance between independence and dependence in relationships is sought. What makes relationship issues so complex is the fact that at any given time, two individuals struggle with this balance internally and interpersonally. If both individuals are particularly needy or dependent at a given time, can their needs be met within the context of their relationship? Or if both are highly independent and struggling to preserve self-disclosure, what happens to the quantity of shared experience?

Obviously, some of this potential difficulty is alleviated with the large number of relationships that most individuals have concurrently. This allows for many potential sources of need gratification.

A further factor affecting relations with others is the nature of one's *interactional skills*, particularly observation and communication. One needs a means of collecting and sharing information, and negotiating issues of responsibility, if a relationship is to develop and progress. How else are decisions to be made about the respective needs of individuals and whether or how they can be met?

Finally, the *social context* can also influence an interpersonal relationship. Do married couples behave the same way publicly in the United States and in India? Do two persons relate in the same way if, when introduced, they are labeled as coworkers rather than as supervisor and subordinate?

> *T*he ability to use external cues and interpersonal feedback can profoundly influence the nature and course of a relationship.

MEMORY JOGS

Predictable chronological phases occur as any relationship develops. Generally, initial contacts between two people allow for some sharing of information and personal exposure. If a level of trust can be established here, then the sharing process is likely to continue in a mutually agreed upon manner. It is at this working level or phase that the potential for increased growth and mutual gratification can best be achieved. Finally, termination occurs in all relationships; sometimes because of imposed external circumstances and sometimes based upon the decisions of those involved. Ideally, the successful completion of this process fosters the growth and further development of each participant.

> *H*uman relationships progress through initial, working, and termination phases.

The *therapeutic nurse–patient relationship* constitutes a specialized form of interpersonal relationship. How does this relationship differ from others? First, its formation often occurs under somewhat unusual circumstances. In the initial phase, the focus of information sharing is often upon the patient's experience, past and present. Relatively little information about the nurse of a personal nature is shared with the patient. Further, the focus of the relationship is often on meeting specific needs of the patient that the patient is presently unable to meet. The patient is *not* expected to meet the nurse's needs.

There is also the expectation that the relationship itself be facilitative. In other words, in addition to meeting the identified health needs of the patient, the experience of a therapeutic relationship and interactions is to be validating and growth-producing. By definition, the nurse–patient relationship is goal-oriented and limited in scope and duration. The nurse is expected to be cognizant of these issues and evaluate the status of the relationship in an ongoing fashion.

> *T*he therapeutic relationship between nurse and patient can be used as a tool in fostering growth and/or facilitating change.

Principle

Prerequisites to satisfying interpersonal relationships are basic trust and a sense of self as separate from, but related to, others

Illustration of Principle

In order to form mature and mutually rewarding relationships with others, an individual must trust that the interpersonal world is basically a safe and good place. He or she must have had past relationships that were more good than bad or more gratifying than disappointing. Otherwise, uncertainty and anxiety will color any contacts with others and leave little energy available to the self for adequate functioning or adaptation to changing circumstances, let alone the risk taking that relationships require.

It is only through the prolonged process of psychological growth and development that one begins to formulate an understanding of one's self. This includes a sense of what is unique to the individual (likes, dislikes, interests, capabilities, strengths, and weaknesses) and what is shared in common with others. One also needs to know what can be given to others as well as what can be obtained from them. If these things are achieved, the quality of relationships improves.

Past delay or arrest in emotional development, and subsequent alteration or impairment in the self, will become visible in patient behavior. This includes the nature of interpersonal relationships. Conversely, experiences in the interpersonal sphere and in relationships continue to influence internal psychic development throughout the life span.

Thus, the nurse has obvious tools available in meeting the emotional health needs of patients. First, assessment of the nature of a given individual's relationships and the observation of how the patient relates to the nurse provide some possible clues about past experiences and unmet needs. Observation of behavior also gives clues about the nature of the patient's perceptions, thoughts, feelings, and actions. Difficulties in any of these areas are then amenable to nursing intervention.

Evaluation of the patient's responses to nursing interventions may demonstrate that change has occurred. And through more therapeutic and gratifying interactions and relationships with the nurse and others, it is hoped that further individual growth can take place.

> *H*ow we behave influences how others respond to us and our relationships. Our relationships influence how we behave.

MEMORY JOGS

Recall that the nurse–patient relationship is often based upon and developed around our ability to meet needs that the patient cannot meet alone. Like other relationships, to be satisfying, the nurse–patient relationship also must be based upon trust. Trust is the cornerstone in the nurse–patient relationship. Without it, little can be accomplished. Interestingly, *how* we meet the needs of patients can do much to build or destroy that trust.

Further, the self of both patient and nurse enter into the therapeutic relationship. In many instances, the self of the patient is either deficient (particularly in psychiatric settings) or temporarily threatened and vulnerable (e.g., the mastectomy patient who experiences a change in body image). The self of the nurse is often used as a tool in aiding patients. Thus, the nurse must be knowledgeable about the patient *and* the self, and will therefore be assessing both selves in an ongoing fashion by a review of behavior and introspection.

MEMORY JOGS

*T*he nurse must demonstrate self-awareness and an ability to examine the nurse's own behavior.

Principle

The quality and quantity of one's interpersonal network may augment or diminish the ability to cope with stress

Illustration of Principle

As a social being, man is clearly more than a biological organism. Other humans provide us with a vast number of possibilities for the gratification of our needs. Even if we are not dependent upon others for help in meeting survival and safety needs, our need to belong or become self-actualized, as articulated by Maslow, is highly dependent upon experiences with others.

Research tells us that relationships—their absence or presence—influence our chances of survival, not just in the sense of physical safety, but also in terms of coping with stress and adversity. Those who experience the loss of a significant relationship are subsequently at greater risk for illness, injury, and death for some period of time. According to statistics, those who are married live longer. Thus, the availability of others and our contacts with them serve to aid us in making the adaptations required in life.

How are others beneficial to us? They provide comfort and nurturance. They validate us and our experiences. They allow us to give and receive. We can bond together to achieve a common purpose or share a sorrow.

Without others and relationships, we often behave differently. Do you always dress the same way? Does the priority placed on comfort when selecting clothing vary depending on whether you plan to stay home alone or are expecting company? Probably. Similarly, our inner experience may well change when our contacts or relationships with others are disrupted. The phenomenon of winter "cabin fever" illustrates what even a brief change in contacts with others can do to our emotional state.

> *T*he quality of an individual's relationships has an impact on emotional health. Conversely, the state of one's emotional health influences the nature of relationships.

Reasoning Exercises: *Interpersonal Relationships*

A 24-year-old man is ordered by the court to undergo psychiatric evaluation after arrest for robbery and assault. During admission to the unit he comments to the nurse, "Don't worry, sweetie, I'll only be here a short time. This was all my lawyer's idea, but it sure beats jail."

1. These statements would *best* illustrate the defense mechanism of
  A. Rationalization
  B. Regression
  C. Sublimation
  D. Splitting

Intended Response: **A.** The patient provides a "logical" explanation for his inappropriate behavior.

2. The patient's tentative diagnosis is sociopathic personality disorder. What factors in the patient's history would be *least* consistent with this diagnosis?
  A. Early childhood deprivation and neglect
  B. Previous incarceration for stealing and vandalism
  C. Prior diagnosis of childhood conduct disorder
  D. Symptom onset following an identifiable loss

Intended Response: **D.** All of the other factors are positively correlated with the subsequent diagnosis of sociopathy.

3. In light of his diagnosis, the nurse should anticipate that the patient's interactions with other patients will be characterized by which of the following?
  A. Attempting to monopolize conversations and being intrusive
  B. Being superficially pleasant and appearing interested in them

   C. Avoiding most contact and refusing to join in group activities

   D. Demonstrating poor social skills and little awareness of the milieu

Intended Response: B. Contrary to most lay expectations, sociopaths are often superficially pleasant and quite popular with other patients. They demonstrate keen awareness of the environment at the obvious and subtle levels. They may assume "leadership" roles within the patient group and appear sensitive and supportive to peers.

4. In developing an effective nurse–patient relationship, the nurse should

   A. Anticipate that with support and nurturance he may well recognize the degree of his illness

   B. Expect attempts to test limits and recognize their importance for him

   C. Capitalize upon his highly developed intelligence and level of insight

   D. Allow him a high degree of autonomy and self direction to increase motivation

Intended Response: B. Sociopaths are rarely insightful or genuinely interested in change because they do not share the same values as most of society. Adherence to rules is often only accomplished because of the consistent reinforcement of consequences associated with violation. Limits should be set firmly and consistently without punitive or personal investment.

5. A man is brought to an acute psychiatric facility by his family, who describe him as a "loner" who seems "out of time with the rest of the world." Past psychiatric records indicate that he has been hospitalized 13 times since age 19 for treatment of psychiatric illness. The patient has never followed up with outpatient care. His current diagnosis is schizophrenia, chronic undifferentiated type. The patient is placed on Prolixin (fluphenazine) and is to be discharged to a structured group home in the community. After he learns he has been accepted for placement, the nurse notices he begins to regress and becomes very dependent upon the staff. What should the nurse do first?

   A. Postpone discharge until he appears ready

   B. Describe the observed behavior and discuss it with him

   C. Suggest to his physician increasing his dosage of medication

   D. Ignore the behavior unless he comments on it himself

Intended Response: **B.** The patient deserves feedback about his behavior and an opportunity to share his perceptions, thoughts, and feelings. This approach validates his improved functional ability and autonomy.

6. A 68-year-old retired teacher is admitted to psychiatry for treatment of depression. The patient isolates herself in her room for much of the day. She is quiet and somewhat disheveled in appearance. When approached by the nurse during her first hospital day she makes no eye contact. In attempting to address issues of grooming and hygiene, the nurse might best say:

    A. Here are your linens. Now go clean up before lunch.

    B. You look a mess. Let's do something about that right now.

    C. I think you'll feel better after you have a chance to bathe and dress. I'll help you.

    D. Why haven't you gotten dressed? It's after 10 o'clock.

Intended Response: **C.** The nurse is offering assistance to the patient in a respectful way. This response is most likely to engender beginning trust.

7. Which of the following responses by the patient, when the nurse arrives 10 minutes late for a planned "talk," suggests that trust has been established?

    A. Oh, you're here. What were we going to do again?

    B. I didn't think I'd ever see you again, nurse.

    C. I thought you'd come as soon as you could.

    D. Who are you? I forgot your name.

Intended Response: **C.** The patient is expressing confidence in the nurse and also the belief that she is important enough for the nurse to honor their commitment.

8. As the time for the patient's discharge approaches, she and the nurse begin to discuss the termination process. Which of the following statements by the patient would increase the nurse's confidence that their relationship has been helpful?

    A. How will I ever manage? No one out there will want to bother with me like you have.

    B. Nothing is going to be different. I'll come back to see you, and you can come and see me.

C. Oh nurse, you've been so wonderful. I'll be lost without you.

D. I feel so much better now. Help me figure out how I've done it so I can stay out of here.

Intended Response: **D.** As part of the termination process, it is helpful for both nurse and patient to review the course of the relationship and to identify the work accomplished and future goals. Additionally, a therapeutic relationship should be validating and enabling, not one creating unnecessary dependence or artificial independence.

Growth and Development

CYNTHIA A. LEVY

Principle

Biological growth is very rapid during the first 12 months of life. Motor development follows specific patterns (cephalocaudal, proximal-distal)

Illustration of Principle

The overall increase in the size of the body and the continual maturation of body systems during infancy are remarkable. During each of the first 6 months of life, an infant will gain approximately 1 1/2 pounds, thereby doubling the body weight in 6 months. Weight gain decreases somewhat during the second 6 months. Yet, by 12 months of age, she will have tripled in body weight. Increases in length or height will be confined to the trunk primarily.

The most remarkable developmental changes are related to the nervous system, as evidenced by the progressive fine and gross motor developments that occur during this stage.

Principle

Infants must develop a sense of trust. This is established through the relationship(s) with the primary caregiver(s)

Illustration of Principle

A consistent, loving, protective, and responsive primary caregiver is essential for the development of trust. Yet, the infant also has a strong role to play and must

281

be loving and responsive to the caregiver as well. Each must provide the other with positive feedback for the relationship to develop. Through a complex process of displaying his needs and having them met in a gratifying way, the infant develops a sense of trust in his primary caregiver (usually parent), and in his environment.

Very early on, the infant will begin to make associations between her needs and actions that lead to the fulfillment of those needs. As the infant grows and develops, she will make increasingly more complex associations between needs and their fulfillment. For example, when the newborn infant feels uncomfortable because she is hungry, she will cry. Crying will bring a nipple to her mouth. She soon will associate hunger and crying with the satisfaction gained from sucking. Later, she will recognize that when she cries, she not only gets the nipple, but she will hear her mother's voice. Her voice soon will be associated with the comfort and security she feels in her arms. As this process continues to be reinforced, she will begin to accept and trust that this cycle will occur whenever she expresses her needs. Although this is a simple example, it illustrates a process that will be built upon throughout the first 12 months (Table 21–1; Table 21–2).

Table 21-1. Gross motor development

Newborn	Maintains head control for short periods
4 months	Lifts head and upper body to bear weight on forearms Can roll onto either side
5 months	Can roll from front to back with ease
6 months	Lifts head and upper body to bear weight on hands Can roll from back to abdomen from prone position
7 months	Adds to the upright position mastered at 6 months by being able to bear weight with one hand while exploring with the other Can sit alone now, often leaning forward onto hands for support
8 months	Has mastered skill of sitting alone Will begin to actively explore surroundings Will use both hands now (falls over frequently)
9 months	Can pull self upon furniture
10 months	Will be able to achieve sitting position from prone position by herself Crawls well When standing with support, will try to step with one foot
11 months	Will walk along furniture
12 months	Can walk while holding hands with caregiver

Table 21-2. Fine motor development (developing increased dexterity, learning to use hands and fingers to explore self and environment)

Newborn	Is not aware of own hands or fingers, unless by accident they reach his or her mouth Grasp is reflexive
1 to 5 months	Discovers hands, fingers, feet and plays with them Will replace primitive, reflexive grasp with purposeful, voluntary grasp by 5 months Purposeful grasp at 5 months is usually two-handed
6 months	Level of skill with hands is greatly increased Can hold items easily (bottles, cookies, toys) Can only handle one object at a time Actively uses hands for exploration
7 months	Will be able to transfer objects between hands Likes to bang objects Learns to use fingers for increased exploration
10 months	Pincher grasp is established
11 to 12 months	Likes to manipulate objects Enjoys putting things into larger objects (the beginning understanding of the concept of object permanence)

Principle

Infants learn through participation with their primary caregivers and by actively exploring themselves and their environments

Illustration of Principle

Cognitive development during the first 24 months is referred to as the sensorimotor phase. The first four stages take place from birth to 12 months. During this phase, the infant will learn that he is separate from other objects and beings within the environment, the groundwork for the concept of object permanence will be laid, and he will begin to equate symbols with mental images (i.e., "bye-bye" means someone is leaving).

During the first few months of life, the infant learns through the use of reflexes. Through repetition, the infant will begin to recognize the development of patterns. Recognition of these patterns sets the stage for the replacement of reflex behavior with voluntary actions. From 1 to 4 months, reflexes become deliberate efforts to gain a desired response. Until approximately 8 months, the infant will continue to test her new abilities in a variety of ways. As a result of her experiments, she will begin to develop a sense of causality. Intentions will become more deliberate as she begins to see himself as separate from her environment and from her parents.

Expanding upon the example given in the Principle, one can see how patterns developed from reflexive behavior will be tried and tested until a sense of cause and effect is developed. Once again, when a newborn is hungry, he cries and is given a nipple. Soon, an association is made between the nipple and the comfort of the satisfaction of a need. As this process is repeated time and again, the infant will begin to recognize the development of a consistent pattern. When he begins to add the element of the loving caregiver to this pattern, he will begin to test the reflex in order to gain the comfort of his mother even in the absence of hunger. At this point, reflexive behavior is replaced by voluntary actions. In other words, actions become deliberate—he cries, his mother comes.

The groundwork for the development of object permanence is laid during infancy. The infant begins to first recognize that the removal of something from sight doesn't necessarily mean that it is gone forever through his interaction with parents. This is illustrated best by reviewing the attachment and separation process. The process of attachment begins at birth and continues throughout the first year. The infant will develop a sense of attachment and separation by progressing through *overlapping* stages.

1. From birth until approximately 2 months of age, the infant will respond to anyone and everyone.

2. From 8 to 12 weeks, infants will respond primarily to parents. Although the infant enjoys the comfort of the mother, most others are perceived as equally comforting and loving. At this stage, because the primary caregiver is always readily available to meet his every need, the infant does not perceive himself as separate.

3. At 6 months of age, infants will show a definite preference for their mothers. Between 4 and 8 months, an infant will begin to have an awareness of himself as separate from mother. This is the point at which anxiety will be evident whenever mother and baby are separated. Infants begin to learn about object permanence as a result of sight; they will protest desperately, believing that if mom is out of sight, mom is gone forever. Yet, when she reappears and anxiety subsides, the infant's concept of her predictability and permanence will be reinforced.

4. By about 7 months, the infant will begin to show preference for other familiar family members or consistent caregivers. During this stage, he will begin to recognize the differences between the familiar and the unfamiliar. Protest and anxiety will begin to be displayed when the infant is confronted with strangers.

Special Needs and Problems

1. Love, comfort, and security (trust)
2. Adequate nutrition for growth
3. Prevention of injury
   a. Foreign object aspiration
   b. Suffocation
   c. Falls
   d. Poisoning
   e. Burns
4. Immunization administration

Nursing Considerations

1. Emotional support to family
2. Education and guidance
3. Maintenance of infant–parent trust relationship

MEMORY JOGS

Principle

Biological growth is slower and steadier during the toddler years, compared with the months of infancy. Body organs achieve more mature functioning. Improved motor skills create many new opportunities for the toddler

Illustration of Principle

Overall growth is much slower at this time. By 2 1/2 years of age, most toddlers will have quadrupled their birth weights. Increases in height are also less dramatic. Most of the height increase will be a result of an increase in the length of their legs. Toddlers will gain approximately 3 inches in height each year. Growth of the head is also slower and steadier. The anterior fontanel will close between 12 and 18 months. Chest circumference will continue to increase and will surpass head circumference.

Most body systems are relatively mature by the end of the toddler years. One of the most obvious body system changes is related to the gastrointestinal system. Most children can successfully achieve voluntary control over elimination between 18 and 24 months.

Studies made at this time in both fine and gross motor development can be seen in all that the toddler does.

Increased fine motor control is evidenced by increased dexterity. Toddlers can hold and release (throw) arms at will, open doors, pick up tiny objects and examine them closely, and put their little fingers into the most impossible places.

Increased gross motor control is evident by the rapid progress made in locomotion. From 15 months to 2 years, the toddler progresses rapidly from walking with ease to running fairly well. By 2 years of age, most toddlers will have mastered the stairs, one foot at a time. The 2 1/2-year-old can jump and stand on one foot for brief periods of time. By the age of 3 years, the toddler can stand on tip toe, climb stairs by alternating feet, and stand on one foot at a time with ease.

Principle

Cognitive development at this stage is related primarily to language development, primitive reasoning, and trial and error experimentation

Illustration of Principle

Much of the language development is accomplished through liptation and imitation. For example, as parents continue to use the word "up" every time they pick up their child, the toddler soon learns to say "up" whenever he wants to be held. Much to the dismay of many parents, the egocentric toddler also enjoys the selective use of the words that he has mastered. "No" and "mine" are two perfect examples. From 12 to 24 months, toddlers usually have developed a vocabulary of approximately 300 words. By 2 years of age, the toddler is able to group words into simple sentences to convey a meaning, such as "Me outside" or "Grandma go bye-bye." More remarkable than their vocabularies, though, are their levels of comprehension. They are able to understand much more than what they can say.

An illustration can be made by picturing the toddler who has wandered away from mother momentarily to explore the kitchen cabinets alone. Upon hearing the familiar rattle of the pots and pans, Mom yells, "Hey, what are you doing in there?" from the other room. The toddler will stop instantly and think to himself, "Who, me? I'm just checking out the cabinets. Are you yelling at me or just asking? Okay, just a minute. Here I come." Certainly these sentences are more complex than he's capable of, but they illustrate the complexity of his level of comprehension.

The toddler's level of reasoning is quite primitive. It is described as transductional. He makes generalizations and applies them loosely. For example, he reasons that if one's sweater is scratchy, therefore all sweaters are scratchy. So, whenever his parents try to dress him in a sweater, he will protest violently. Another example of such reasoning can be illustrated by examining the typical mealtime behavior of the toddler. After crying for one-half hour for something to eat, the toddler is finally served dinner. With four things to choose from on his plate, he'll try the most appealing item first. If it happens to be something that he doesn't like, he'll immediately assume that everything will taste just as bad and refuse everything despite all efforts from his parents. This is transductional thinking—making generalizations from particular to particular.

The toddler's approach to learning and discovery is one of trial and error. The memory of the toddler is very short, and he frequently will have to learn the same lesson over and over again. Because he has a high level of understanding of the concept of object permanence, the toddler will now know that if something is missing, it may be located in any number of possible hiding places. He will set out, using a trial and error approach, until he locates the missing item.

Principle

The toddler must develop a sense of autonomy

Illustration of Principle

The activities of the toddler are directed toward the exploration of and control over the environment. The daily mission of the toddler is to explore and learn as much as he possibly can. This is evidenced by the fact that toddlers are into everything—almost always at once. They play in the water of the toilet, rummage through closets, put their fingers into the darnedest places, and are almost always creating a mess. That is how they learn, and of course it is also how they frequently get themselves into a hundred jams. All of this activity is also helping them to learn to be less dependent upon their parents. As they venture out into their world, they become less concerned about separation from their parents, yet they still need visual and verbal reassurance of their parents' closeness. For example, a 2-year-old can play alone with his toys for extended periods of time. As long as the parent is still there each time he looks up, he is content.

Usually at this stage they are very fearful of strangers, particularly when their parents are present.

During the toddler years, independence must be balanced with appropriate guidance. Limit setting by parents should be constructive and encourage self-control, reasonable autonomy, and independence. Discipline may be necessary. If so, it should be carried out in an appropriate, consistent, and timely fashion.

**MEMORY
JOGS**

*S*pecial Needs and Problems

1. Temper tantrums
2. Negativism
3. Sibling rivalry
4. Toilet training
5. Dental hygiene
6. Prevention of injury
   a. Drowning
   b. Burns
   c. Poisoning
   d. Falls
   e. Aspiration

*N*ursing Considerations

1. Helping parents to learn to "set limits"
2. Accident prevention

Principle
Rate of physical growth stabilizes. Motor skills are refined

Illustration of Principle

The preschooler is characteristically more slender, stands more erect, and is more graceful than the toddler. Average weight gain is approximately 5 pounds per year. As with the toddler, the preschooler adds 2.5 to 3 inches per year to his height, with most of it occurring in the legs rather than in the trunk.

Advances in motor development are related chiefly to continued refinement of all skills.

Principle

Preschoolers learn through a more advanced exploration of the environment. These are the "why" years, during which they develop a sense of initiative

Illustration of Principle

The preschooler is best described as an inquisitive, creative, aggressive, foolhardy ball of energy. These characteristics can be seen easily whenever preschoolers are seen at "work"—exploring! To them, the world is full of wonder and magic. The environment offers many new and wonderful experiences and opportunities for discovery, and the preschooler intends to see and experience them all. He develops a sense of himself and his world through this exploration and a seemingly endless string of questions. *Why* is the key word of the preschooler's vocabulary.

As the preschooler sets out on his own to conquer the world, he learns many lessons. Because he doesn't know his own limits, the preschooler will often get into more mischief than he can handle. He begins to develop a sense of good versus bad, and right versus wrong. These principles are the foundation of the development of a sense of conscience. He will constantly test the limits set by his parents in order to determine what is good or bad behavior. At this stage, the child remains quite self-centered and will worry about the consequences of his actions only in reference to himself. He has little use for the concerns of others except for his parents. He fears the disapproval of his parents and usually will do things or not do them in order to stay in their good graces. Children of this age group strive to be cooperative and responsible members of the family.

Principle

Thinking is prelogical and magical

Illustration of Principle

Conceptual thinking can be described as prelogical in that the preschooler is unable to perceive parts in terms of the whole. They only understand what they can see. For example, if two glasses of different sizes contain the same amount of juice, the preschooler will believe that the larger glass has more. To him, bigger means more. By the same token, a small, fat candy bar will never be as satisfactory as a large, thin one.

Children at this age have a very poor sense of body boundaries. For example, they wholeheartedly believe that if they have a cut or have an injection that the "hole" must be covered in order to prevent anything from escaping from their bodies. Boundaries are a critical necessity for the injured preschooler.

The preschooler can understand time only in relation to events. For example, when separated from his parents, the preschooler is calmed much more easily with the comment, "Your mother will be home after Mr. Rogers," than from "She'll be here at 2 pm."

Because the preschooler depends upon his parents for answers to his questions, this is a time when parental fears can be transferred easily to the child—for example, fear of the dark, or fear of the cellar. The child often will use magical thinking in an attempt to control fears or to solve mysteries. The preschooler believes that thinking or wishing for something will make the event occur. The preschooler will create "special friends" to take the blame for his actions. Only a preschooler can see the monster in the closet or under the bed. Children of this age delight in the magic of Santa.

MEMORY JOGS

Special Needs and Problems

1. Consistency in limit setting

2. Sleep disturbances (nightmares)

3. Prevention of injury, falls, or poisoning

4. Communicable diseases

5. Child abuse or neglect

Nursing Considerations

1. Protection of body image

2. Helping parents prepare for day school or preschool

3. Concrete answers to questions

Principle

Throughout the school years, physical growth remains slow and steady

Illustration of Principle

Between the ages of 6 and 12 years, physical growth will proceed at a slow yet steady pace. Children will gain approximately 2 inches per year in height and will have doubled their weight over the 6-year period. Toward the end of these school-age years, girls will begin to surpass boys in height and weight. Shedding of the primary teeth occurs at this time.

Characteristically, school-age children appear leaner and taller, with improved posture, when compared with preschoolers. They become more graceful as their coordination and motor skills improve.

Principle

During this developmental stage, children must develop a sense of industry

Illustration of Principle

Throughout the school-age years, children will be struggling with developing a sense of industry. Failure to do so will result in feelings of inadequacy or inferiority. The developmental tasks of the child in this age group are met through the challenges and conflicts encountered at school and through the development of peer group relationships. With each new experience, the child will be developing a sense of self-worth (self-esteem and body image), evaluating family and social values, and learning to cope with a variety of failures and successes.

Principle

Through formal education, children will achieve a sense of personal competence by gaining knowledge and technical skills

Illustration of Principle

The entrance into school marks a period of significant change for children. They are entering a new world. They leave the security and freedom of the home and family environment and enter a system that is very structured, one with new rules and regulations. They must learn to respect and obey adults other than their parents. Teachers exert a great deal of influence over children. Hero worship is typical during this stage.

During this developmental stage, children are very active and eager intellectually. They enjoy new experiences and delight in the acquisition of new abilities and skills. They are excited to discover the answers to the many unanswered questions of the previous developmental stage.

Piaget describes this developmental stage as one of *concrete operations*, which is the process of using thoughts to experience work and to describe actions or events. In other words, children learn to "think" through a process, and can perform it in their minds rather than having to act out the actual activity. This skill will become refined with increased use throughout the school years.

For example, a 4-year-old child can find his way to the park six blocks from home after having been there several times. Simply stated, he has learned the way—he can act it out. Yet an 8-year-old can think of going to the park, and in his mind he can find his way. Furthermore, when asked the way to that same park, he can give directions easily; he can perform the task mentally.

Principle

Children are faced with making their first true commitments to relationships outside the home. Peer group versus family values are often a source of conflict

Illustration of Principle

Between the ages of 6 and 12, children will seek independence from their parents by increasing their identification with the peer group. The peer group exerts a tremendous amount of influence over the daily activities of the school-aged child.

During these years, children are in the process of laying the groundwork for the development of self-esteem and self-worth. This is accomplished as they integrate family and peer group values. Quite often, they are faced with a conflict of standards. It is not always easy or desirable to defy their parents in order to conform to the pressures of the group. As a result, children are faced with the task of self- and social evaluation. These are the wonderful years of best friends, blood buddies, secret places, clubs of exclusive memberships, and rigid group rules. Peer relations dictate how the group members walk, talk, and dress. Roles frequently are assumed according to group standards.

Children often will modify their behavior and beliefs in order to conform to peer group values and pressures. Yet, when in serious conflict with the values taught by parents, family values almost always will prevail.

**MEMORY
JOGS**

Special Concerns and Problems

1. Dishonest behavior
   a. Cheating
   b. Lying
   c. Stealing

2. Latch-key children

3. Need for sexual exploration

4. Injury prevention (often sports-related)

(continued)

Special Concerns and Problems

5. Dental hygiene

6. Skin disorders

7. Behavior disorders (attention deficit disorder—ADD)

8. Learning disabilities

Nursing Considerations

1. Reinforce positive body image perceptions

2. Support educational needs while hospitalized

Principle

Physical growth and bodily changes are dramatic and visible during adolescence

Illustration of Principle

The physical changes that occur in adolescence are caused by hormones. Sexual maturation is also closely associated with a dramatic increase in physical growth. The "growth spurt" occurs over a relatively short period of time—2 to 3 years. During adolescence, children will achieve the remainder of their linear growth, and body systems will reach full maturity. The onset of puberty is variable for both sexes and is widened by the development of secondary sex characteristics.

Girls

Puberty can begin at any point between the ages of 8 and 14 years. Once puberty begins, all physical changes are usually completed within approximately 3 years. The onset of menstruation usually occurs about 2 to 2 1/2 years after the onset of puberty.

Boys

Puberty begins later for boys than for girls, usually with its onset between 10 and 16 years of age. Major developmental changes for boys are related to increases in height and musculature, maturation of the gonads, and the development of secondary sex characteristics.

Principle

The task of adolescents is to develop a sense of identity

Illustration of Principle

As a result of the onset and rapid development of physical growth and sexual maturation, adolescents must face many new and unfamiliar feelings about themselves and their bodies. This is a time when children are confronted with an increased sensitivity to peer approval and acceptance.

The adolescent will strive for a sense of self and separation from the family. This is a complex process that involves an intense need for peer identity, which leads ultimately to the development of self-identity.

Principle

Cognitive growth at this stage is related to the development of abstract thinking. This is the period of formal operations

Illustration of Principle

Piaget's fourth stage of cognitive development is the period of *formal operations*. During this stage, adolescents will develop the capacity for abstract thinking. They will become capable of scientific reasoning and formal logic. They can begin to direct their thoughts to the future, to the possibilities that lie ahead of them. By using these new abilities and thought processes, they can begin to plan the future and see themselves and others—the world—in a much more realistic fashion.

Principle

Concerns related to body image are of paramount concern to the adolescent

Illustration of Principle

As a result of the rapid growth and sexual development of their bodies, adolescents typically suffer from difficulties in adjusting to their new appearances. Depending upon their personal perceptions and the perceptions of their peers, adolescents may attempt to hide their bodies or, on the other hand, may flaunt them. Peer acceptance of their appearance is very important to adolescents. They are constantly comparing themselves with others. They will make judgments about themselves and about what is normal based on peer standards and norms. This process eventually will influence their perceptions of personal body—perceptions that they will maintain throughout the remainder of their lives.

MEMORY JOGS

Special Problems or Concerns

1. Protection from injury (motor vehicles, firearms)
2. Substance abuse (smoking, alcohol, drugs)
3. Sports-related injuries
4. Acne
5. Alterations in maturation
   a. Short stature, tall stature
   b. Precocious puberty
   c. Dysmenorrhea
6. Adolescent pregnancy
7. Sexually transmitted diseases

Nursing Considerations

1. Nutrition guidance
2. Sexual counseling
3. Personal hygiene
4. Contraception

Concept: Social Development in Childhood

Social development throughout childhood is closely linked to interaction with people (peers, parents, and family) and to play activities.

Principle

Play is the work of a child

Illustration of Principle

Infant

Infant play activities are centered primarily around the body. The infant finds pleasure in these play activities, which are the major source of sensory stimulation for infants. A great deal of intrapersonal contact during play is of the greatest importance to infants, more so than the quality of the toys. For example, paper to crumple is just as stimulating as a colorful rattle; likewise, wooden spoons and plastic bowls are very entertaining.

Toddler

The toddler requires a higher level of intrapersonal interaction during play. The toddler is capable of parallel play, or playing beside another child. One of the most characteristic elements of toddler play is the toddler's use of vivid imagination. He can paint the house for hours with a brush and a pail of water, and can "keep house" as well as any parent. For the toddler, falling is a very important means of play. He enjoys radios, television, and reading stories.

Preschooler

Preschoolers particularly enjoy "associative play." Most characteristic of the preschooler, though, is imitative play. They enjoy dress up, playing house, doctor kits, or any activity in which they can pretend or act out adult roles. Preschoolers have a difficult time separating reality from fantasy. This is particularly evident when their imaginary friends stay for dinner after the play activity has ended. The development of imaginary friends or playmates is normal and quite useful for children of this age. They can keep a child company when no one else has time, suffer many misfortunes, and take the blame without protest when called upon.

School-Aged Child

Play at this stage is a total reflection of the child's developmental growth. It is more organized, intelligent, and creative. Play in peer groups of the same sex is most particular to children of this developmental age group. "Team play" teaches the child many lessons: taking turns, respect for rules, support of team goals, team success or failure, an the nature of competition.

Adolescent

Play activities are related primarily to peer group activities, which may be organized school activities, sports, or just "hanging out" in groups. Adolescents enjoy games and activities that test their intellectual abilities as well as their physical abilities.

Reasoning Exercises: *Growth and Development*

1. The pediatric nurse is examining Daniel, age 12 months, as part of a wellness check-up. Which of the following assessments of Daniel would suggest to the nurse a lag in expected growth and development for this child?

   A. Daniel has doubled his birth weight.

   B. Daniel cries when his mother leaves the examination room.

   C. Daniel tries to pull himself up to a standing position.

   D. Daniel sits upright on the examination table without support.

Intended Response: **A.** At age 12 months, it is expected that a child will have tripled his birth weight, which suggests a lag in growth and development. The remaining responses are all appropriate to standard growth and developmental norms for a child this age.

2. The parents of 26-month-old Jason explain to a pediatric clinic nurse that they have provided a number of instructions to their child regarding safety. Which of the following instructions provided to Jason should the nurse discuss in greater detail with the parents?

   A. "We have all our cleaning supplies locked in a high kitchen cabinet."

   B. "Jason knows that he should not cross the street without a grown-up."

   C. "We've placed safety covers on all of the unused electrical outlets in our home."

   D. "I've told Jason to dial 911 on the phone in case of emergency."

Intended Response: **D.** As accidents are a common concern during the toddler years, the parents in this situation are to be recognized and supported for their efforts to teach their child regarding his safety. However, a child at this age cannot think abstractly, and would not comprehend the concept of "emergency." Thus, instructing Jason to dial 911 in an emergency is inappropriate at this developmental level. The remaining responses are all appropriate safety interventions for a child during the toddler years.

3. A three-year-old child has achieved all of the following developmental skills. Which of these was likely achieved most recently?
   A. Holds a large ball in both hands.
   B. Able to feed "finger foods" to himself.
   C. Uses simple language in short phrases.
   D. Alternates feet when climbing stairs.

Intended Response: **D.** The most recently acquired skill, alternating feet, requires both gross motor control and coordination, indicating increasing development of neuromuscular control.

4. A toddler hospitalized for the past three days stands up in his crib and pulls back and forth on the bedrails, crying loudly at frequent intervals. This noisy behavior is distressing other children on the unit. Which of the following interventions would be most appropriate in meeting the needs of the toddler?
   A. Divert him to a quiet, passive activity.
   B. Place soft protective "mittens" on his hands.
   C. Place his upper extremities in soft wrist restraints.
   D. Provide him with a coloring book and crayons for scribbling.

Intended Response: **D.** The toddler is expressing his anger over separation from his mother, as well as frustration with the limitations of hospitalization on autonomy. Providing the child with a play activity which sublimates his anxiety is appropriate to help him cope with his feelings. The physical activity of scribbling will be helpful in reducing the emotional stress and anxiety. Quiet, passive activities **A** will not allow him to "vent" his feelings. Although providing protective equipment **B, C** may reduce risk of self-injury, neither is beneficial to the child in expressing his emotions.

5. The nurse may evaluate a child's development of object permanence using which of the following techniques?
   A. Asking the child to transfer an object from one hand to the other.
   B. Playing "peek-a-boo" with the child.
   C. Asking the child to mimic waving "Bye bye."
   D. Playing with colored ring stacking toys.

Intended Response: **B.** Object permanence has developed in a child when he realizes that the removal of something from his sight doesn't necessarily mean that it is gone forever. When playing peek-a-boo, the child realizes that although he cannot see (however temporarily) the person playing with him, that person does not disappear forever.

6. A preschool-age child has been hospitalized for the past three days. The child asks the nurse, "When is my Mommy coming to see me?" The nurse is aware that the child's mother visits him daily in the mid-afternoon hours. Which of the following responses of the nurse would be most appropriate to the child's developmental level?

   A. "She'll be here very soon."

   B. "I'll let you know shortly before she is due to arrive."

   C. "I believe she told me she would be here around 2:00."

   D. "After your lunch and nap, your Mommy should be here."

Intended Response: **D.** As the preschooler is not yet capable of abstract thinking, he can understand time only in relation to concrete realities, such as events. None of the remaining responses connect the expected time of the mother's arrival with a concrete reality the child can understand.

7. The nurse is preparing to teach a preschooler scheduled for abdominal surgery about pre- and post-op care expected with the procedure. Which of the following interventions would be most likely to both enhance the child's understanding of the teaching and decrease his fear regarding the surgery?

   A. Showing pictures of the operating room and any special equipment that may be used.

   B. Using a doll having a surgical incision and surgical dressings for the child to look at and "take care of."

   C. Relating stories of other children who have undergone similar surgery.

   D. Describing the important information using simple, friendly terms such as "Dr. Good" and "Nurse Nice."

Intended Response: **B.** Use of a doll having a surgical incision and surgical dressings provides the preschool-age child with a concrete image that he can see and thus better understand. Encouraging the child to interact with the doll and "take care of" the doll provides the child with a sense of autonomy and empowerment, a developmental need for this age. Although Response A also provides concrete images, the pictures will be of an environment too foreign for the child to understand or accept. Relating stories of other children does not address the need for empowerment and autonomy. Terms such as "Dr. Good" are value-laden, and thus inappropriate.

8. The nurse is leading a class discussion on prevention of pregnancy and sexually transmitted diseases with a group of sexually active adolescent girls. Which of the following comments by members of the group would indicate the need for further teaching?

   A. "I won't say yes to sex unless my boyfriend agrees to wear a condom—every time."

   B. "My periods are pretty irregular. Trying to time sex for the safe times just doesn't work well for me."

   C. "I'm not worried about getting HIV. I take my birth control pills faithfully—every day."

   D. "I've decided I just want to wait for a while. I don't think I'm ready for a sexual relationship."

Intended Response: **C.** Although faithful use of oral contraceptives is an effective measure for birth control, it provides no protection against the transmission of sexually transmitted diseases, including gonorrhea, chlamydia, and HIV/AIDS.

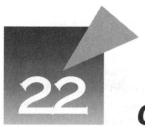

Children's Health

PATRICIA HUGHES

The focus of this chapter is the structure and organization of children's health deviations. It is critical to view children's health issues within the developmental framework outlined in the previous chapter. This chapter will review the major body systems, emphasizing the elements that are unique to the nursing care of children, while drawing parallels to the areas that are similar to adult nursing care. You will find that the nursing care of children is not based upon principles foreign to adult care; rather it adds another dimension to the nursing principles upon which all care is based.

Principle

Children exist and function within a multitude of groups. The nurse must assess, plan, implement, and evaluate care in the context of the group structures within which the child exists.

Illustration of Principle

A child's family is his or her primary group. The child forms one support beam in the structure of the family, and the other members of the family form the remainder of the supports. If one support is weakened by illness, the remainder of the supports must work harder to maintain the integrity of the family structure. A child's family and/or primary caregivers are the groups with the greatest significance to the child. Children derive physical and emotional support from their primary caregivers (typically the family). This support becomes a vehicle for development, and the cornerstone of a child's coping mechanisms. When caring for a child, the nurse must appreciate how intimately entwined the lives, hopes, dreams, and fears of the family group are. The nurse is truly caring for the family rather than the child as an individual.

Parents or primary caretakers have their roles altered when the child entrusted into their care becomes ill. They are required to exert greater energy toward the ill child, letting other responsibilities go. They may sense their caretaking roles being taken from them if their child is in need of hospitalization. They can no longer provide for their child fully. Parents often express helplessness as intravenous medicines and dressings seem to offer the sustenance for their ill child's life—a responsibility that was previously theirs. Siblings are also affected by a child's illness. Siblings' daily routines are altered as parents struggle to meet the different needs of the ill and well children. Siblings may express jealousy over the greater attention that the ill child receives.

The nurse's role is to view the entire family as "the client." By focusing care on the family as a unit, the nurse truly provides holistic care to the child.

Principle

Children and adults have anatomically similar bodies, but the maturity and efficiency of body organs and functions are different

Illustration of Principle

One of the most significant differences between adults and children is the difference in their metabolic rates. The infant's metabolic rate is twice that of an adult. This means that children and infants will consume a greater amount of fuel in proportion to their body size. The body fuels are oxygen, water, and calories. You can remember this metabolic fact by visualizing the child as a gas guzzling car versus the adult as an energy efficient car model. The child's rapid growth rate, along with higher heart and respiratory rates, are visible clues to the child's faster metabolic rate.

Principle

The body tries to maintain a balance between the supply and demand for fuels

Illustration of Principle

Anything that will increase a child's metabolic rate will increase the need for fuels. If a body is stressed by illness, disease, or injury, the body's ability to meet the demands for fuels may be compromised. Situations that may increase the demand for fuel are physical activity, pain, anxiety, altered body temperature, wound healing, and infections. A major goal in nursing care is to assist in balancing the supply and demand of fuels. After a complete assessment, the nurse plans and implements strategies that increase the supply of fuel, and assists the child in decreasing the demand for fuel.

> *I*nterventions that decrease the demand for fuels are found by addressing situations that increase the child's metabolic rate. Interventions that will increase the supply are typically found by addressing the illness state.

MEMORY JOGS

Oxygenation

Using the fuel of oxygen, we can highlight the balancing of supply and demand. The body can be viewed as a factory. Each of the machines (body organs) in the factory requires oxygen as fuel to run. This process of manufacturing is called aerobic metabolism. Our brain is the boss of our factory; it will try to keep the factory running smoothly by making sure there are proper supplies and fuels for the factory to function—or in the case of our scenario, a proper amount of oxygen for our tissues and organs to survive and perform their functions. When a factory runs short of fuel the first reaction of the boss is not to shut down and send its workers home; but rather, to figure out how to keep the factory running and producing.

The boss will make decisions to compensate and continue production. Often it means that the workers must pull together and work harder. The same is true for the body when faced with the lack of oxygen. The body compensates with tachycardia and tachypnea. The heart and lungs are called to work a little harder. This compensation may do the job. When faced with a prolonged reduction in oxygen, the body may ask for more workers to help carry out the jobs. The body can produce more red blood cells, which is termed polycythemia. Visualize this process by thinking of the heart as an engine, and the cardiovascular system as a conveyor belt. On the conveyor belt are baskets (hemoglobin) to carry oxygen to the tissues.

Polycythemia is merely the body compensating by adding more baskets to the conveyor belt. A potential side effect of this compensatory action is that the blood will become thick and sluggish (the conveyor belt is overfilled with baskets) creating an increased risk for thrombus. If our compensatory mechanisms are not adequate, the body will still not shut down its factory; but rather, it will change its method of metabolism. The body changes to an anaerobic or low oxygen metabolism. The by-product of this method of metabolism is acid. Acid in our serum will lower our pH, leading to metabolic acidosis, organ damage, and eventually death, if uncorrected.

After a thorough assessment of the child, focusing especially on the cardio-respiratory systems, the nurse plans and implements strategies that help return the balance of supply and demand. When tissues are at risk from an altered state of oxygen, or from any cause, it is important not to challenge the body further. Interventions that will reduce the demand for oxygen are interventions that will not promote an increase in the metabolic rate.

Nursing Management for Oxygenation Framework

Balancing Demand

1. Decreasing physical activity (possibly full bed rest)
2. Addressing the child's pain
3. Addressing the child's anxiety
4. Keeping the child normothermic
5. Treating any other physical problems that would increase the metabolic rate (i.e., infections or wounds).

Interventions to help increase the supply of oxygen can be found by addressing the illness state. The basic nursing interventions for any child experiencing altered oxygenation, whether from a respiratory cause, a hematalogic cause, or a cardiac cause, can be found if the nurse keeps the following concept in mind. Not all interventions will be used in each situation, but the nurse can use this concept as a framework to select interventions.

Balancing Supply

1. Open Airway (Assess for patency)
   Position for optimum ventilation.
   Keep airways clear with suctioning, and/or coughing and deep breathing.
   Facilitate clearing of lower airways through chest physiotherapy.
   Assess responses of ordered respiratory medications.
   Bronchodilators will be used when there is smooth muscle constriction.
   Steroids will be used to reduce inflammations of the respiratory tree.
2. Oxygen
   Oxygen may be ordered to supplement the supply.

3. Fluids

   Humidified air and adequate fluids help liquify secretions.

   Adequate fluids can help promote a more fluid circulatory system when the child is at risk for "sluggish blood" from hemoconcentration or polycythemia.

4. Transfuse

   Transfusions are given when a child has a deficit in oxygen carrying capacity and other efforts prove inadequate by themselves.

> *S*ituations that substantially decrease circulating red blood cells or alter their function are times when transfusions are considered. Hemolytic anemia, hemorrhages, or large losses of blood through surgical drains are examples of situations in which you may expect a physician's order for packed red blood cells to increase the oxygen carrying capacity.

MEMORY JOGS

5. Medications or treatments that address the disease that alters O_2
   Sometimes the disease state that challenges the supply of oxygen is not respiratory in origin. The nurse should have a clear idea of the origin after a complete assessment. By treating the disease state itself, the supply of oxygen will improve. Examples:

   Digoxin will improve the heart's contractility, thus improving the circulation of oxygen throughout the body.

   Diuretics are prescribed to decrease fluid excesses that may challenge a child's heart affected by a congenital heart defect. Easing the workload of the heart can improve circulation and perfusion of oxygen to tissues.

   Surgery may repair anomalies such as congenital heart defects and tracheoesophageal fistulas; remove foreign bodies that may have been aspirated or tumors that may be present; or treat complications such as pnuemothorax.

Illustration of Principle

Larngotracheobronchitis

Larngotracheobronchitis is a viral inflammation of the larynx, trachea, and bronchi. The inflammation causes varying degrees of spasm in the larynx and bronchi. Its common name is croup. Croup strikes many young children each year. Because it is a respiratory virus, the clinical assessment would typically find a young child (usually 3 months to 3 years) with a history of cold symptoms (increased secretions, rhinorrhea, cough, and possible low grade fever). The inflammation in the upper airway causes a characteristic stridor followed by a barking cough. Stridor and coughing episodes frequently increase in intensity at night.

Application of principle and framework

1. **Open Airway:** Position the child for optimum ventilation (high Fowler's). Aspirate via bulb syringe the nose and mouth of infants to help clear secretions.* Bronchodilators may be used if bronchospasm is noted. Corticosteroids are commonly ordered to reduce the inflammation, and racemic epinephrine by aerosol can offer transient symptom relief.

2. **Oxygen:** Oxygen may be ordered at the hospital if the child's dyspnea does not improve quickly.

3. **Fluids:** Humidified air from a cool mist humidifier or steam from a hot shower can reduce laryngospasm, assist in reducing inflammation, and keep secretions liquified. This is the first line of action prescribed for home treatment for the child in mild distress. Typically the humidity, or humidity coupled with cool air, relieves the obstruction.

MEMORY JOGS

> *S*team vaporizers are not recommended because of the high risk for injury.

4. **Transfusions:** Not needed

5. **Medications or treatments for the disease:** Croup is typically viral in nature; therefore, treatment focuses on symptom relief and comfort. Less frequently, croup will be bacterial in origin. In this case, antibiotics will be prescribed to directly address the disease state.

6. **Decrease activity:** A child who appears in distress should be kept quiet.

7. **Pain:** The child may be uncomfortable from the cold symptoms, or fever. Acetaminophen or ibuprofen are the drugs of choice to alleviate these symptoms.

---

* The child requiring hospitalization may need medication to open the airway.

8. **Anxiety:** Children as well as parents may be full of anxiety when faced with symptoms of difficulty in breathing. The child's panic for air may further inhibit the child's breathing patterns. The nurse can use developmentally appropriate therapeutic communication skills, distraction, and play to reduce anxieties.

9. **Normothermic:** Fevers can be treated with acetaminophen or ibuprofen, in addition to sponging and dressing lightly.

Sickle Cell Anemia

Sickle cell anemia is an autosomal recessive trait that is found most frequently in people of African descent, and to a lesser extent, Mediterranean descent. A child with sickle cell anemia does not form normal hemoglobin (Hgb). These children have a decreased oxygen transport ability. The normal hemoglobin A is replaced by hemoglobin S. Hemoglobin S lacks the affinity for oxygen.

The process of sickling begins when the body has an increased demand for oxygen. Triggers causing sickling are infection, dehydration, extreme temperatures, stress, heavy exercise, or high altitudes. Under these conditions, the Hgb S sickles the red blood cells (RBCs) into a crescent shape. In addition to the sickled cells lacking the affinity for oxygen, the crescent shaped red blood cells clump together and impede blood flow in small vascular areas. The blockage of vessels and the reduced oxygen carrying capacity of the blood leads to tissue ischemia. Left untreated, the ischemia can lead to organ damage or even death. The disease creates a vicious cycle as the sickling creates a new demand on the oxygen balance, which in turn causes more sickling.

Use the oxygen supply and demand framework to assist you in developing your nursing management plan. The key nursing goal is to assist the child in balancing the supply and demand for oxygen. To reduce the demand from activity, the child will be placed on bed rest. A mixture of narcotics and nonsteroidal anti-inflammatory medications, as well as warm heat are used to treat the severe pain from tissue ischemia. Antibiotics are prescribed for infections and are also part of a prophylactic treatment for infections in the child. Fever is kept under control. To increase the supply of oxygen, oxygen is administered. Fluids are critical to the treatment of sickle cell vaso-occlusive crisis. Fluids are aggressively pushed to keep the circulatory system fluid and to avoid clumping of the sickled cells. If the blood becomes sluggish, the tissues will be greatly deprived of oxygen, perpetuating the vicious cycle and continuing the intense pain from tissue ischemia. Transfusions may be needed to replace the damaged red blood cells, and to improve oxygen carrying capacity. Other treatments that address the diseased state include iron and folic acid supplements, and a diet rich in iron and ascorbic acid.

Fluids

Principle

Fluids play a vital role in the homeostasis of the body

Illustration of Principle

The functions of fluids in the body include transportation of energy sources, cellular stability, cooling, lubrication, and removal of wastes. Fluids are regulated by many systems in our body—the renal, gastrointestinal, integumentary, and, to a lesser extent, the respiratory system. Continuing with the analogy of our body as a factory, we can easily gain an appreciation of the significant role fluids play in the child's body. The functions of fluids in the body parallel the uses of fluids within a factory. The factory may use water to transport needed energy sources throughout its machines (transport medium). It may be needed to buffer and protect vital machine components (cellular stability). It may be needed to maintain the machine at proper working temperature, so as not to burn out any components (cooling). Water can be used to lubricate and protect the machine from movement or friction (lubrication). Finally, water is often used to flush out unwanted by-products of manufacturing from the system, or to clean out the system (removal of wastes).

Principle

Infants and young children are the most vulnerable to alterations in fluids and electrolytes

Illustration of Principle

There are some unique differences between children and adults that put children at greater risk from fluid loss. Water is the highest component in the infant's and in the child's body. It is expressed as a percentage of total body weight. Water may make up 80% of the infant's weight, 65% of the toddler's, and 60% of the adolescent's. The majority of a child's fluids are extracellular, and therefore have a higher susceptibility to loss. There are also other developmental factors that make the infant and young child at higher risk for fluid alterations.

The infant and younger child have higher demands for fluids because of higher metabolic rates. The infant uses about 15% of body weight in fluids each day. The infant and child have high skin surface to body weight ratios, increasing their susceptibility to insensible losses or losses through any alteration of skin integrity. The infant's kidneys are immature and fail to concentrate urine even when faced with a deficit state of fluids. Finally, infants and young children often lack the communication skills needed to express their thirst.

Principle

The role of the nurse is to assist the child in balancing the supply and demand for fluids

*W*ater loss is influenced by illness, injury, activity, altitude, intake ability, medicines, and insensible losses.

MEMORY JOGS

Nursing Management for Fluid Framework

Think supply and demand. Ask yourself, what factors are increasing the need for fluids? Your answer may be the nature of the disease state itself, or it may be activity, which increases the metabolic rate and further stresses the supply and demand ratio. If it is the disease, look for nursing actions that will help treat the disease and fluid losses. If it is excess activities, assist the client to limit these. Next, ask yourself what you can do as a nurse to improve the supply of fluids the client has to work with. It may be that you need to add fluids, or you may need to focus on retaining the fluids the child already has, and prevent losses, or both.

Steps to take in developing your nursing management plan:

1. Assess/identify the cause.
2. Treat the cause.
3. Treat the deficit.
4. Limit other excess demands for fluids.

Illustration of Principle

Vomiting and diarrhea are two of the most common causes of dehydration in infants and children. Remember your goal is to balance the supply of water with the demand for water.

1. **A complete assessment:** Remember fluids are regulated by almost every system in your body, so be sure to assess them all to determine the degree of deficit. In our example, our assessment would lead us to identifying vomiting and diarrhea as the cause.

2. **Treat the cause:** (Decreasing demand). If the cause can be addressed, then you are taking the first step in controlling the deficit. For example, if the diarrhea is bacterial in origin, administering the prescribed antibiotics will begin the process of resolution. If the cause of vomiting is assessed to be a possible milk intolerance, removing all milk-based products from the diet will remove the irritation so that healing can begin.

3. **Treat the deficit:** (Increasing supply). Frequent small amounts of clear fluids are tolerated best by the child with vomiting and diarrhea. Oral rehydrating solutions are beneficial in treating not only the fluid loss, but also the electrolyte losses that children with vomiting and diarrhea will experience as well. For older children and adolescents, Gatorade may be given. When an oral rehydration solution is unavailable, decarbonated soft drinks or diluted soft drinks are often tolerated when trying to rehydrate a child who is vomiting, but can cause further irritation due to their high carbohydrate gram count.

MEMORY JOGS

*R*eintroduce bland soft solids slowly. (Increasing supply). It is advisable to wait 4–6 hours before reintroduction of solids after vomiting. Most products may not be tolerated at first by the child after diarrhea, because of a transient lactose intolerance. Formulas should be introduced at 1/4 strength, then increased as tolerated. Another option is to switch to a soy or hydrolysate formula temporarily. Breast fed babies can continue breast feeding.

4. **Limit excess demands for fluids:** (Decrease demand). Look for things that would increase the metabolic rate, such as activity, fever, and infections. Then explore other factors that may challenge the demand for fluids, such as the use of diuretics.

Illustration of Principle

Fluids are not always lost from the baby, but sometimes are shifted within the body, leaving the child in a dehydrated state. Nephrotic syndrome is an example of this shifting of fluids. Nephrotic syndrome is caused by a viral agent that increases the glomerular permeability to plasma proteins. The glomerulus is similar to a sorting machine in your factory. It sifts out what products are injected and will become waste, and what products will continue down the line for use by the factory. Plasma proteins are needed by the body and should be retained. A simple way to conceptualize the pathophysiology of nephrotic syndrome is to visualize the glomerulus (the sorting machine) becoming damaged by a viral intruder, and made unable to control the losses of the plasma proteins. The proteins are lost in the waste product line (the urine). The result is a low-serum protein and proteinuria.

> *P*roteins hold fluids in the vasculature by their osmotic pull.

MEMORY JOGS

When there is a loss of serum proteins, the osmotic gradient is shifted. Fluids in the vasculature are no longer in balance with the electrolytes and proteins. The fluids shift out into the tissues to find balance there. The body senses a fluid loss and turns on its compensatory systems to save water (renin-angiotensin-aldosterone mechanism), but this water is lost to the tissues in a vicious cycle. The net result is that the child becomes dehydrated, yet experiences massive edema.

> *E*dema in children is usually first seen as periorbital edema.

MEMORY JOGS

> *I*ndividuals experiencing edema must have meticulous assessment and care of their skin.

MEMORY JOGS

To treat this type of loss we can use the same framework:

1. **Assess/identify:** Assess client and determine degree of dehydration. The cause of fluid shifts in nephrotic syndrome is a protein loss.
2. **Treat cause:** Steroids are used to induce remission. You can think of the steroids as assisting to patch the holes in the broken sorter. Our goal here is to reduce further losses.

3. **Treat deficit:** With nephrotic syndrome there is a large quantity of fluid in the body, but it is maldistributed. Treating the deficit will involve redistribution of fluids. Albumin will help pull fluids back into the vasculature and diuretics will help achieve balance and reduce the risk of fluid overload from the shifting fluids. A high protein, no added salt diet is sometimes recommended to further help achieve balance.

4. **Limit excess demands for fluids:** The child's activity will be restricted during the acute stages and early convalescence. Fevers and infections should be assessed and treated.

MEMORY JOGS

*R*elapses of nephrotic syndrome are common, so patient and family education is important. Explanations of the uses and side effects of steroids are needed, as well as instruction on how to test for urine protein.

Principle

Energy is derived from food; the intake and uptake of food stuffs is what allows for energy expenditure

MEMORY JOGS

A child is at risk for failure to thrive, electrolyte and vitamin deficiencies, growth delays and developmental delays, and activity intolerance if there is a negative balance of calories and nutrients supplied to the child's body.

Illustration of Principle

In reconsidering our body as a factory, it is the calories (measured in kilocalories) and nutrients from foods that are the true energy sources that keep the machines running. Food can be thought of as providing not only the spark but the current upon which our machines run. If there is a lack of energy from a calorie fuel deficit, the machine may sputter, slow down, or work less efficiently. To compensate for a low supply or high demand for calories and nutrients, our body will use lean mass and fat stored for energy.

Principle

Infants' and children's energy requirements vary according to age, health status, body size, body composition, developmental stage, and activity level

Illustration of Principle

Developmental Variance

Infants have the most rapid growth and therefore require the greatest amount of kilocalories per kilogram per day. An infant may need over 100 kcal/kg/day, whereas children by mid-school age may need an average of 50 kcal/kg/day. Infants have a high requirement for fats. Fats are needed to myelinize the neural pathways. An infant needs to consume over 30% fat from his or her diet for proper neural development. The consumption of whole milk, versus reduced fat milk, after the first year of life, helps provide the fat needed in the diet. Breast milk supplies the proper balance of nutrients and calories.

> *A*n infant begins solid foods around 6 months of age. At this time, he has lost his protrusion reflex and can begin swallowing. There is the emergence of primary teeth, the child is beginning to be able to sit with support, and the child shows some skill with his or her hands, including a palmar grasp.

MEMORY JOGS

As a child grows, kilocalorie/kilogram requirements decrease, yet the total calorie requirement increases. The growing child becomes more active and muscle mass increases, which increases the child's requirements for calories and proteins.

> *D*uring the toddler/preschool time, a child may refuse to eat any variety of foods, possibly accepting only a few items to eat, requesting them over and over.

MEMORY JOGS

School-ager's energy needs depend on activity and body size. The increasing muscle mass and frequent sports activities will increase the need for calories.

MEMORY JOGS

*S*chool-agers as well as adolescents are at risk for obesity if they are sedentary.

High levels of calories are needed during the adolescent's growth spurt. The adolescent may appear like a bottomless pit, yet the high food consumption is the body's way of balancing the supply and demand ratio during the rapid growth spurt at this age.

Health State Variance

Many illness factors can upset the supply and demand balance of calories and nutrients. Illness states can reduce the caloric and nutrient supply:

Examples affecting the supply of calories and nutrients:

· Illnesses that impair intake
· Ingestion problems
· Digestion problems
· Malabsorption problems

MEMORY JOGS

*P*hysical limitations or altered perception or taste of food will impair intake.

MEMORY JOGS

*D*emands for fuel are determined by the metabolic rate. When a child has an increased metabolic rate, the need for fuel increases. For example, the metabolic rate of a child recovering from burn wounds may be six times the baseline, and a child's healthy baseline is typically twice that of an adult. The recovering burn victim will need foods dense in calories and high in protein.

Examples affecting the demand of calories and nutrients:

- Growth
- Activity
- Tissue repairs
- Fever
- Infections

Principle

The nurse's role is to assist the child in restoring a balance between the supply for calories and nutrients and the child's demand for these same calories and nutrients

Illustration of Principle

To improve supply, efforts need to focus on improving the child's intake, retention, and absorption of food in reference to the child's health status. To decrease the demand for calories, the nurse must identify those factors that are placing extra stress on the supply of caloric fuel.

Nursing Management for Nutrient Framework

1. **Assess caloric needs:** What are the maintenance needs plus any additional caloric needs from growth, wound healing, health status, or activity levels? A 3-day diet recall is a useful tool to determine the child's intake patterns.
2. **Enhance nutrition:** The goal is to improve the quantity and quality of intake, or improve its retention and absorption. Small frequent feedings of calorie-rich, nutrient-rich meals are typically the intervention of choice. Sometimes it is important to supplement oral feedings with tube feedings during the sleeping hours. Placing the child in an upright, or upright sidelying position will improve food retention and gastric emptying. Infant seats can be used to position young children.

> *A*dding instant breakfast powders to drinks or serving pudding for snacks are just a couple of ways to increase the caloric density of foods while maintaining the nutritional status.

MEMORY JOGS

3. **Treat illness state:** If the illness state can be improved, the nutritional state will follow. Often the illness states can be improved through the administration of ordered medications. Metoclopramide is used to improve gastric emptying in the child suffering from gastroesophageal reflux. Pancreatic enzymes can allow for the absorption of proteins and fats in the child with cystic fibrosis. Fat-soluble vitamin replacements can also help restore the deficits the child with cystic fibrosis experiences. Sometimes surgical intervention may be needed, as seen with the infant with pyloric stenosis. Still other times, nutritional status will improve with careful adherence to a diet plan. The effect of a careful diet can be examined when considering the gluten-free diet that a child with celiac disease follows. By eliminating wheat, rye, oats, and barley from the diet, a child with celiac no longer experiences a malabsorptive process.

4. **Limit demands:** Careful consideration should be given to reducing any unnecessary demands on the metabolic rate. By reducing any excess demands for calories, the child is able to use the calories at hand for healing or growth.

Principle

Children are susceptible to many threats to their body's integrity and functioning

Illustration of Principle

Childhood is a time of health risks from communicable disease, injuries, and poisonings. Think of the child's body as a factory. These threats can be thought of as vandals who invade the factory, break machines, impair the work force, or even threaten the ability of the factory to survive. Consider, for example that a communicable disease or poison is a vandal, or a loose invader without authorization to be in the body (factory). The nurse's role is likened to law enforcement's role when an intruder trespasses into a building. The police would assess the building, evaluate the damage, and identify the perpetrator. The police would try to prevent the spread of further vandalism. Finally, the police would try to prevent complications from the attack, and then support and educate the victims. These are the same steps the nurse carries out when caring for a child facing a threat to body integrity.

Nursing Management for Body Threats Framework:

1. **Assess:** For balance
2. **Identify:** Identify the threat to body integrity or function through analysis of history and physical assessments.

3. **Prevent spread/terminate exposure:** Limit or stop further threat, i.e., remove poison or isolate communicable children.
4. **Prevent complications**
5. **Provide comfort**
6. **Support and educate**

Illustration of Principle

Varicella

Young children are prone to acquiring communicable diseases because of poor hand washing habits, and because of the close contacts with others made in schools and daycare centers. The major focus of prevention of many communicable diseases is during the infant through preschool years, and prevention is achieved through the use of immunizations. Immunizations provide protection from some of the most serious communicable diseases.

Varicella or chickenpox is a common childhood communicable disease that usually passes without incident, and is typically managed at home. Using the steps outlined in the body threats framework, see if you can develop your plan of care. When you are done, try developing plans of care for other communicable diseases, such as lice infestation, or for ingestion of poisonous substances such as lead or acetaminophen.

1. **Assess:** Assess child for baseline, and to obtain any history that might point to recent known exposures.
2. **Identify:** The history and physical exam for varicella would show exposure to chickenpox during the two- to three-week incubation period. The child usually has a slight fever, general malaise, and a characteristic rash. The rash starts out macular, and then progresses to papule, vesicle, and scabbing. All phases of the rash are present at the same time.
3. **Prevent spread:** To prevent the spread of chickenpox, the child should be isolated until crusts have formed. The period of communicability is one day before the lesions appear to six days after the first vesicles have scabbed (typically 7–10 days). Chickenpox is spread through respiratory droplets and drainage from erupted vesicles.
4. **Prevent complications:** The nurse can assist the child or parents in reducing scratching. Children should have their nails clipped short, and even have mittens applied if scratching persists.

5. **Provide comfort:** Lessening the pruritus will provide great relief; methods include tepid oatmeal baths, application of calamine lotion, or administration of Benadryl (diphenhydramine) and Tylenol (acetaminophen) as ordered to relieve fever and itching.

6. **Support and educate:** Any illness of a child can cause great concern and anxiety within a family. Chickenpox, although typically benign, causes considerable inconvenience for the family. Caring for the ill child may mean the loss of a parent's work hours for a week. Siblings may be exposed to the virus, potentially starting the cycle again. The use of the new varicella vaccine may help lessen family disruptions by preventing the disease. Varicella is an optional vaccine that is administered at 18 months of age or later.

Illustration of Principle

Injuries

Each developmental age brings with it a high risk for injuries. Causes of injuries range from the falls of a new walker to the risky stunts taken by a new teenage driver. The nurse will always be faced with physical injuries when caring for children. You can use the body threats framework to organize your care for the injured child. **Assess** the child for a baseline, and to establish the extent of injury. **Prevent spread** of the injury by proper immobilization, or removal from the source of danger. **Treat the injury** itself. This may mean anything from wound care to traction set-ups. **Prevent complications** through careful monitoring of the injury. **Provide support and comfort** to the child and parent. Injuries are not only painful—they also may be frightening to both children and parents. Great emphasis needs to be placed on **educating** children and families about high risk behaviors. Without education we cannot reduce the threats to children. Education is the best means of childproofing the environment.

Reasoning Exercises: *Children's Health*

1. Patrick's mother complains that he seems to have a poor appetite and eats very small meals. Which of the following suggestions by the clinic Z nurse would be most helpful in improving Patrick's nutritional intake?

    A. Allow Patrick to eat whenever he wishes during the day

    B. Serve Patrick's foods on special plates and in bowls with cartoon decorations

C. Encourage Patrick to taste a few bites of a large variety of new foods

D. Supplement Patrick's intake at meals with several snacks throughout the day

Intended Response: **B.** Foods served on special dinnerware is likely to seem much more attractive to the 5-year-old. Appetite and intake vary widely in this age group, and the parents should expect that their child will go through periods when he simply does not wish to eat certain amounts or types of foods. However, the parents should not allow the child to eat frequent snacks or have meals whenever he chooses. Likewise, the child should not be encouraged to try a large variety of new foods, with small bites of each, because he will probably rebel and instead choose not to eat at all.

2. Patrick receives a DPT booster injection. The physician has ordered him to receive 15 mg of Tylenol per kg of body weight at home if fever develops. Patrick weighs 36 lb. The nurse calculates the total dosage to be

A. 180 mg

B. 220 mg

C. 240 mg

D. 260 mg

Intended Response: **C.** Since 1 kg = 2.2 lb, Patrick's kilogram weight is approximately 16 kg. 16×15 mg = 240 mg total dosage.

3. Mrs. Kathy Murphy calls her son Danny's pediatric nurse practitioner with concern over her son's difficulty with respirations and his "barking" cough. The PNP suspects laryngotracheobronchitis (LTB). The characteristic "crowing" sound of respirations in LTB is

A. Stridor

B. Rhonchi

C. Wheeze

D. Rales

Intended Response: **A.** A characteristic sign of LTB is a loud, crowing sound with respirations termed stridor (response A), caused by a narrowing of the air passageways.

4. The nurse practitioner recognizes that the primary goal of treatment of LTB is airway dilation. This goal is best achieved by instructing Mrs. Murphy to do which of the following?

   A. Place Danny in a hot, steamy shower stall

   B. Position Danny for sleep sitting up in a comfortable chair

   C. Place a cool, moist humidifier in Danny's room

   D. Administer an over-the-counter cough suppressant

Intended Response: **C.** Cool, moist humidification of room air is the ideal method of dilating airway passages. Placing a child in a steamy bathroom is an acceptable alternative; but, to reduce the risk of burns, the child should never be placed in a shower stall or tub with hot running water.

5. Kevin Lewis, a 3-year-old attending preschool daily, complains to his mother that he is feeling tired, achy, and warm. She notes an elevated temperature and a few reddish blisterlike lesions on his chest. Kevin's mother suspects chickenpox. Which of the following clusters of symptoms would support a diagnosis of chickenpox (varicella)?

   A. Chills, headache, and malaise

   B. Nausea, vomiting, and diarrhea

   C. Koplik's spots, photophobia, and fever

   D. Sore throat, chills, and fever

Intended Response: **A.** The symptoms listed in response **B** are typical of influenza, and these gastrointestinal complaints are not typical of chickenpox. The symptoms in response **C** characterize measles. Response **D** describes respiratory symptoms typical of upper respiratory infections.

6. Which of the following home care measures should the clinic nurse instruct Mrs. Lewis to use for Kevin?

   A. Avoid bright indoor lights or sunlight for 2 weeks

   B. Isolate Kevin from siblings and playmates for 2 to 3 weeks

   C. Administer Benadryl as ordered for its antihistamine effect

   D. Administer Tylenol 10 grains, every 4 hours as needed for fever and aches

Intended Response: **C.** Since the lesions of chickenpox cause itching, the child has a tendency to scratch the lesions, exacerbating his condition and leading to potential scarring. The administration of Benadryl is desirable for its anti-itching effect.

Response **A** typifies management of the child with measles. Isolation of a child for a period of 2 to 3 weeks, response **B,** is unnecessary and undesirable. Tylenol may be given for symptomatic relief, but the dosage in response **D** is 10 grains (600 mg), an adult dosage.

7. Michael Washington is a 14-year-old with sickle cell anemia. Diagnosed at birth, this is his 23rd admission for sickle cell disease. The nurse caring for Michael should have which of the following understandings about the etiology of sickle cell disease?
   A. It is related to fetal trauma during the birthing process.
   B. It is usually caused by an acute viral infection.
   C. It is a genetically linked disorder inherited from parents.
   D. It is associated with poor nutritional intake of iron.

Intended Response: **C.** Sickle cell disease is a genetically linked disease inherited from parents who either have the disease or carry the trait for the disease. For this reason, couples with a history of sickle cell disease are encouraged to seek genetic counseling prior to conception of future offspring.

8. Michael is in sickle cell crisis. All of the following signs and symptoms would suggest crisis except
   A. Acute abdominal pain
   B. Fatigue and shortness of breath
   C. Severe joint pain
   D. Anorexia and weight loss

Intended Response: **D.** Anorexia and weight loss, response **D,** are not typically associated with sickle cell crisis. The vaso-occlusive changes that occur as a result of the bunching of sickle red blood cells cause the remaining three symptoms: abdominal pain, joint pain, and shortness of breath.

9. In preparing a plan of care for Michael during crisis, the nurse recognizes that his most immediate need is for which of the following?
   A. Hydration
   B. Pain control
   C. Prevention of joint contracture
   D. Emotional support

Intended Response: **A.** Because Michael is experiencing vaso-occlusion from the sickled cells, hydration, typically by means of IV therapy, is the priority measure in sickle cell crisis. The remaining responses, though important, are of secondary importance to hydration.

23

Surgical Intervention

NANCY KORCHEK

Principle

The primary goal for the immediate postoperative patient is to establish physiological balance

Illustration of Principle

Surgical intervention presents a major insult to the normal functioning of the body's systems.

Critical assessment of the immediate postoperative patient includes:

· Patency of airway
· Vital signs—values and qualities
· Adequacy of peripheral circulation
· Regulation of core body temperature
· Fluid status and regulation
· Level of consciousness and orientation

Nursing Management

Optimally, all data gathered from these assessment criteria would indicate a return to normal state, evidencing a reestablishment of physiological balance. Since surgical patients are cooled to reduce risk for bleeding, the nurse should note a steady increase in body temperature to normal or slightly elevated levels. Recovering patients should show an increase in level of consciousness and awareness, becoming able to orient themselves correctly to the postsurgical environment. Respirations should become spontaneous, unlabored, and adequate as the effects of anesthesia dissipate.

Assessment data that indicate a movement *away* from normal parameters should alert the nurse to possible postoperative complications. Accelerating respiratory rates may indicate inadequate oxygenation; precipitous falls in arterial blood pressure may signal fluid loss or hemorrhage. The nurse should remain alert for any such indications and take appropriate action to ensure the postoperative well-being and safety of the patient.

Principle

Surgical intervention inherently places the patient at risk for infection

Illustration of Principle

Because most surgical procedures involve the opening of skin layers, the body's first line of defense against the invasion of microorganisms and contaminants is compromised, placing the surgical patient at risk for the development of infection. Additionally, surgical intervention compromises defense against infection in the following ways:

- Surgery may involve the opening of sterile body cavities, such as the lung, bladder, uterus, or peritoneum.
- Surgery places an additional stress on the body, possibly decreasing its resistance to infection.
- Postoperative convalescence may influence risk for infection secondary to anorexia associated with discomfort or anesthesia, bed rest associated with decreased circulation, or contamination of the wound associated with handling during dressing changes and irrigations.

Nursing Management

Because of these risks, the nurse must have an ongoing awareness of the patient's immune status following surgery, focusing on signs of developing infection:

- Elevated body temperature
- Elevated white blood cell count
- Increase in severity of pain at the surgical site
- Increase in swelling, redness, or tenderness at the surgical site

- Change in wound drainage from the expected (sanguineous, or serosanguineous) to purulent

The nurse should assess the patient's operative site routinely for evidence of progress in healing. Wounds healing in the expected manner should have the following characteristics:

- Wound edges in close approximation (first intention healing)
- Sutures or staples intact, with no evidence of pulling or gaping of the wound edges
- Absence of redness, swelling, or tenderness at wound site
- Absence of foul odor or purulent drainage from surgical wound

The nurse should plan interventions aimed at preventing or containing postoperative infection, such as careful handling of dressing materials, use of sterile technique in wound care, and observance of isolation restrictions for wound drainage, should they apply. The most valuable method for infection management, however, is the simplest—*thorough hand washing* before and after contact with the patient.

> *B*ecause surgery involves the opening of skin layers, the body is at risk for infection from invading microorganisms. The nurse should conscientiously use hand washing before and after contact with the patient to reduce the patient's risk of developing postoperative infection.

MEMORY JOGS

Principle

The stress of surgical intervention increases the body's nutritional needs to effect healing

Illustration of Principle

Nutritional factors play a significant role in timely and complete postoperative healing. Typically, the recovering patient requires the following:

- Increased protein for tissue repair
- Increased carbohydrate to be used by the body for energy, thus sparing the protein for tissue repair

- Increased fluids as allowed to flush out residual anesthesia and reduce risk for postoperative fluid and electrolyte imbalance
- Increased vitamin C for tissue healing

Nursing Management

The nurse should assess the readiness for oral intake of foods and fluids, guided by physician order and the patient's ability to swallow and retain intake following surgery. Mild, transient anorexia can be expected in the early recovery period and can be managed by offering the patient small, frequent feedings rather than full meals. Oral fluids should be encouraged as early as possible and permitted. If the patient enjoyed a healthy nutritional status prior to surgery, a general (regular) postoperative diet will provide ample amounts of the above nutritional requirements to promote healing. However, if the patient was in a poor nutritional state preoperatively, as evidenced by significant weight loss, poor skin turgor and repair, and pale coloring, then additional nutritional snacks and supplements are indicated. Hyperalimentation (parenteral nutrition) is indicated as a therapy to counteract serious malnutrition that could compromise healing during the recovery period.

MEMORY JOGS

*P*ostoperative patients should have ample sources of protein, carbohydrates, fluids, and vitamin C to promote effective and timely healing in the recovery period.

Principle

Processes or measures that slow or halt peristalsis decrease the body's ability to metabolize and absorb foods

Illustration of Principle

This principle is readily applied to the surgical patient because general anesthesia markedly decreases or halts the process of peristalsis in the gastrointestinal tract, thus negatively influencing the body's ability to metabolize, absorb, transport, or eliminate foods. For this reason, patients who have undergone surgery with general anesthesia, patients who have experienced prolonged surgeries, or patients who have had abdominal surgery should be assessed carefully for readiness for and tolerance of oral intake.

Nursing Management

In view of this effect of anesthesia and surgery, the nurse caring for the postoperative patient should include as a *routine* assessment the activity of peristalsis by the auscultation of bowel sounds. Absence of bowel sounds is common after surgery and is an indication that the patient is *not* ready for oral intake. This patient should remain NPO until peristaltic activity is noted, and then may be advanced to ice chips and clear fluids gradually. Presence of bowel sound activity in all four quadrants indicates a readiness for oral intake.

Typically, oral fluids for postoperative patients are advanced from clear fluids such as ice chips, water, or juices to more complex foods and fluids steadily as oral tolerance is verified. Patients who experience severe nausea or vomiting with oral intake should be reversed back to NPO status until oral tolerance is assured.

Providing complex foods to a patient with inadequate peristalsis places him or her at risk for a number of complications, including constipation, fecal impaction, bowel obstruction, and paralytic ileus. It is evident from this list of possible complications that postoperative diet is an important consideration for the nurse.

It is important to note that continuous use of narcotic analgesia for pain management in the postoperative phase may precipitate constipation, with abdominal firmness and bloating, abdominal fullness and discomfort, and decreased or absent passing of flatus and stool. Because narcotics significantly reduce peristaltic activity in much the same way as general anesthesia does, the nurse caring for the postsurgical patient receiving narcotic pain medications should monitor elimination patterns and subsequent readiness for oral intake.

> *B*ecause perioperative anesthesia can slow or halt peristalsis, the nurse must check for the presence of active bowel sounds before allowing the postoperative patient foods or fluids.

MEMORY JOGS

Principle

Postoperative pain decreases with each successive day after surgery

Illustration of Principle

Unlike the chronic pain associated with arthritis or advanced malignancy, postoperative pain diminishes in its intensity and frequency with each successive day following surgery. Typically, the patient will experience his or her most severe or acute pain on the first postoperative day, with diminution of pain as recovery progresses. In light of this principle, postoperative pain management typically is initiated with medication of greater strength and duration, such as narcotic analgesia. Intravenous or intramuscular routes are selected most often to enhance pain management. Analgesia is then slowly tapered with each successive day, and the patient will likely be placed on oral analgesia of less potency as recovery progresses.

Nursing Management

Prior to administering pain medication, the nurse should assess the patient's pain for the following characteristics:

- Location (helpful to ask patient to *point* to source of pain)
- Type (dull, aching, sharp, stabbing, or burning)
- Severity (on a scale of 1 to 10, with 10 being most severe)
- Frequency (how often pain recurs following medication)
- Success of previous management (pain relief with previous medication)

Following administration of medication, the nurse should observe for relief of pain as well as any side effects of the medication, such as drowsiness, lethargy, disorientation, hypotension, and so on. The nurse may enhance pain relief with medication by using measures to calm and reassure the patient, because anxiety exacerbates the pain experience. The patient should receive instruction on measures that will decrease postoperative pain, such as splinting the abdomen for coughing, moving after abdominal surgery, or lying in the lateral position to facilitate expulsion of flatus.

It is evident, then, that if the patient's pain does *not* seem to be decreasing with each successive postoperative day, the possibility of physiological or psychological factors that could exacerbate pain should be explored. For example, if the patient continues to complain of acute pain by the fourth and fifth days after an appendectomy, the possibility of a physiological problem such as peritonitis or a psychological problem such as anxiety should be ruled out to determine the cause of the continued pain.

> *P*ostoperative pain is an expected occurrence that should decrease as each postoperative day passes. Nurses should anticipate using stronger, typically narcotic, analgesia the first few days, tapering the strength and frequency of medication as pain subsides.

MEMORY JOGS

Principle

The process of surgical intervention potentiates changes in both the body image and role perception of the surgical patient

Illustration of Principle

Depending on the type and involvement of surgery, a patient may be faced with significant changes in perceptions about his or her physical appearance, attractiveness and desirability, and concepts of gender roles and work roles in employment as well as in a family structure. A patient with bowel obstruction facing the surgical creation of a temporary colostomy is confronted with changes in his or her body image, and potential anxiety over physical appearance and attractiveness. A male patient undergoing prostate surgery may feel ill at ease about exposure of his genitals to a predominantly female nursing staff. A middle-aged female could easily fear hysterectomy surgery, not only for the physical changes this surgery will cause, but also for the interruption in daily living that the postoperative convalescence will bring about. Finally, even minor surgery such as the removal of a mole may cause anxiety for a patient if there is a question about the possible malignancy of that mole tissue.

Nursing Management

The nurse caring for the surgical patient routinely should include questions in a preoperative assessment that will provide information about the patient's background, work and family roles, and perceptions of self. The nurse should anticipate typical questions the patient may have, and plan to address any concerns that most surgical patients have when facing upcoming surgery, knowledge specifically correlating to the type of surgery. For example, most surgical patients will have questions about the length of their postoperative recovery period, restrictions they may have after surgery, any dietary modifications they may need to make, and how postoperative pain will be managed. The nurse caring for the patient undergoing a total abdominal hysterectomy, then, should share with the patient preoperatively that the expected hospitalization will be approximately 4 to 6 days following surgery, during which time her diet will be advanced slowly as tolerated. The patient may expect some limitations on her physical activity (heavy housework, or stair climbing) and on sexual intercourse for a period of 4 to 6 weeks postoperatively. Pain will be managed with narcotic injections and then with oral analgesics.

Preparation of the patient in such a manner helps to decrease preoperative fears and anxieties, which should in turn make the recovery period less difficult and more predictable. Likewise, providing the patient with answers to questions will reduce the unknowns of the surgical experience and will foster greater understanding and cooperation between patient and nurse.

Principle

The ideal management of the unknowns in the surgical experience is the provision of adequate and timely preoperative patient teaching

Illustration of Principle

As discussed in the illustration of the previous principle, informational preparation of the patient undergoing surgery is a critical nursing intervention. The patient facing surgery will undergo a number of changes in normal day-to-day functioning that will be foreign or unknown to him or her. For example, the patient may have concerns about the exposure of his or her body in the surgical suite or may fear exposing himself or herself emotionally because of a loss of inhibitions under anesthesia's influence. Patients may cling to erroneous old wives' tales about medical interventions that could cause them unnecessary anxiety. If the patient believes that receiving a blood transfusion means that he is critically ill or close to death, for example, he may unnecessarily fear administration of blood products before, during, or after surgery. Informational instruction pertinent to the type of surgery and explained in simple, concise terms will help dispel misconceptions and thus reduce the patient's preoperative anxiety over the "unknowns" related to the surgical procedure.

It is presumptuous and foolhardy for the nurse to believe that patients are medically aware and enlightened, and that they thus understand the general concepts and procedures involved in their surgeries. For example, if the nurse tells the patient that he or she will be held *NPO* prior to surgery, there is an underlying belief that the patient will have an appreciation of the meaning of that abbreviation and its application to preoperative management. Because all patients are unique and have different levels of education and awareness, the nurse is wisest to evaluate the patient's level of knowledge, rather than assume that he or she possesses a set level of knowledge, no matter how simple the principles, concepts, or procedures involved.

Some predictable unknowns that can be managed effectively through adequate and timely preoperative teaching include the following:

- The need for turning, coughing, and deep breathing after surgery to mobilize lung secretions and prevent pneumonia
- The role of early ambulation in preventing complications associated with immobility (e.g., venous stasis, thrombus)
- The purpose of NPO and diet advancement orders
- The purpose and function of tubes or drains postoperatively (Penrose drain, Jackson-Pratt, IV tubing, endotracheal tube)
- Methods of pain management, including medication, positioning, and transcutaneous nerve stimulator units

MEMORY JOGS

> *T*imely and appropriate preoperative teaching is a valuable way to reduce postoperative anxieties and complications.

Reasoning Exercises: *Surgical Intervention*

1. Another nurse is preparing to assist in a surgical procedure. Which of the following actions of the nurse would require correction?
    A. Hair is tucked completely under a surgical bonnet
    B. Jeweled rings are covered by sterile gloves
    C. Scrub top is tucked into waist of the scrub pants
    D. Sterile gloves cover the wrist bands of the surgical gown

Intended Response: **B.** Because surgical patients are at risk for acquired infection, the goal of the use of surgical attire such as the gown and mask is to prevent transfer of microorganisms to the surgical patient and surrounding environment. Wearing jewelry in a surgical (sterile) environment increases the risk of microorganism transfer in a number of ways:

- The jewelry itself is contaminated with bacteria
- Jewelry increases sloughing of skin tissue due to friction
- Jewelry may cause perforation of a surgical glove

Thus, jewelry should not be worn in sterile environments, even if covered by a surgical (sterile) glove.

2. A nurse caring for a postoperative patient is performing hand washing prior to a sterile dressing change. Which of the following would be an appropriate action?
   A. Hands are held down into the bowl of the sink
   B. A circular motion is used to wash hands and wrist area
   C. Extra water droplets are shaken off hands prior to drying
   D. Both hands are dried simultaneously with one paper towel

Intended Response: **B.** Surgical intervention inherently places the patient at risk for infection; thus, hand washing for procedures requiring sterile technique assumes special importance. When performing hand washing for a sterile procedure, hands should be held up higher than the elbows so that water will run down from the cleanest surface (hands) to the most contaminated surface (elbows). Shaking of water droplets increases the risk for spread of microorganisms from the skin. Each hand should be dried with a separate towel in order to prevent transfer of microorganisms from one hand to the other. Circular motion in hand washing helps remove microorganisms mechanically.

3. While performing a sterile procedure, the nurse inadvertently drops an object needed for the procedure onto the floor. Which of the following actions should the nurse take?
   A. Use a sterile forceps to pick up the object and place it back into the sterile field
   B. Remove one sterile glove to pick up the object and place it back onto the sterile field
   C. Ask an individual assisting with the procedure to pick up the object and place it back onto the sterile field
   D. Ask an individual assisting with the procedure to replace the dropped object with a second sterile one

Intended Response: **D.** The goal of sterile technique is to eliminate to the highest degree possible the risk of transmission of microorganisms. A sterile object dropped to the floor is no longer sterile. Brought back onto the sterile field, the object may then contaminate all other objects on the field, and defeat the purpose of sterile technique.

4. Which of the following steps should be taken **first** by a nurse preparing to change a dressing on a patient's surgical wound?

    A. Wash hands

    B. Apply gloves to hands

    C. Open all dressing packages and kits

    D. Pour into containers fluids needed to cleanse wound

Intended Response: **A.** An intact skin layer is the body's first defense against infection. Because a surgical wound opens the body to potential infection, hand washing is especially important. Hand washing remains one of the most effective mechanisms in the prevention of transmission of microorganisms.

5. A patient who has developed postoperative pneumonia has congested respirations and needs to be suctioned. When performing nasopharyngeal suctioning, the nurse should wear which barrier protection?

    A. Sterile gloves; mask and goggles

    B. Sterile gown and mask

    C. Nonsterile gloves and goggles

    D. Particulate respirator (HEPA) mask

Intended Response: **A.** Because the lower respiratory tract is considered sterile, suctioning of the respiratory tract is a sterile procedure, requiring sterile gloves. A mask and goggles should be worn to protect the nurse from potential exposure to a spray of secretions from the respiratory tract. A particulate respirator mask would only be needed if the patient were diagnosed with tuberculin disease.

6. Which of the following changes in the lab values of a patient postoperative from colon resection would alert the nurse to the probability of infection?

    A. Increase in red blood cells above normal range

    B. Decrease in hemoglobin below normal range

    C. Increase in white blood cells above normal range

    D. Decrease in platelets below normal range

Intended Response: **C.** Because white blood cells are immune bodies, an increase in the white blood cell count above normal range suggests the presence of infection. Red blood cells are hemoglobin function in oxygen transport. Platelets are associated with clotting.

7. The nurse monitoring a postoperative patient for development of hypovolemic shock should assess for a **decrease** in which of the following vital signs?

   A. Temperature

   B. Pulse

   C. Respirations

   D. Blood pressure

Intended Response: **D.** In early stage hypovolemic shock, compensatory mechanisms are activated in the body's effort to maintain homeostasis. Both respiratory and pulse rates increase in order to enhance cellular oxygenation. Blood pressure begins to fall as less circulating fluid volume exerts less pressure on the arterial walls. Changes in temperature are not associated with hypovolemic shock.

8. An elderly patient recovering from open reduction of an ankle fracture has been receiving Tylenol #3 three to four times daily for the past two days. Which of the following assessments of the patient would alert the nurse to a side effect of this narcotic medication?

   A. Firm, round, and distended abdomen

   B. Excessive thirst and polyuria

   C. Edema and tenderness of lower extremities

   D. Excessive itching and diffuse rash

Intended Response: **A.** A common side effect of any narcotic medication is decreased peristalsis and constipation, indicated by firmness and distention of the abdomen. Excessive itching and rash would indicate an allergic reaction to the medication—not an expected side effect. Neither fluid deficit (thirst) nor fluid excess (edema) is associated with narcotics as central nervous system depressants.

9. Which of the following assessments of a postoperative patient's lower right extremity would alert the nurse to a possibility of thrombophlebitis?

   A. Diminished or absent pulse

   B. Delayed capillary refill

   C. Localized redness, swelling, and warmth

   D. Paresthesia

Intended Response: **C.** The suffix "itis" relates to inflammatory processes, indicated by the classic clinical signs of redness, warmth, swelling, pain, and loss of function.

10. Another nurse is reinforcing teaching of a patient on the second post surgical day following mastectomy. Which of the following instructions would require **correction?**

    A. Coughing and deep breathing every two hours

    B. Maintaining head of bed in semi-Fowler's position

    C. Elevating affected arm on pillows

    D. Anticipating clear serous drainage in surgical Hemovac

Intended Response: **D.** Drainage in the surgical Hemovac would likely be sanguineous (deep red) or serosanguineous (reddish-pink) and not clear serous. If the patient were expecting a clear drainage, the presence of a deep red drainage in her Hemovac drain would likely cause her undue alarm and concern. Responses **A, B,** and **C** are appropriate interventions to prevent postoperative complications. Response **A** serves to decrease the risk of stasis pneumonia, response **B** to enhance ventilation capacity and lung expansion, and response **C** to reduce postoperative edema in the affected extremity.

24

Comfort

LESLIE RITTENMEYER

Principle

Pain is a subjective human experience. The meaning and interpretation of the pain experience is highly individualized. Pain cannot be objectively measured

Illustration of Principle

No two people experience pain exactly alike. The concept of pain is often difficult to communicate clearly because the interpretation of another's pain is often vulnerable to preconceived judgments and value systems. The only person who can adequately describe his or her own pain experience is the individual experiencing the pain.

> *P*ain is whatever the experiencing person says it is, existing whenever he or she says it does (McCaffery, M. 1979, p. 11).

WINNING THOUGHTS

> *I*t is of vital importance that nurses understand the individualized nature of the pain experience and provide nursing care that reflects that understanding.

MEMORY JOGS

Principle

Pain is a complicated process involving physiological, psychological, and behavioral responses

Illustration of Principle

Dealing with pain requires energy. The physiological responses to pain occur either to provide that energy or they occur as a result of the prolonged stress caused by pain. Pain of low or moderate intensity causes sympathetic stimulation, and severe, prolonged pain results in parasympathetic stimulation.

Sympathetic Responses

- Respirations increase to provide greater O_2 intake
- Heart rate increases to provide greater O_2 transportation
- Blood pressure (BP) elevates in order to shift blood supply to the skeletal muscles and brain
- Muscle tension increases in order to prepare muscles for action
- Diaphoresis occurs to control body temperature during stress
- Blood glucose level increases in order to provide additional energy
- Gastrointestinal motility decreases to free energy

Parasympathetic Responses

- Increased muscle tension results from fatigue
- Decreased heart rate and BP results from vagal stimulation
- Rapid, irregular respirations result from the prolonged stress of pain
- Nausea and vomiting result from return of GI function
- Weakness is caused by depletion of physiological resources

A myriad of factors influence the physiological responses caused by the pain experience. An individual's previous experiences with pain, sociocultural background, age, and degree of health all influence the physiological response.

MEMORY JOGS

Psychological responses often tend to intensify the pain experience.

Common Psychological Responses

- Fear
- Anxiety
- Frustration
- Anger
- Hostility
- Feelings of powerlessness and hopelessness
- Restlessness
- Withdrawal
- Stoicism
- Depression

> *A* wide variety of behaviors can be seen as responses to pain. These responses vary from individual to individual. The nurse can use the richness found in these individual behaviors to assist in understanding how his or her client is experiencing pain.

MEMORY JOGS

Principle
The experience of pain is often a lonely, frightening experience

Illustration of Principle

Clients are frequently frightened by the experience of pain. It is not unusual for individuals to have difficulty describing their pain to others, which makes them vulnerable to developing feelings of loneliness and isolation. The fact that hospitalization takes them away from family and familiar environments adds to this problem. When a client is forced to depend on strangers to control the environment and the outcome of events, he or she often feels an acute loss of personal autonomy. How each individual client copes with this experience depends on the available resources he or she brings to the situation. If there is evidence that the client has a limited repertoire of coping skills, the nurse can be invaluable in helping him or her develop new coping strategies.

**MEMORY
JOGS**

> *I*t is most important that the client in pain feels understood and trusts that the nurse can competently work with him or her to influence outcomes.

Principle

Nurses have an ethical and legal responsibility to provide safe, effective pain relief.

Illustration of Principle

Clients have a right to expert, effective pain relief measures. Nurses have an ethical and legal responsibility to listen to their clients' statements about pain, carry out comprehensive assessments, and address problems in a timely, competent fashion. Clients also have the right to receive education about their pain. The client who is well informed is likely to display better coping behaviors than a client who is not informed.

Pain Patients' Bill of Rights

You have the right to:

- Have your pain prevented or controlled adequately
- Have your pain and pain medication history taken
- Have your pain questions answered freely
- Develop a pain plan with your doctor
- Know what medication, treatment, or anesthesia will be given
- Know the risks, benefits, and side effects of treatment
- Know what alternative pain treatments may be available
- Sign a statement of informed consent before any treatment
- Be believed when you say you have pain
- Have your pain assessed on an individual basis
- Have your pain assessed using the 0 = no pain, 10 = worst pain scale

- Ask for changes in treatments if your pain persists
- Receive compassionate and sympathetic care
- Receive pain medication on a timely basis
- Refuse treatment without prejudice from your doctor
- Seek a second opinion or request a pain care specialist
- Be given your records on request
- Include your family in decision making
- Remind those who care for you that your pain management is part of your diagnostic, medical, or surgical care (Batten, M. 1995, p. 80).

Principle

Assessment is an essential process in understanding the pain experience

Illustration of Principle

When performing a pain assessment, data are gathered about the following characteristics of pain:

- The client's description of the pain
- The duration of pain: How long has the pain been going on?
- The location of pain: Where is the pain?
- The quantity and intensity of pain; degree or amount of pain on a scale of 1–10
- The quality of pain; words client uses to describe pain
- The chronology of pain: How does the pain develop and progress?
- Aggravating factors: What makes the pain occur or get worse?
- Physiological indicators of pain; signs of sympathetic and parasympathetic stimulation
- Anxiety; evident signs of anxiety
- Behavioral responses; postural, facial, and verbal expressions, depression, withdrawal, hostility, anger, crying, moaning, and grimacing

In addition to the above characteristics, it is also important to explore the degree to which the pain interferes with the client's life, the perception of pain and its meaning to the client, the coping mechanisms that are used by the client, and the expectations the client has for pain relief.

Principle

The nature of the pain and the extent to which it is affecting the client's life will determine the type of actions taken by the nurse

Illustration of Principle

All nursing actions are aimed at assisting the client to achieve pain relief and to be able to report a sense of well-being and comfort. The nurse should employ a variety of pain relief measures, and implement strategies that complement prescribed treatments. A therapeutic relationship based on mutual trust is essential to achieve maximum pain relief. The nurse must be able to convey to clients that he or she believes the clients are the "experts" on their own pain. Mutual goal setting should occur as the client and nurse explore the client's feelings and expectations.

**MEMORY
JOGS**

A variety of nursing strategies should be employed to complement prescribed treatments.

- Control the client's environment (positioning, temperature, and noise)
- Provide pain relief measures before pain becomes severe
- Choose pain relief measures based on the severity of the pain
- Provide cutaneous stimulation (massage, warm bath, application of liniments, hot and cold therapies, or TENS)
- Use guided imagery and relaxation
- Provide music
- Provide modification of anxiety
- Use biofeedback
- Provide diversion
- Provide pharmacological therapy

> *E*ach nurse has a moral and ethical responsibility to develop and maintain a current knowledge base in all areas of pain management.

MEMORY JOGS

Principle
Evaluation is an essential component in the achievement of effective pain relief

Illustration of Principle

As pain relief measures are employed, it is necessary to implement ongoing evaluation strategies. Evaluation ensures that the mutual goals set by the nurse and the client are being achieved. The client is the best source for evaluating pain relief measures. Clients should be able to report a continued sense of well-being and comfort, as well as the perception that they are being understood and listened to. The family may also be useful in providing feedback to the nurse. If pain relief measures are ineffective, additional assessment, goal setting, intervention, and evaluation are needed.

Reasoning Exercises: *Comfort*

1. The nurse is concerned about managing the pain of a highly anxious preoperative client after he returns from surgery. Which one of the following principles best validates this concern?

   A. Clients with low pain tolerance are difficult to manage postoperatively.

   B. Psychological responses often tend to intensify the pain experience.

   C. Clients who are highly anxious tend not to report their pain honestly.

   D. Clients who are highly anxious are in greater danger of becoming dependent on pain medication than other clients.

Intended Response: **B.** Anxiety is a psychological response that tends to intensify the pain experience. None of the remaining responses are true statements.

2. The nurse is caring for a very ill postoperative client who is reporting severe pain at the incisional site. She understands that effective pain management is essential for the client's comfort, but it is also important because:

   A. Dealing with pain requires energy that would otherwise be available for healing.
   B. The nurse will have more time to do other activities.
   C. The nurse must determine whether the pain is actually present.
   D. The nurse must determine whether the pain is physiological or psychological.

Intended Response: **A.** Severe pain uses psychic and physiologic energy that might better be used for healing. Response **C** is incorrect because pain is what the individual says it is, and **D** is incorrect because it is almost impossible to differentiate between physiological and psychological variables.

3. A client shares with her nurse that she is very frightened by the thought that she will be in pain, because as a child she was badly burned and experienced severe pain. Which response by the nurse would indicate that the nurse understands the significance of this statement?

   A. "Don't worry about that. What happened way back then doesn't influence how you will respond now."
   B. "That experience will only make you stronger now."
   C. "Why don't you try to forget your past experience and deal with things as they come."
   D. "Those must be frightening memories for you. You and I can work together to handle any pain that you might have."

Intended Response: **D.** The nurse recognizes that pain is a frightening experience for some individuals, that past experiences with pain do affect how a person responds to pain, and that the client needs to feel understood. The remaining responses are incorrect because they do not take into account the individualized nature of the pain experience.

4. The nurse suspects that a client is in severe pain even though he denies it and refuses pain medications. The nurse understands that he or she may be dealing with a person who:

   A. Uses stoicism as a psychological response to pain
   B. Is angry and hostile
   C. Gets needs met by being a martyr
   D. Has a psychological need to punish himself

Intended Response: **A.** Stoicism is a common psychological response to pain, particularly in some cultures. The remaining answers are assumptions that cannot be made with this amount of information.

5. The nurse is working with a client who is complaining about pain despite the fact that he is receiving his pain medication every four hours. Which one of the following responses by the nurse would be most appropriate?
   A. "Show me the location of your pain."
   B. "On a scale of 1–10, how severe is your pain?"
   C. "This must be frustrating for you, tell me more about what you are feeling."
   D. "Do you think your pain medication should be increased?"

Intended Response: **C.** It relates to the feelings of the client and is meant to make the client feel understood. The remaining responses might help to obtain valuable assessment data, but do not deal with the individual response to pain.

6. The nurse asks a client how her pain develops and progresses. This information assesses:
   A. The quantity of pain
   B. The quality of pain
   C. The chronology of pain
   D. The duration of pain

Intended Response: **C.** How pain develops and progresses is the definition of the chronology of pain. Quantity is the degree or amount of pain. Quality refers to the words clients use to describe pain. Duration is how long the pain has been present.

7. Which one of the following actions by the nurse illustrates the principle that evaluation is an essential component in the achievement of effective pain relief?
   A. Administering pain medication to her client promptly
   B. Practicing guided imagery with her client
   C. Determining the quantity and quality of pain
   D. Returning to the client 20 minutes after pain medication has been administered to assess effectiveness

Intended Response: **D.** This nursing action evaluates the efficacy of the pain medication. The remaining answers illustrate assessment and intervention strategies.

25 Pharmacologic Intervention and Medication Dosage Calculation

KATHLEEN KICK

Principle

The first step in calculating a prescribed medication dosage is to communicate

Illustration of Principle

When we think about the process of communication, we think about the use of language in order to relay a message. Indeed, the process of calculating correct dosages of medication requires the same process—that is, the use of language. The languages used in medication administration are the three systems of weights and measures used in medical practice in the United States. Each system has unique words, symbols, and abbreviations to describe the same ideas, just as three different languages would. For example, fluid measurements of medications can be communicated in terms of drams, teaspoons, or milliliters, and can be symbolized as dr, tsp, or mL. In order to administer the correct dose of a prescribed medication, the nurse must be "fluent" in the three systems of weights and measures, or measurement languages, so that the "translation" of words and symbols used in each of the three different systems will be performed correctly.

Household System

The system of weights and measures that is probably most familiar to the American nurse is the household system, because this system is used in America to measure most food products, liquids, gasoline, and ingredients for recipes.

Key measures of the household system include the following:

Volume

teaspoon (tsp) (t)

tablespoon (tbs) (T)

cup (c)

ounce (oz)

pint (pt)

quart (qt)

gallon (gal)

drop (gtt)

Weight

pound (lb)

ounce (oz)

Amounts of medication are expressed in whole numbers and fractions, such as "2 tsp" or 1/2 tbs.

Apothecary System

Used in ancient times for the distribution of medicinal potions and treatments, its measures are foreign to Americans, and are now used exclusively in medical and pharmaceutical practice; these measures are slowly being phased out.

Key measures of the apothecary system include the following:

Volume

minim (m)

fluid dram (fl dr)

fluid ounce (fl oz)

Weight

grain (gr)

dram (dr)

Amounts of medication are expressed in terms of the Roman numeral system, either in small case or in upper case. For examples, *gr* X means 10 grains and dram ii means 2 drams. Fractions of whole numbers are expressed as such, that is, "gr 1/6" or "one sixth of a grain."

Metric System

The third and final system is also the simplest and most exact system of measurement—the metric system. This system is based on the number 10 and its multiples. For example, the prefix *milli* in milligram expresses *one-thousandth* of a gram. Fractions of whole numbers are expressed in terms of decimals in the tenths and hundredths. In this system, very small quantities of medications can be measured much more accurately than in the other two systems, because decimals are far more precise than are the fraction dosages used in the household and apothecary systems. It is the exactness, then, of the metric system that makes it the system most ideal and valuable for medical practice. It is also the system used in many other countries and it allows us to communicate in one language.

Key measures of the metric system include:

Volume

liter (L)

milliliter (mL)

cubic centimeters (cc)

Weight

kilogram (kg)

gram (Gm) (gm) (g)

milligram (mg)

microgram (mcg) (μg)

Amounts of medication are expressed in whole numbers or decimals of whole numbers, such as "1000 mL," "1.5 cc" or "0.5 mg."

The first step in calculating the correct dosage of a medication, then, is to identify which system, or "language" is being used in the medication order, compared with the language of the medication label—to communicate between what the order asks and what the medication label states.

Consider the example below:

Order: Tylenol gr × Q4 hours PRN for temp over 100 degrees F.

Label: ASA 325 mg = 1 tablet

In the example above, the nurse notes that the physician's order "Tylenol 10 grains for temperature greater than 100 degrees F" is written in the apothecary language. The medication label, however, indicates that the medication weight, milligrams, is measured in the metric language.

In this first step, then, the nurse communicates between the order and label.

Principle

*Medication calculations cannot be completed when unlike systems of measure are being used. The nurse must **convert** the units of measure used in the medication **order** to the units used on the medication **label***

Illustration of Principle

Remembering that the systems of measurement are like three different languages, the nurse must be able to translate the meanings of words and symbols used in one system to another system, so that both the **order** and the medication **label** are "speaking the same language."

Consider the sample below:

Physician order: Morphine sulfate gr 1/6 IM STAT

Medication label: Morphine sulfate 10 mg = 1.0 mL

Because the order is written in the apothecary system and the label is in the metric system, the nurse, prior to dosage calculation, must convert or translate the units of measure in the physician's order to the units of measure stated on the medication label.

In order to convert the units of measure in the physician's order from the apothecary system into the unit of measure on the medication label, the metric system, the factor labeling method of problem solving can be used.

Factor labeling uses conversion factors that change the unit of measurement from one "language" or system into another "language" or system.

Factor labeling enables the nurse to set up a problem correctly before calculating the answer. It uses conversion factors to convert one unit of measurement to another unit of measurement without changing its value.

A conversion factor is an equivalent factor that can produce a change in the form or "label" without changing its value.

In the above medication order, gr 1/6 must be converted into mg; because gr 1 is equivalent to 60 mg, we can write it in a different form, or "label" it, without changing its value. For example: gr 1 = 60 mg can be written in fraction form without changing its value.

$$\frac{\text{gr } 1}{60 \text{ mg}} \text{ or } \frac{60 \text{ mg}}{\text{gr } 1}$$

Principle
The next steps in determining the correct dosage of a medication are to set the problem up correctly and to calculate

Illustration of Principle

Once the nurse has communicated between the medication order and the label, the nurse must set the problem up in the correct fashion and then proceed to calculate the correct dosage to be administered.

In the above problem, the physician has ordered morphine sulfate gr 1/6. The medication label reads morphine sulfate 10 mg = 1.0 mL. We will need to calculate how many mL of the morphine we will administer. In order to do this calculation, we will use the **factor labeling** method of dosage calculation.

Factor labeling consists of 4 steps:

Step #1. What is the problem asking?

For example: How many tablets?

How many milliliters?

How many teaspoons, etc.?

In factor labeling, x represents the unknown number. In the above problem, we need to know how many mL are needed to administer morphine sulfate gr 1/6.

x mL = gr 1/6?

Step #2. What conversion factors are needed to solve the problem? When calculating the correct dosage, the form the drug comes in from the manufacturer is considered a conversion factor. In the above problem, the conversion factors needed are:

60 mg = 1 gr.

1.0 mL = 10 mg.

Step #3. Set up the problem so that all unwanted labels can be canceled, and you are left with only the label needed in the numerator.

$$x \text{ mL's} = \text{gr } 1/6 \times \frac{60 \text{ mg}}{\text{gr } 1} \times \frac{1.0 \text{ mL}}{60 \text{ mg}}$$

Step #4. Cancel the unwanted labels and do the required math. Multiply the numbers in the numerator, multiply the numbers in the denominator, and divide the numerator by the denominator.

$$x \text{ mL's} = \text{gr } 1/6 \times \frac{60 \text{ mg}}{\text{gr } 1} \times \frac{1.0 \text{ mL}}{10 \text{ mg}} = 1.0 \text{ mL of morphine}$$

Therefore, the calculation of correct dosage is as simple as the 3 C's—Communicate, Convert, Calculate.

Because the NCLEX examination requires mathematical conversions from one system of measurement to another from memory and without assistance from charts or conversion tables, we recommend that candidates for the examination learn the following conversion equivalents.

Volume

1 mL = 1 cc
1 dram = 5 mL = 1 tsp
15 mL = 1 tbs = 3 tsp
1 ounce = 30 mL
1 liter = 1000 mL

Weight

1 gr = 60 mg
1 gm = 1000 mg
1 mg = 1000 mcg
1 kg = 2.2 lb

Reasoning Exercises

Try to recall the equivalencies for the conversions below:

1. 1 L = _____mL

2. 2 drams = _____mL

   3. 30 mL = _____tbs

   4. 10 gr = _____mg

   5. 1 tsp = _____dr

   6. 250 mL = _____L

   7. gr 1/6 = _____mg

   8. 1 gm = _____mg

   9. 15 mL = _____oz

   10. 10 kg = _____lb

The correct responses for the above conversions are:

   1. 1000

   2. 10

   3. 2

   4. 600

   5. 1

   6. 0.25

   7. 10

   8. 1000

   9. 0.5

   10. 22

Principle

Flow rates of IV fluids may be expressed in terms of **milliliters per hour** *or* **drops per minute.**

Illustration of Principle

The mathematical calculations required to determine flow rates for IV fluids are relatively simple and can be calculated using the same **factor label** method of calculation.

Consider the example below:

Order: 1000 cc of D5W are to infuse in 8 hr. How many mL per hour are necessary to infuse this IV?

Because the nurse is aware that cubic centimeters is an equal measure for milliliters, the flow rate of milliliters per hour is easily calculated using the step method.

Remember that your answer must be in the numerator and the denominator in this case and that unwanted labels must be canceled.

Step #1. What is the problem asking? In this example, we need to know how many mL per hour are necessary to infuse 1000 mL in 8 hours.

$$\frac{x \text{ mL}}{\text{hr}} = \frac{1000 \text{ mL}}{8 \text{ hr}}$$

Step #2. What conversion factors are needed to solve the problem? Because the labels needed in the answer are already in the problem, no conversion factors are necessary.

Step #3. Set the problem up so like labels can be canceled and you are left with only the label the problem is asking for in the numerator and denominator. In this problem, the labels are already set up correctly.

$$\frac{x \text{ mL}}{\text{hr}} = \frac{1000 \text{ mL}}{8 \text{ hr}} = 125 \text{ mL per hour}$$

In order to calculate the drops per minute, two new conversion factors must be added to the equation. The drop factor, i.e., the number of drops per milliliter that the IV tubing delivers, and the number of minutes that equal 1 hour (60 minutes = 1 hour).

Step #1. What is the problem asking for? In the above problem, how many drops per minute are needed to infuse 1000 mL in 8 hours?

$$\frac{x \text{ gtt}}{\text{min}} = \frac{1000 \text{ mL}}{8 \text{ hr}}$$

Step #2. What conversion factors are needed to solve this problem?
10 gtt = 1 mL
60 minutes = 1 hour
These are the two conversion factors needed to calculate this problem.
Step #3. Set up the problem so like labels can be canceled and you are left with only the label the problem is asking for in the numerator and the denominator.

$$\frac{x \text{ gtt}}{\text{min}} = \frac{1000 \text{ mL}}{8 \text{ hr}} \times \frac{10 \text{ gtt}}{1 \text{ mL}} \times \frac{1 \text{ hr}}{60 \text{ min}}$$

Step #4. Cancel the unwanted labels and do the required math.

$$\frac{x \text{ gtt}}{\text{min}} = \frac{1000 \text{ m\!\!\!/L}}{8 \text{ h\!\!\!/r}} \times \frac{100 \text{ gtt}}{1 \text{ m\!\!\!/L}} \times \frac{1 \text{ h\!\!\!/r}}{60 \text{ min}} = 20.8 \text{ gtt/min} = 21 \text{ drops/min}$$

Because 0.8 of a drop is too small to measure, the number must be rounded to the nearest whole number, 21 drops/min.

Principle

When a set dosage of medication is added to IV fluids, the flow rate should be calculated in terms of the amount of medication infused rather than the amount of IV fluids infused

Illustration of Principle

A physician may order a client to receive a set concentration or dosage of medication by IV drip route; this requires that the nurse focus attention on the amount of medication infusing per hour or per minute, rather than the amount of IV fluids infusing.

Consider the example below:

The physician has ordered a client to receive a total dosage of 20,000 units of heparin in 500 mL of IV fluid. The client is to receive 1000 units/hr. The drop factor is 10 drops per milliliter. How many drops per minute will the client receive?

We can determine the drops per minute for this problem by using the **factor labeling** method.

Step #1. What is the problem asking for? How many drops are necessary per minute to infuse heparin at 1000 units per hour?

$$\frac{x \text{ gtt}}{\text{min}} = \frac{1000 \text{ U}}{\text{hr}}$$

Step #2. What conversion factors are needed?
20,000 units of heparin in 500 mL of fluid
10 drops = 1 mL
60 minutes = 1 hour
Step #3. Set up the problem so like labels can be canceled and you are left with only the label the problem is asking for in the numerator and denominator.

$$\frac{x \text{ gtt}}{\text{min}} = \frac{1000 \text{ U}}{1 \text{ hr}} \times \frac{500 \text{ mL}}{20,000 \text{ U}} \times \frac{10 \text{ gtt}}{1 \text{ mL}} \times \frac{1 \text{ hr}}{60 \text{ min}}$$

Step #4. Cancel the unwanted labels and do the required math.

$$\frac{x \text{ gtt}}{\text{min}} = \frac{1000 \cancel{\text{ U}}}{1 \cancel{\text{ hr}}} \times \frac{500 \cancel{\text{ mL}}}{20,000 \cancel{\text{ U}}} \times \frac{10 \text{ gtt}}{1 \cancel{\text{ mL}}} \times \frac{1 \cancel{\text{ hr}}}{60 \text{ min}} = 4.1 \text{ gtt/min or } 4 \text{ gtt/min}$$

Reasoning Exercises: *Pharmacologic Intervention and Medication Dosage Calculation*

Try to apply the principles for medication and IV fluid calculations in the reasoning exercises below.

1. The physician has ordered the patient to receive Atropine, gr 1/150 preoperatively. The label indicates that atropine 0.4 mg = 1 mL. How many mL should the nurse administer?

    A. 0.5 mL

    B. 0.8 mL

    C. 1.0 mL

    D. 1.2 mL

    Intended response: **C.** Because the medication order is in the apothecary system and the label is in the metric system, a conversion of order to label is necessary in this situation.

    $$x \text{ mL} = \text{gr } 1/150 \times \frac{60 \text{ mg}}{1 \text{ gr}} \times \frac{1 \text{ mL}}{0.4 \text{ mg}} = .99 \text{ or } 1 \text{ mL}$$

2. Mr. Davis is to receive phenobarbital gr 1 ss PO BID. The label reads phenobarbital 100 mg = 10 mL. How many mL should the nurse administer per dose?

    A. 5 mL

B. 7 mL

C. 9 mL

D. 11 mL

Intended Response: **C.** Again, a conversion from the apothecary system to the metric system is required before a calculation of dosage can be completed.

gr 1 ss = gr 1 1/2, because the symbol "ss" stands for "half" in the apothecary system.

$$x \text{ mL} = \text{gr } 1 \ 1/2 \times \frac{60 \text{ mg}}{1 \text{ gr}} \times \frac{10 \text{ mL}}{100 \text{ mg}} + 9\text{mL}$$

3. If a multidose vial of heparin contains 20,000 units in 10 mL, how many mL should the nurse administer to a patient who requires a 5000 unit dose?

A. 2.0 mL

B. 2.5 mL

C. 3.0 mL

D. 3.5 mL

Intended Response: **B.** Because both the order and the label are written in the same system (units), a conversion from one system to another is not necessary.

$$x \text{ mL} = 5000 \text{ U} \times \frac{10 \text{ mL}}{20,000 \text{ U}} = 2.5 \text{ mL}$$

4. One liter of IV fluid is to infuse in 8 hours. The drop factor of the IV equipment is 10 drops/mL. How many drops per minute will the IV infuse?

A. 16 drops/min

B. 19 drops/min

C. 21 drops/min

D. 23 drops/min

Intended Response: **C.**

$$\frac{x \text{ gtt}}{\text{min}} = \frac{1 \text{ L}}{8 \text{ hr}} \times \frac{1000 \text{ mL}}{1 \text{ L}} \times \frac{10 \text{ gtt}}{1 \text{ mL}} \times \frac{1 \text{ hr}}{60 \text{ min}} = 20.8 \text{ gtt/min or } 21 \text{ gtt/min}$$

5. The physician orders 1 gm of lidocaine in 500 mL 5% D/W to infuse at 4 mg/min per pump. How many mL/hr should the patient receive?

A. 80 mL/hr

B. 100 mL/hr

C. 120 mL/hr

D. 140 mL/hr

Intended Response: **C.**

$$\frac{x\text{ mL}}{\text{hr}} = \frac{4\text{ mg}}{\text{min}} \times \frac{500\text{ mL}}{1\text{ gm}} \times \frac{1\text{ gm}}{1000\text{ mg}} \times \frac{60\text{ min}}{1\text{ hr}} = 120\text{ mL/hr}$$

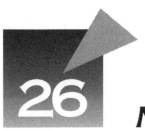

26 *Nutrition*

DIANE BLACK

Principle

Carbohydrates are the human body's fuel source

Illustration of Principle

Much as a car needs gasoline to run, the human body needs carbohydrates to carry out its functions. Carbohydrates are needed for the following functions:

Energy source

Cellular nutrition

Maintaining body temperature

Sparing use of proteins and fats

Promoting lower GI functioning

Maintaining blood glucose levels

When a car increases its speed, its gasoline requirements are greatly increased. Likewise, the human body needs carbohydrates in increased amounts in the presence of fever, hyperthyroidism, excessive exercise, and pregnancy. When the body does not receive an adequate supply of carbohydrates, it must use other sources, such as proteins and fats, resulting in a loss of weight.

*C*arbohydrates are the most readily usable form of energy for body metabolism.

MEMORY JOGS

Sugars, starches, and fiber are the main forms in which carbohydrates occur in food. Sugars and starches are the main source of energy for the body. Food sources of starches are plant foods, vegetables, breads, cereals, and grains.

Examples include:

Potatoes

Macaroni

Rice

Food sources of sugars are fruits.
Examples include:

Honey

Molasses

Grapefruit

Apples

Fiber, another plant component that is a carbohydrate, does not furnish energy but is needed for lower GI functioning.

Carbohydrate deficiency is manifested clinically as a loss of weight, with protein sources being used for energy as fats are broken down to produce a state of ketosis. Prolonged carbohydrate deficiencies can lead to liver damage. Decreased fiber in the diet can lead to constipation and diverticulosis, and may increase the occurrence of hemorrhoids, varicose veins, and hiatal hernias by increasing pressure in the colon.

Clients that present with carbohydrate deficiency may be anorexic or bulimic.

Clinical manifestations of the overconsumption of carbohydrates are the opposite of those of carbohydrate deficiency. Excessive intake of starches and sugars can lead to obesity and dental caries.

Other clients at risk for impaired carbohydrate metabolism are clients with diabetes mellitus, an illness in which carbohydrates are not metabolized because of a deficiency in insulin production by the pancreas.

Principle
Proteins are the building blocks of the body, which break down into amino acids

Illustration of Principle

Proteins are the fundamental components of cells, much as a brick is the fundamental block of a building. The body is constantly under construction—with new cell and tissue production. Therefore, the body requires protein throughout the lifespan, and particularly during periods of rapid growth (e.g., pregnancy [baby under construction], and infancy to young adulthood).

Proteins are present in the human body in a number of forms, and perform various functions. One type of protein is an enzyme. Enzymes are proteins that break down other proteins. Another type of protein, albumin, helps maintain fluid balance in the body. Antibodies are proteins, as are hormones such as thyroid and insulin. Proteins known as lipoproteins act as transport mechanisms. One important protein is collagen, which helps develop scar tissue.

MEMORY JOGS

> *P*roteins are the major nutrients for cellular and tissue growth and repair.

It is important to remember that when increased proteins are needed for tissue repair, increased carbohydrates are required to meet the body's energy needs and thus spare the protein for tissue repair.

Protein sources containing essential amino acids are those foods of high biological value, such as eggs, milk and dairy products, meat, fish, and poultry.

The client who lacks protein in the diet in sufficient amounts will appear weak and apathetic, with poor fat stores under the skin. The skin may appear patchy and scaly, the hair loses its color, and wounds fail to heal.

Proteins are lost in the drainage of open wounds and in urine. Increased protein intake is needed to promote tissue growth and repair when damage or injury occurs in the body (e.g., decubitus ulcers, surgery, and preeclampsia). Protein is also needed when bodies are in states of catabolism, such as in clients with anorexia, cachexia, or malnutrition (kwashiorkor and marasmus).

On the other hand, protein is not needed when the by-products of protein metabolism (nitrogen) cannot be excreted or used, as in renal failure (urea cannot be excreted) and cirrhosis of the liver (nitrogen binds with hydrogen to form ammonia, leading to hepatic encephalopathy).

Principle
Fats are the body's fuel and energy storage systems and its "cushions" for protection

Illustration of Principle

Much like a gas station, which stores gasoline until it is pumped into cars, fats are the repository of fuel for the human body. Excess carbohydrates are turned into fats and stored for later use. Fats are also protein-sparing, which means they reduce the need to use protein for energy. Fat has several other functions, such as maintaining body temperature by acting as insulation, cushioning vital organs, and facilitating absorption of the fat-soluble vitamins A, D, E, and K.

MEMORY JOGS

> *F*ats are stored forms of energy that need carbohydrates for complete oxidation.

Fats are also classified as lipids. Those that are liquid are considered oils, while those that are solid are considered fats, which break down into triglycerides and fatty acids. Fatty acids are classified as saturated or unsaturated. Saturated fatty acids tend to be solid at room temperature (i.e., a steak left on a table will begin to show white patches of fat as it reaches room temperature). Thus, animals are the greatest source of saturated fat.

The following are examples of saturated fats:

Beef

Pork

Poultry

Milk and milk products

Butter

Ice cream

Egg yolk

Unsaturated fats do not solidify at room temperature. Vegetable oils are largely unsaturated fats. Examples of unsaturated fats are:

Safflower oil

Corn oil

Soybean oil

Essential fatty acids are needed by the body for normal nutrition but cannot be synthesized.

Cholesterol is a fat-soluble substance that is synthesized and stored in the liver. It is found in the blood and serves as a transporter of fat and a producer of vitamin D and hormones. Sources of cholesterol are egg yolk and animal brain. Other sources include butter, cream, cheese, and organ meats (liver, heart, and kidney).

If there is inadequate fat in the body, there is no fuel for energy, no cushion, and no insulation. For example, a premature infant cannot regulate body temperature or meet the body's energy demands. Consequently, the infant is put under a radiant heater for thermoregulation and given high-calorie nutrition intravenously to meet energy demands.

On the other hand, too much intake of fat in the form of triglycerides and cholesterol can lead to obesity and various problems, such as atherosclerosis, leading to myocardial infarction, cerebrovascular accident, peripheral vascular disease, or rupture of an artery.

Other clients at risk with the intake of fats would include those with gallbladder dysfunction or pancreatitis. Bile is produced in the liver and stored in the gallbladder. Bile aids in emulsifying fats or breaking down fats into small particles for digestion and absorption. Thus, if the common bile duct is blocked or liver disease is present, the client must restrict the intake of fat. If such a client eats fat, digestion is blocked, but the client's hunger is satiated. Fat is then excreted as fatty acids along with vitamins A, D, E, and K. Therefore, this type of client needs supplementary intake of fat-soluble vitamins with an increased intake of carbohydrates.

Principle

Vitamins are nutrients necessary for life and growth processes. Vitamins facilitate the use of energy nutrients, the regulation of some body functions, and the maintenance of body structures. Vitamins are classified as either fat-soluble or water-soluble

Illustration of Principle

The fat-soluble vitamins are vitamins A, D, E, and K. These vitamins are soluble in fats and are absorbed from the intestinal tract in much the same way as fats.

> *B*ile is needed to emulsify fats; therefore, bile is necessary for absorption of fat-soluble vitamins.

MEMORY JOGS

These vitamins are stored in the body, mostly in the liver. Each vitamin has its own food sources, function, and symptoms of deficiency.

Vitamin A aids in the adaptation of vision to dim light, maintenance of skin and mucous membranes, and the formation of bones and teeth. Food sources high in vitamin A include yellow carotene foods and green leafy vegetables. Other sources are fish liver oil and animal liver. A deficiency of vitamin A can lead to night blindness and lowered resistance to infection.

Vitamin D aids in the absorption and mobilization of calcium for the development and maintenance of bones and teeth.

MEMORY JOGS

> *V*itamin D is called the "sunshine vitamin."

Fortified milk is a food source rich in vitamin D. A diet deficient in this vitamin will parallel a deficiency of calcium, leading to rickets and osteomalacia.

The functions of vitamin E are to protect vitamin A from oxidation in the intestines and to guard the red blood cells from hemolysis. Vitamin E also increases the structural integrity of the cell membrane. Food sources include whole grains, nuts, and salad oils. A deficiency can lead to increased hemolysis of red blood cells.

Vitamin K, the blood-clotting vitamin, is needed for the formation of prothrombin. Food sources include green leafy vegetables. Vitamin K can also be synthesized by intestinal bacteria. A deficiency of this vitamin can lead to hemorrhage from lack of prothrombin.

MEMORY JOGS

> *V*itamin K injections are routinely given to newborns to enhance prothrombin production and prevent hemorrhagic disorders.

Clients who develop problems with fat absorption will also develop problems associated with fat-soluble vitamin depletion. Cholelithiasis with blocked ducts inhibits bile use, continued intake of mineral oil prevents absorption of nutrients, and celiac diseases prevent fat absorption. Clients who develop steatorrheic stools eventually will manifest signs and symptoms of fat-soluble vitamin deficiencies.

MEMORY JOGS

> *A*ny interference with fat absorption in the GI tract will also interfere with the absorption of fat-soluble vitamins.

Illustration of Principle

Water-soluble vitamins are the B and C complex vitamins. These vitamins are soluble in water and absorbed in the small intestines. Once the body has attained maximum saturation, the excess is excreted in the urine.

Vitamin C, also known as ascorbic acid, has a significant role in the formation of collagen. It also functions in the metabolism of amino acids, the absorption of iron, and the conversion of folatin to folinic acid.

> *V*itamin C is needed in increased amounts during growth phases and in tissue healing.

Vitamin C is found in citrus fruits such as strawberries, oranges, and grapefruits. Dark green leafy vegetables are also high in vitamin C.

A deficiency of ascorbic acid can result in scurvy, a disease characterized by easy bruising, sore mouth and gums, and joint tenderness due to the disruption of cartilage.

Vitamin B complex includes 12 fractions, the major ones being thiamine, riboflavin, niacin, B_{12}, folacin, pantothenic acid, and biotin. The major function of these vitamins is to aid in metabolism to provide energy (Table 26–1).

Table 26-1. Vitamin B complex

Vitamin	Food Sources	Deficiency
Thiamine	Dry yeast, wheat germ, pork, enriched bread	Beriberi (nervous system manifestations)
Riboflavin	Organ meats, green leafy vegetables	Cheilosis (scaly skin, cracked lips)
Niacin	Meat, poultry, fish, enriched products	Pellagra (dermatitis)
B_6 (pyridoxine)	Organ meats, legumes, nuts	CNS abnormalities
B_{12}	Organ meats, milk, fish	Pernicious anemia (lack of intrinsic factor)
Pantothenic acid	Organ meats, eggs, yeast	
Folacin	Green leafy vegetables	Macrocytic anemia
Biotin	Organ meats, peanuts	Anemia

Alcoholism, prolonged fasting (anorexia), and gastric carcinoma predispose clients to water-soluble vitamin deficiencies.

Reasoning Exercises: *Nutrition*

1. Which of the following vitamins would be most essential to effect healing of multiple decubitus ulcers in an immobilized patient?

   A. Vitamin A

   B. Vitamin C

   C. Vitamin D

   D. Vitamin K

   Intended Response: **B.** Vitamin C is needed in increased amounts to effect tissue healing. Vitamin A also affects skin condition, but not as significantly as Vitamin C.

   Vitamin D is needed for skeletal integrity. Vitamin K is essential for normal clotting processes.

2. Which of the following would decrease the need for carbohydrates as a fuel source for body cells?

   A. Rest and sleep

   B. Stress

   C. Infection and fever

   D. Sexual activity

   Intended Response: **A.** The metabolic rate of the body decreases during rest and sleep, causing a decreased need for fuel for the cells. Factors that increase metabolic rate, such as responses **B, C,** and **D,** cause an increased need for fuel, demanding an increased carbohydrate metabolism to provide cellular energy.

3. To help maintain a patient's bowel regularity, the nurse should encourage an increased intake of fluid and which of the following?

   A. Fiber

   B. Protein

   C. Iron

   D. Fat

   Intended Response: **A.** Foods rich in fiber, such as fresh vegetables and fruits, aid in forming the bulk of the stool and in stimulating bowel evacuation. Fluids are increased if possible to keep stool softer and easier to pass in a bowel movement.

4. Deficiency of which of the following would correlate most to a compromised immune response?

    A. Fat

    B. Carbohydrate

    C. Protein

    D. Fiber

Intended Response: **C.** Antibodies, the cells of the immune response, are proteins. Deficient protein intake, then, could result in compromised immunity. Although deficiencies in other nutrients, such as carbohydrates, could cause malnutrition associated with impaired immunity, inadequate protein is more significant to altered immune function.

5. The nurse would likely restrict protein intake for which of the following patients?

    A. An elderly patient with stasis ulcers on heels and ankles

    B. A teenage patient recovering from abdominal surgery

    C. A middle-aged patient with advanced cirrhosis of the liver

    D. An adult patient hospitalized for exacerbation of COPD

Intended Response: **C.** Persons with liver failure require restriction of protein intake because nitrogen by-products of protein metabolism form ammonia, a toxin to the neuromuscular system. Patients in responses **A** and **B** would require increased protein intake to effect healing. The patient in response **D** would benefit from increased protein intake to enhance general nutritional status.

6. A nurse is providing dietary modification instructions to a patient with gallbladder dysfunction. The nurse should advise the patient to avoid which of the following foods?

    A. Citrus fruits

    B. Breads and cereals

    C. Dairy products

    D. Green leafy vegetables

Intended Response: **C.** Persons with gallbladder disease may experience significant pain or difficulty in digestion with dietary intake of fats. All remaining foods are acceptable in this patient's diet.

7. Which of the following is a concern for persons whose gallbladder dysfunction causes impaired metabolism of fats and fat-soluble vitamins?

    A. Potential for bleeding
    B. Increased risk for infection
    C. Potential for delayed healing
    D. Increased risk for thrombus

Intended Response: **A.** Patients who develop problems with fat absorption will also develop problems associated with fat-soluble vitamin depletion. Gallbladder dysfunction may lead to impaired absorption of vitamin K, a fat-soluble vitamin. Because vitamin K is essential in clotting processes, a depletion of vitamin K causes potential for bleeding.

8. The clinic nurse is developing a plan of care for a patient with calcium and vitamin D deficiencies. Which of the following nursing diagnoses should be given priority?

    A. Fatigue
    B. High risk for infection
    C. Constipation
    D. High risk for injury

Intended Response: **D.** Deficiencies in calcium and vitamin D render bone more fragile, placing the patient at risk for pathologic (spontaneous) fracture. Fatigue may be associated with the deficiency of iron, because iron is essential in the formation of oxygen-carrying hemoglobin and red blood cells. An increased risk of infection may be associated with deficiency in protein and/or vitamin C. Constipation may be associated with deficient intake of fluid and fiber.

Comprehensive Examination

LEAD ITEM WRITER: *Nancy Korchek*

CONTRIBUTORS: *Diane Black, Ann Filipski, Karen Gousman, Patti Hughes, Kimberly Jezek-Tisch, Barbara Murphy, Lori Pacura, Scott Sabbish, Marry Williams*

EDITOR: *Marian B. Sides*

1. The nurse is caring for an elderly patient receiving an IVPB nephrotoxic antibiotic for treatment of sepsis. Which of the following laboratory values should the nurse monitor more closely?

    A. RBC and platelet count

    B. Serum sodium and potassium

    C. BUN and serum acetone

    D. Creatinine and creatinine clearance

2. A patient c/o persistent cough, low grade fever, and night sweats is to be transferred from an outpatient clinic to the hospital for admission. The admission diagnosis is suspected active tuberculosis. The admitting nurse should plan to place this patient in which of the following?

    A. Semi-private room, contact isolation

    B. Enteric precautions

    C. Private room, AFB isolation

    D. Respiratory precautions

3. A patient newly admitted to the emergency room with multiple internal injuries following a motor vehicle accident is to be monitored for evidence of internal bleeding and possible hypovolemic shock. Which of the following clinical manifestations would be most significant?

    A. Patient c/o severe pain in lower chest and abdomen

    B. Decrease in blood pressure from 102/58 to 88/40

    C. Patient c/o increasing lightheadedness and weakness

    D. Increase in pulse rate from 68 to 80 beats per minute

4. A patient in early stage hypovolemic shock is hyperventilating with a respiratory rate of 38 bpm. Which of the following nursing actions is indicated for this patient?

    A. Place the patient in semi-Fowler's to sitting position

    B. Administer oxygen per nasal cannula at 2–3 L/min

    C. Instruct the patient to cough and deep breathe at frequent intervals

    D. Request a physician's order for sedative medication

5. Which of the following clinical manifestations could increase a patient's risk for the development of respiratory acidosis?

    A. Repeated episodes of vomiting

    B. Crackles auscultated in lower lung fields bilaterally

    C. Acute pain in the lower abdomen and pelvis

    D. Rapid and deep "blowing" respirations

6. A patient with chronic obstructive pulmonary disease had the following ABG values upon admission:

    ph 7.27; pco_2 66 mEq/L; HCO_2 27 mEq/L; po_2 74

    Which of the following changes in blood gas values would indicate to the nurse that management of the patient's acid–base imbalance has been effective?

    A. pco_2 increased

    B. Hco_2 decreased

    C. pH increased

    D. po_2 decreased

7. A physician has written the following order for a patient who is hyperventilating during an acute anxiety attack:

    Valium 5 mg PO STAT and PRN for anxiety/agitation

    The nurse should clarify this order with the physician based upon which of the following?

    A. Valium as a narcotic analgesic is contraindicated for anxiety management

    B. The frequency for administration of the medication is not specified

    C. The abbreviation mg could stand for either milligrams or micrograms

    D. The dosage of the medication is not specified

8. A newly admitted elderly patient is scheduled for a stat magnetic resonance image (MRI) examination. Which of the following questions should the nurse ask the patient prior to this diagnostic testing?

   A. "Are you allergic to shellfish?"

   B. "Do you have a history of high blood pressure?"

   C. "When was the last time you had anything to eat or drink?"

   D. "Have you had joint replacement surgery in the past?"

9. The clinic nurse notes a patient's most recent hemoglobin value is 8.6 g/dL. The nurse should seek further information from the patient concerning which of the following?

   A. Easy or unexplained bruising

   B. Fatigue and shortness of breath on exertion

   C. Periodic cramping pain in the lower extremities

   D. Recurrent infections or low grade fevers

10. Which of the following is of priority in the care of a patient immediate post-procedure following sternal bone marrow aspiration?

    A. Administration of analgesia

    B. Application of pressure at the puncture site

    C. Frequent assessment of vital signs

    D. Placement of patient in high-Fowler's position

11. A patient is to receive a transfusion of two units of packed red blood cells. During the administration of the transfusion, the nurse should monitor the patient for which of the following?

    A. Oliguria

    B. Hemoptysis

    C. Urticaria

    D. Ecchymosis

12. While performing a sterile procedure, the nurse inadvertently drops an object needed for the procedure onto the floor. Which of the following actions should the nurse take?

    A. Use a sterile forceps to pick up the object and place it back onto the sterile field

    B. Remove one sterile glove to pick up the object and place it back onto the sterile field

C. Ask an individual assisting with the procedure to pick up the object and place it back on the sterile field

D. Ask an individual assisting with the procedure to replace the dropped object with a second sterile one

13. Which of the following elements of a urine analysis should be monitored by the nurse to determine changes in the fluid status of a patient hospitalized with fluid volume deficit?

A. Ketones

B. Specific gravity

C. Occult blood

D. Culture

14. Which of the following urine laboratory test values would provide the most valuable information to the nurse caring for a patient complaining of urinary frequency, urgency, and dysuria?

A. Ketones

B. Specific gravity

C. Occult blood

D. Culture

15. Which of the following interventions should the nurse include in a plan of care for a patient with renal insufficiency?

A. Push oral fluids

B. Assess blood pressure q 8 hours

C. Monitor strict intake and output

D. Assess body weight weekly

16. A nurse has included all of the following interventions in a plan of care for a patient with increased intracranial pressure secondary to closed head injury. Which intervention would require correction?

A. Maintain dim lighting in the patient's room

B. Limit painful or noxious stimuli to the patient

C. Maintain the head of the bed at a 45 degree angle

D. Monitor and restrict fluid intake

17. Which of the following nursing diagnoses would be of priority for a patient newly diagnosed with Parkinson's disease?

A. High Risk for Injury

    B. Impaired Verbal Communication

    C. Self Care Deficit

    D. Ineffective Individual Coping

18. The nurse notes that a patient's continuous cardiac monitor indicated ventricular tachycardia (VT). Upon arriving at the patient's bedside, which action should the nurse take first?

    A. Position the patient supine with head of bed flat

    B. Prepare an immediate administration of atropine

    C. Assess the patient's carotid pulse

    D. Secure a manual resuscitation (Ambu) bag at bedside

19. A patient having continuous cardiac monitoring demonstrates the following 6 second ECG monitor pattern

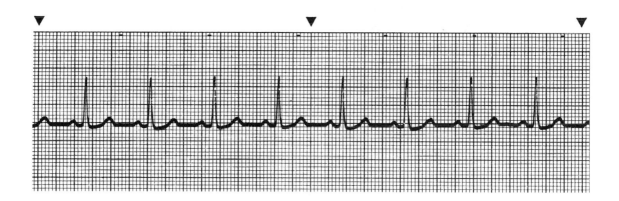

    Which of the following actions should the nurse take related to the patient's cardiac monitor pattern?

    A. Record the monitor strip in the patient's chart

    B. Position the patient on his left side

    C. Prepare an intravenous administration of atropine

    D. Activate the EMS and initiate CPR

20. Which of the following patients should the nurse identify as at risk for the development of hypokalemia?

    A. A patient whose urinary output is averaging 500 mL/24 hours

    B. A patient with lactose intolerance

C. A patient receiving loop diuretic therapy for fluid volume excess

D. A patient maintaining a low fat, low cholesterol diet

21. A patient who will remain NPO for several days following colon resection is ordered to receive potassium supplements IV drip. Prior to initiating an administration of potassium, the nurse should assess which of the following clinical parameters?

    A. Level of consciousness

    B. Urinary output

    C. Blood pressure

    D. Lung sounds

22. The nurse performing glucose monitoring notes that a patient's glucose reading is 48 mg/dL. Which of the following should the nurse administer to this patient?

    A. Apple juice

    B. 2 or 3 cookies

    C. A slice of toast

    D. 2 or 3 saltine crackers

23. The nurse has admitted a patient diagnosed in acute diabetic ketoacidosis (DKA). Which of the following serum lab values should the nurse most closely monitor during the treatment of diabetic ketaocidosis?

    A. Blood urea nitrogen (BUN)

    B. Potassium (K^+)

    C. Hematocrit (Hct)

    D. Sodium (Na^+)

24. Which of the following interventions should the nurse include in a plan of care for a patient with thrombocytopenia?

    A. Encourage oral fluid intake

    B. Instruct all visitors to wear a gown and mask

    C. Limit use of sharps

    D. Provide for frequent rest periods

25. The nurse is instructing a group of middle-aged women anticipating mammography as part of a cancer screening program. Which of the following instructions should the nurse provide to the group members?

    A. "You should have nothing to eat or drink after midnight before your scheduled mammogram."

B. "You should not wear deodorant or talc the day of your mammogram."

C. "An intravenous infusion will be started at a low flow rate just prior to your scheduled mammogram."

D. "You should not wear a bra or constrictive clothing for several hours following your mammogram."

26. Which of the following topics should be incorporated into a discharge teaching plan for a patient recovering from surgical implantation of a pacemaker?

A. Restriction of fluid intake to 500 mL/daily

B. Need to perform daily self-assessment of pulse

C. Restriction of sexual intercourse for 2–3 months

D. Need to perform daily measurement of urinary output

27. Which of the following prescribed interventions assumes priority in the immediate care of a patient experiencing an acute myocardial infarction (AMI)?

A. Scheduling of a 12-lead ECG

B. Administration of intravenous analgesia

C. Obtaining a blood sample for cardiac enzymes

D. Insertion of an indwelling urinary catheter

28. Which of the following clinical manifestations would suggest to the nurse that a patient recovering from acute myocardial infarction has developed left heart failure?

A. Sinus bradycardia noted on cardiac monitor

B. Distended neck veins and peripheral edema

C. Crackles noted on auscultation of lung fields

D. Polyuria and excessive thirst

29. A nurse is providing care for a patient receiving intravenous heparin therapy for treatment of a deep vein thrombosis in the left calf. Which of the actions by the nurse would require correction?

A. The nurse monitors IV heparin therapy dose with the patient's daily PTT value

B. The nurse measures the circumference of each calf with a tape measure

C. The nurse reapplies antiembolism (TED) hose after bathing the patient's lower extremities

D. The nurse assists the patient in ambulating to the bathroom

30. Which of the following nursing diagnoses assumes priority in the care of a patient with syndrome of inappropriate antidiuretic hormone (SIADH)?
    A. Body Image Disturbance
    B. Pain
    C. Fluid Volume Excess
    D. Altered Nutrition: Less Than Body Requirements

31. A clinic nurse is providing health teaching for a patient newly diagnosed with gastroesophageal reflux disease (GERD). Which of the following instructions should be discussed with the patient?
    A. Change of dietary pattern to small frequent feedings and bedtime snack
    B. Restriction of alcohol intake to two evening servings daily
    C. Use of magnesium carbonate (Gaviscon) prior to each meal
    D. Avoidance of bending, stooping, or slumping posture

32. Which of the following clinical manifestations would indicate that a patient experiencing recurrent bouts of nausea and vomiting has developed a fluid volume deficit?
    A. Full, bounding pulse
    B. Increase in blood pressure
    C. Poor skin turgor
    d. Increase in central venous pressure

33. The nurse readying a patient for surgery notes all of the following preoperative findings. Which should be reported to the patient's surgeon prior to the scheduled surgery?
    A. Oral temperature 101.2°F
    B. Serum glucose 128 mg/dL
    C. Blood pressure 136/63
    D. Serum potassium 3.8 mEq/L

34. Which of the following interventions would be beneficial in maintaining effective nutrition for a patient experiencing nausea and vomiting secondary to anticancer chemotherapy?
    A. Position the patient upright for 1–2 hours after meals
    B. Offer the patient small, frequent feedings
    C. Limit oral intake of fluids with meals
    D. Administer prescribed antiemetic medication at regular intervals

35. The nurse caring for a patient diagnosed with dysfunctional uterine bleeding should most closely monitor which of the following serum laboratory values?

  A. Sodium and potassium

  B. Red blood cells and hemoglobin

  C. Blood urea nitrogen and creatinine

  D. White blood cells and sedimentation rate

36. Which of the following nursing diagnoses should be included in a plan of care for a patient experiencing an acute exacerbation of gouty arthritis?

  A. Impaired Physical Mobility

  B. High Risk for Infection

  C. Alteration in Urinary Elimination

  D. High Risk for Altered Peripheral Perfusion

37. The nurse may conclude that skeletal traction is exerting a therapeutic effect when a patient with a fractured femur evidences which of the following findings of the affected limb?

  A. Decreased muscle spasms

  B. Increased arterial perfusion

  C. Decreased sensation to temperature and touch

  D. Increased muscle strength and mass

38. A patient recovering from open reduction of a hip fracture is suspected of having thrombophlebitis in her left calf. Which of the following clinical findings in the patient's lower left extremity would support the suspected diagnosis?

  A. Sudden onset of severe pain

  B. Absence of pedal pulse

  C. Localized redness, swelling, and warmth

  D. Increasing sensations of numbness and tingling

39. Which of the following complaints by an immobilized male patient would **most** likely suggest the possibility of renal calculi?

  A. "I feel a burning sensation when I urinate."

  B. "I noticed some blood in my urine the last time I used the urinal."

  C. "I noticed that my urine has a foul odor."

  D. "I've been feeling feverish and achy since last night."

40. A patient with a plaster of Paris cast on his right upper arm and forearm for 3 days c/o a new onset of severe pain in the casted extremity. Which of the following additional clinical findings would support a diagnosis of osteomyelitis for this patient?

A. WBC = 5000

B. Oral temperature = 101.8°F

C. Hgb = 12.4

D. Paresthesia of the right upper extremity

41. A 35-year-old woman is 28 weeks pregnant with her first child. She has been diagnosed with gestational diabetes following an abnormal 3-hour glucose tolerance test. During the patient's first visit to the diabetes and pregnancy clinic, the nurse completes a comprehensive assessment. Which of the following assessment strategies will best assist the nurse and patient in planning an appropriate diet and treatment plan?

A. Assessment of the patient's previous medical history, including family history of both preexisting and gestational diabetes

B. 24-hour diet recall by the patient, including her likes and dislikes

C. Exploring with the patient her feelings and fears about her diagnosis

D. Assessment of the patient's weight gain and estimated fetal growth

42. During a routine prenatal visit, the woman states, "My aunt told me that babies of diabetic mothers sometimes die before they are born." The nurse's best response is:

A. "That's true for women who are insulin-dependent diabetics before they become pregnant, but not for those women with gestational diabetes."

B. "There is a higher incidence of intrauterine fetal demise in diabetic pregnancies as they get close to term, so your doctor will probably induce you before your due date."

C. "If you follow your treatment plan closely and maintain your blood glucose levels in a normal range, research has shown that you have no greater chance of having your baby die before birth than any other normal, pregnant women."

D. "That's an old wives' tale. Diabetic pregnancies have no greater incidence of intrauterine fetal demise than any other pregnancy."

43. The diabetic woman receives instruction on diet and self-monitoring of blood glucose. When she returns to the clinic a week later, the nurse notes that her blood glucose results 1–2 hours after dinner have been mildly elevated. The nurse's first action should be:

A. Review the patient's diet record to see whether any of her food choices may have contributed to the post-dinner blood glucose elevations

B. Instruct the patient to take a vigorous walk for at least 1 hour after completing her evening meal

C. Inform the patient that she will need to begin insulin administration, and set up an appointment with her physician

D. Have the patient return-demonstrate her blood glucose self-monitoring technique to ensure accuracy

44. Which of the following findings indicates that a gestational diabetes treatment plan is not having the desired effect?

A. Absence of fetal lung maturity at 35 weeks, as evidenced by an amniotic fluid L/S ratio of < 2/1 and the absence of PG factor

B. Maternal weight gain of 3–5 lb/week, in the last 3 weeks of pregnancy

C. Patient's uterine fundal height measured approximately 32 cm at 32 weeks' gestation

D. Fasting blood glucose results consistently in the range of 90–100 mg/dL

45. A 28-year-old is admitted to the labor and delivery unit at 35 weeks' gestation with preeclampsia. She is started on an intravenous infusion of magnesium sulfate for seizure prophylaxis. Which of the following interventions is most important once magnesium sulfate toxicity has been identified?

A. Provide emergency equipment at the bedside, including suction, oxygen, and airway management devices (e.g., oral airway)

B. Assess patient for signs of magnesium toxicity, including respiratory depression, absence of deep tendon reflexes, and decreased level of consciousness

C. Make sure the magnesium sulfate is being administered via intravenous infusion pump

D. Administer intravenous calcium gluconate, per physician's order

46. A G1 P0 is in active labor at 5 cm dilation. Her husband is at the bedside assisting her in Lamaze breathing. The client requests medication to help her relax. Meperidine (Demerol) 25 mg is given slow IV push. With your understanding of the pharmacokinetic properties of this medication, which of the following observations would necessitate intervention due to the side effects of this medication?

A. The client complains of an urge to push

B. The fetal heart rate shows variable decelerations

C. The newborn's respirations are 24

D. The client's blood pressure has decreased below her baseline

47. A 16-year-old client has been diagnosed with pregnancy-induced hypertension. She is currently on magnesium sulfate to prevent seizures. Which of the following assessments would necessitate immediate intervention?

A. Respiration rate of 18

B. Deep tendon reflexes of +2

C. Urine output of 27 cc

D. Client's perception of warmth; client appears flushed and complains of shortness of breath

48. A 30-year-old G2 P1 requests an epidural analgesia for pain relief in the active phase of labor. Nursing care during this time includes 500–1000 cc bolus of saline solution prior to the procedure, and left lateral position after the procedure. Which of the following do these nursing interventions intend to prevent?

A. Hypertension

B. Fetal distress

C. Increased discomfort from the procedure

D. Venous stasis

49. A G4 P1 is admitted to the labor and delivery suite at 28 weeks' gestation. She has a previous history of preterm labor and is now contracting every 5 minutes. Ritodrine is infusing at 100 mcg/min per protocol. The patient is agitated and concerned about her daughter at home. What is the best response by the nurse?

A. "Your daughter is fine; you need to be concerned about this baby right now."

B. "I am sure your family will be all right. You can have your parents watch your daughter."

C. "Your daughter can come to see you."

D. "I hear that you are concerned about your daughter."

50. A client is started on Methergine (methylergonovine maleate) by mouth every four hours to control postpartum bleeding. Which of the following in the patient's intrapartum history would make this medication contraindicated?

A. History of twin gestation

    B. History of gestational diabetes

    C. History of pregnancy induced hypertension

    D. History of hypotonic labor and Pitocin (oxytocin) augmentation

51. A client calls the clinic for medication to alleviate her nasal stuffiness. Which of the following is not an appropriate intervention to suggest?

    A. Use of cool air vaporizer or humidifier

    B. Use of moist towel on the sinuses

    C. Decrease fluid intake

    D. Massage sinuses

52. A G6 P5 has just precipitously delivered a 2500-g newborn. During the initial nursing history on substance abuse, the patient denied use of cocaine and marijuana, but confided that others do use these substances while she is in the room. Which newborn assessment would make you suspicious of substance abuse during pregnancy?

    A. Short stature and smaller head circumference; muscular rigidity and increased irritability

    B. Low set ears, mongolian spotting, and subconjunctival hemorrhages

    C. Cephalohematoma, hyperactive bowel sounds, and tremors

    D. Irritability, disturbed sleep pattern, high pitched cry, and drug withdrawal

53. A new client is sent for treatment in the Driving Under the Influence (DUI) program. It is his third DUI offense. When asked why he has sought treatment, the client responds, "I had a fight with my wife. She ran out on me, and I was looking for her. The cop pulled me over so that he could get his quota of tickets for the month." The nurse recognizes that the client is using which of the following defense mechanisms?

    A. Reaction formation

    B. Rationalization

    C. Repression

    D. Sublimation

54. A schizophrenic client removes his clothes and begins pacing after a session with his therapist. The following statement by the nurse would be the most appropriate at this time.

    A. "The unit policy states that clients must be dressed appropriately at all times."

    B. "Tell me why your therapy session has made you so anxious."

C. "Let's walk to your room and see if we can find your clothes."

D. "We are going to need to place you in restraints until you can demonstrate better control."

55. The nurse has worked with her client for several days. Previously he was rather quiet and introspective. Which of the following statements indicates that the client is ready to enter the working phase of the relationship?

A. "I'm glad that you finally realize that my wife is the problem."

B. "I think that the medication is starting to help me feel better."

C. "You are my favorite nurse in this place. No one else understands me like you do."

D. "It seems that I always end up in trouble. What can I do to make sure that it doesn't happen again?"

56. Upon admission assessment, the nurse notes that the client, diagnosed with bipolar disorder, has been prescribed medications by several different physicians. In addition to lithium carbonate, the patient is receiving four other medications. Which of the following medications will raise concern on the part of the nurse because of her knowledge regarding the actions and side effects of lithium?

A. Prolixin Decanoate

B. Lasix

C. Tegretol

D. Antabuse

57. The nurse performs an assessment on a 16 y/o male client who is depressed. As she explores the client's risk for suicide, she recalls that all of the following are true except:

A. Adolescents and older white men have the highest rate of suicide

B. A previous unsuccessful suicide attempt makes future attempts unlikely

C. Giving away valued possessions can be a significant warning of suicide

D. A family history of suicide or attempts is an important factor

58. The nurse understands that it is important for the client to recognize symptoms of lithium toxicity. Client teaching will include all of the following except:

A. Ensure adequate nutrition and rest

B. Encourage exercise

C. Provide information about the plan of care

D. Limit decision making and choices in plan of care

59. A 34-year old woman is admitted with a diagnosis of Major Depression. For 3 months she has demonstrated social withdrawal, feelings of hopelessness, anorexia, insomnia, and poor concentration. The nurse will provide all of the following interventions except:

    A. Ensure adequate nutrition and rest

    B. Encourage exercise

    C. Provide information about the plan of care

    D. Limit decision making and choices in plan of care

60. A 23-year-old intermittently experiences periods of anxiety accompanied by shortness of breath, choking sensations, and a feeling that she will die. The nurse intervenes with the following strategies. Which strategy will be least effective?

    A. Teaching the client relaxation techniques

    B. Discussing the physical effects of anxiety

    C. Using a distraction technique during the next episode of anxiety by bringing the client into a more stimulating environment

    D. Helping the client link thoughts or events with anxious feelings

61. A client diagnosed with obsessive-compulsive disorder has persistent fears and worries about germs in her home and work environment. She washes her hands and cleans the bathroom fixtures for many hours each day. The client's behavior demonstrates which of the following defense mechanisms?

    A. Undoing

    B. Reaction formation

    C. Regression

    D. Displacement

62. The nurse evaluates a client with an acute schizophrenic episode, hospitalized for the first time in a short-term facility. All of the following changes may be seen prior to discharge except:

    A. An increase in reality orientation

    B. An increase in appropriateness and/or range of affect

    C. An understanding of the stressors that produce symptoms in the client

    D. An increase in social skills

63. A 4-year-old is in need of preop teaching for her upcoming ear tube surgery. The best time to do this teaching is:

A. A week or two in advance, so she has time to consider it

B. On the way into the surgery holding area

C. Never; the child is too young to understand

D. One to four hours prior to the procedure

64. A 2-year-old is given the nursing diagnosis Anxiety related to (RT) separation fears. An appropriate outcome for this child would be:

A. The child will not cry when parents leave

B. The child will not cry during nursing care

C. The child will demonstrate attachments to the nursing staff

D. The child calms with familiar comfort items

65. A 12-year-old suffers from sickle cell anemia vaso-occlusive crisis. Nursing interventions that would help alleviate his tissue hypoxia would include all except:

A. Bed rest

B. Encouraging fluids

C. Controlling pain

D. A scheduled exercise routine

66. A 10-year-old boy has come to the hospital for preop teaching. The most appropriate teaching method is:

A. Use of fantasy and medical play

B. Use of nursing and medical books

C. Use of body outline drawings and models

D. Use of research literature

67. A 12-year-old girl is hospitalized for a fractured R femur. She has been in TX 3 traction weeks before being placed in a full hip spica cast. Home teaching for the girl's family should include all but:

A. How to lift and roll her using the support crossbar

B. How to petal the edges of the cast

C. How to use a bed pan

D. How to identify emergency escape routes in their house

68. A 4-year-old girl was diagnosed with celiac disease. If she ingests gluten-containing foods, she will experience:

A. Malabsorption symptoms

B. Neural myelinization problems

C. Dehydration

D. Projectile vomiting

69. A 3-year-old boy is diagnosed with nephrotic syndrome. Which is the expected schedule of symptoms?

A. Proteinuria, mild periorbital edema, hypertension

B. Severe generalized edema, massive proteinuria, and normal to decreased BP

C. Hematuria, periorbital edema, and hypertension

D. Gross hematuria, severe generalized edema, and decreased BP

70. A 2-year-old is placed in a mist tent for laryngotracheobronchitis. An important intervention for children in a mist tent is:

A. Wipe off condensed moisture on tent walls

B. Leave ends of tent loose so air can freely circulate

C. Layer linens on the bed

D. Remove child from tent if child is crying or anxious

71. A 9-year-old was recently diagnosed with cystic fibrosis. His mother has many questions. You conclude that the mother has proper understanding of which health care regimen?

A. Use cough suppressants to deal with episodes of frequent harsh coughing

B. Take pancreatic enzymes with each meal or snack

C. Initiate chest physiotherapy when breath sounds become coarse

D. Use a low-fat diet to control steatorrhea

72. All of these assessments may point to dehydration in an infant or child, except one. Select the response that does not support dehydration.

A. Absence of tears

B. Tachycardia

C. Loss of weight

D. Brisk capillary refill

73. A 4-year-old is postoperative ventricular septal defect repair. You evaluate that more teaching is needed prior to discharge when the child's parents explain that:

A. They would mix her Digoxin (digitoxin) in a favorite food or drink to increase its palatability

B. They would not restrict her play activities once the healing phase was complete

   C. They would call their physician if she began vomiting, refused food, or had bradycardia

   D. They would encourage her to eat lots of strawberries and citrus fruits to maintain normal K+ levels.

74. Nursing interventions for the client receiving chemotherapy include the following:

   A. Restrict fluid intake; monitor CEA lab levels; encourage patient to limit use of pain medications

   B. Push/encourage fluids; monitor CBC; offer pain medication every 4 hours PRN, as ordered

   C. Encourage sun/outdoor activity; high fat diet; bed rest

   D. Monitor for shock and hemorrhage; monitor for phlebitis; apply heat and cold PRN for pain

75. Which of the following are chemotherapeutic drug classifications?

   A. Diclofenac; Meclofenamate; choline salicylate; etodolac

   B. Flurazepam; Diphenhydramine; Alprazolam; Meprobamate

   C. Cytoxan; methotrexate; vincristine; Adriamycin

   D. Antimetabolites; alkalating agents; antitumor antibiotics; plant alkaloids

76. Common side effects of radiation therapy include all of the following except:

   A. Fibrosis

   B. Fatigue

   C. Edema

   D. Skin reactions

77. Which of the following statements indicates that the client has a problem with body image disturbance related to alopecia?

   A. "I can't wait to see my family today. Can you help me apply my makeup?"

   B. "I asked my husband to help me choose a wig that will complement my face and color."

   C. "I just want to go home. I don't want company, and I don't want to go for a walk. It is embarrassing for people to see me looking like this."

   D. "It was nice to get out of the room today to walk to the elevator with my visitors."

78. Which of the following is NOT an appropriate diet for the client undergoing chemotherapy and/or radiation?

   A. High protein, high calorie diet

    B. Small, frequent meals

    C. Nutrition limited to three meals/day with plenty of raw vegetables and fruit accompaniments

    D. Soft, bland, cold foods

79. Which of the following components of the immune system produces antibodies?

    A. Beta lymphocytes (T-4 cells)

    B. T-lymphocytes

    C. Macrophages

    D. White blood cells

80. Which of the following assessments of a client with a new arm cast for a broken wrist should be immediately reported to the physician?

    A. Digital extremities of affected arm warm to touch and mobile

    B. Wrist pain when arm is dependent

    C. Digital extremities of affected arm with slight edema

    D. Bright red bloody drainage on the cast

81. Cast care for the first 48 hours after application includes all of the following except:

    A. Leave cast open to air until dry

    B. Handle the cast minimally while wet/damp, using only the palms of the hands

    C. Elevate casted extremity

    D. Support casted extremity on a hard surface

82. Which of the following activities is contraindicated for the client in Buck's traction for a hip fracture?

    A. Use of overhead trapeze when changing positions

    B. Bedside commode privileges PRN

    C. Isometric exercises with the affected leg

    D. Use of a fracture bed pan for elimination

83. Your patient is postop left total hip replacement surgery and is lying flat on her back. Legs are abducted with 4 pillows. You tell the patient that it is time for her to turn to the right side. The patient refuses to move, stating that she can't see the television lying on the right, and that it hurts too much to move anyway. Your best response to this patient would be:

A. "I can bring your pain medication now, and we can wait 20–30 minutes for it to take effect, but you really must turn off your back for a while to prevent skin breakdown."

B. "You have to turn now because I have six other patients to see, and I don't know when I will be able to return. I'll bring your pain medication after you turn."

C. "What's more important to you, your health and healing or that silly soap opera?"

D. "OK, but if you start to feel a sore, burning sensation or numbness on your back or buttocks, let me know and I will bring your medication, and then you will have to turn."

84. Which of the following nursing interventions are appropriate for the patient with gout?

A. Monitor lactic acid levels; elevate extremity; prescribe an alkaline ash diet and nonsteroidal antiinflammatory drug (NSAID) therapy

B. Monitor uric acid levels; elevate extremity; prescribe an acid ash diet and colchicine (Colsalide).

C. Prescribe high purine diet; wrap affected foot in an elastic bandage; restrict fluids; prescribe ROM exercises for the affected extremity

D. Monitor ascorbic acid levels; prescribe low purine diet, probenecid (Benemid), and increased physical activity and exercise

85. Which diet is best for the client on steroid therapy for treatment of rheumatoid arthritis?

A. Low sodium, low potassium, high carbohydrate diet

B. Low potassium, high carbohydrate, low protein diet

C. High potassium, low carbohydrate, high protein diet

D. Normal sodium, low protein, low carbohydrate diet

86. A 47-year-old male presents to the emergency room with complaints of heart palpitations and chest pain. The patient is diaphoretic, nauseated, and lethargic. During the initial exam the patient loses consciousness. The ECG/monitor shows asystole. Oxygen is in place. Patient's last vitals (3 minutes prior to losing consciousness) are BP 96/54; P 52; R 12. What is your first action?

A. Start two large bore IVs

B. Begin CPR

C. Verify the patient's rhythm

D. Defib at 200 J, 300 J, 360 J

87. A 58-year-old woman presents to the emergency room by ambulance. She is unconscious, pulseless, and nonbreathing. Emergency medical technicians (EMTs) have oxygen 15 L/min in place with a 7.0 ET tube in place. An IV is not yet started. ECG/monitor shows ventricular fibrillation (V-fib). What is your first priority action?

A. Start two large bore IVs

B. Begin CPR

C. Defib at 200 J, 300 J, 360 J

D. Verify the patient's rhythm

88. A 50-year-old man presents to the emergency room with complaints of diaphoresis, irregular pulse at 150 beats per minute (BPM), and a decreasing level of consciousness. During initial assessment, the patient loses consciousness. Oxygen is in place at 15 L/min and an IV 0.9 NS is infusing at 125 cc/hr. What is your first action?

A. Defib patient at 200 J

B. Check pulse vs. pulselessness

C. Intubate patient

D. Begin CPR

89. The patient is a 25-year-old woman who presents to the emergency room. She knows her name, but is unaware of the correct date, day, or year. She is lethargic and has sweet, fruity breath. Accu Check/glucose is 652; P 112/72; P 72; R 16; pH 7.25; CO_2 38 mEq/L; HCO_3 21 mEq/L. Which acid–base imbalance is the patient in?

A. Metabolic acidosis

B. Metabolic alkalosis

C. Respiratory acidosis

D. Respiratory alkalosis

90. An 8-year-old fell from a tree and was taken to the emergency room. When he arrived, he was conscious, but he quickly lost consciousness. After an airway is established, which position is most advantageous?

A. Flat, with feet raised slightly

B. Supine, with head elevated about 30°

C. Flat, with head turned to either side

D. Supine, with head elevated at 90°

91. A patient with head injury remains comatose. On assessment you noted that his pupils suddenly became fixed and nonreactive to light. His systolic blood pressure rises from 110 mm Hg to 160 mm Hg. Your next response should be to:

A. Call the doctor

B. Give oxygen per mask at 6 liters

C. Check his blood pressure and pupils again in 15´

D. Elevate his head to a high-Fowler's position

92. Classic changes in vital signs following head injury are:

A. Irregular respirations; tachycardia

B. Narrowing pulse pressure; bradycardia

C. Low blood pressure; irregular pulse

D. Widening pulse pressure; bradycardia

93. Which of the following medication plans would you anticipate implementing for a closed head injury patient who has decreasing level of consciousness, pupillary changes, and elevated blood pressure?

A. Procardia (Nifedipine) 30 mg orally, followed by Lasix (furosemide) 40 mg IV

B. Mannitol 50 gm IV push, with phenobarbital 30 mg IV

C. 50 gm mannitol IV push over 30–60 minutes followed by Lasix 20 mg IV

D. Reserpine 0.5 mg orally, followed by Decadron (dexamethasone)

94. A 36-year-old was admitted to the hospital with a diagnosis of Guillain-Barré syndrome. The nurse establishes goals for her acute phase. The first priority is to:

A. Maintain adequate respiratory function

B. Reduce anxiety

C. Maintain range of motion of lower extremities

D. Promote adequate nutrition

95. A patient with Guillain-Barré syndrome is placed in mechanical ventilation. After one week she is successfully weaned from the ventilator, but is receiving nasogastric tube feedings. Which of the following assessments would indicate that she might tolerate oral feedings?

A. She states that she is hungry and would like to drink and eat

B. She says that when she swallows she has a tendency to gag

C. She frequently touches the NG tube

D. Her respirations are silent and regular

96. When caring for a client who has lost a body part, it is essential for the nurse to include which of the following measures in the care plan?

A. Encourage immediate independence in self-care

B. Invite the assistance of a person who has had a similar experience

C. Provide information to the client about how to contact community resources

D. Allow adequate time for the client to work through the grief

97. A patient underwent a partial thyroidectomy to correct her hyperthyroidism. Which of the following blood levels would indicate a possible disturbance of the parathyroid glands during surgery?

A. Increase in potassium level

B. Decrease in sodium chloride

C. Decrease in calcium levels

D. Increase in albumin

98. Mrs. Benjamin has a beginning hearing deficit resulting from changes in the ear owing to the aging process. Which of the following nursing approaches would be most appropriate when speaking to her?

A. Raising the voice and accentuating each word

B. Talking slowing and distinctly and using a low frequency voice

C. Using visual speech, such as sign language and gestures

D. Writing out all comments or using flash cards or word lists

99. A patient is admitted to the hospital in a semi-conscious state, apparently suffering from a stroke. He is quite distressed and asks, "Is there any hope?" The most appropriate response by the nurse is:

A. "One should never give up hope."

B. "It's too soon to tell what the outcome will be."

C. "Symptoms are usually worst during the first few days after a stroke occurs."

D. "Try to be patient. These things take time."

100. A CVA patient is placed on heparin therapy. When giving the injection, the nurse should:

A. Squeeze a fold of the skin

B. Rotate sites

C. Inject the thigh

D. Use the Z-track technique

101. When a patient with a pituitary mass produces five or more liters of urine daily, the nurse should suspect:

A. Diabetes insipidus

   B. Graves' disease

   C. Addison's disease

   D. Cushing's syndrome

102. Mr. Jones is a CHF patient on your cardiac unit who has been receiving Lasix
   (furosemide) 40 mg PO every morning. His lab results this morning indicate
   hypokalemia. The doctor has written an order for Mr. Jones to receive potassium chloride (KCL) 20 mg IV. As a nurse preparing to administer the KCl, you
   know:

   A. The KCl can be given IV as received in the medication vial

   B. The KCl can be substituted with an oral dose without a doctor's order
       because it is the same drug and dose as ordered

   C. The KCl must be diluted prior to IV administration

   D. The KCl can be given intramuscularly until the IV is started

103. Which medication should the nurse be prepared to administer when a patient with a high magnesium level has respiratory depression?

   A. Calcium

   B. Corticosteroids

   C. Beta blockers

   D. Vitamin D

104. The laboratory test result that indicates a patient has hypocalcemia is a:

   A. Free calcium level of 5.0 mg/dL

   B. Free calcium level of 7.5 mg/dL

   C. Bound calcium level of 8.0 mg/dL

   D. Total serum calcium level of 7.5 mg/dL

105. What should the nurse tell an athlete who is sweating profusely during an
   activity?

   A. Reduce the exercise level to avoid sweating

   B. Allow the sweat to evaporate naturally

   C. Increase water intake

   D. Drink electrolyte-rich fluids

106. Mr. Jones is a 58-year-old CHF patient who is ready for discharge from your
   unit. His medications include Lasix, 40 mg PO every AM. The dietitian has
   stated that she has completed teaching Mr. Jones about a proper diet. As a
   nurse you determine your patient has a basic understanding of potassium
   replacement when he states:

A. "I don't need to watch my diet. It doesn't affect my potassium levels."

B. "I know my diet affects my potassium, but it's much easier to just take a pill."

C. "I can increase my potassium level by drinking whole milk, and eating cheese, bologna, and canned soups."

D. "I can increase my potassium level by eating citrus fruits, raisins, green leafy vegetables, and baked potatoes."

107. A nurse is preparing to administer Lasix 40 mg IV push as ordered for a patient in heart failure. The nurse notes that the patient's morning K^+ level = 3.8 mEq/L. Which of the following decisions by the nurse would be appropriate?

A. Administer the Lasix 40 mg as ordered.

B. Administer half the dose (20 mg) of Lasix IV push.

C. Administer an oral dose of Lasix 40 mg rather than IV push.

D. Withhold the drug and notify the physician regarding the K^+ value

108. A patient recovering from open heart surgery develops all of the following symptoms. Which most likely indicates that the patient has developed left heart failure?

A. Chest pain

B. Bilateral crackles (rales)

C. Abdominal ascites

D. Extremity edema

109. The nurse monitoring a patient in heart failure for indications of digitalis toxicity should observe the patient for which of the following?

A. Weight gain and dyspnea

B. Weakness and muscle cramps

C. Nausea and vomiting

D. Hypertension and headache

110. The physician has written the orders listed below for a patient diagnosed with acute pulmonary edema. The nurse should contact the physician to question which order?

A. Complete bed rest with head of bed elevated

B. Lasix 60 mg push b.i.d.

C. O_2 per nasal cannula @ 2–3 L/minute

D. 1 L D5/W to infuse @ 150 ml/hr

Comprehensive Exam Item Rationales

1. The intended response is **D**. Creatinine clearance decreases as a function of aging, rendering the elderly patient at high risk for the development of renal insufficiency secondary to nephrotoxic drugs. Although both BUN and serum potassium may increase in renal insufficiency, these lab values are not specific enough to be of greater value in determining renal function. No change in red blood cell values is associated with the onset of acute renal insufficiency.

2. The intended response is **C**. Tuberculosis is a respiratory infection with an airborne mode of transmission. A private room with AFB (acid fast bacillus) isolation is indicated for the patient until either the suspected diagnosis is ruled out, or the patient has been receiving antituberculin therapy. Masks used in respiratory precautions are inadequate for the prevention of tuberculin transmission. Contact isolation is indicated for skin-to-skin mode of transmission. Enteric precautions are indicated for fecal route transmission.

3. The intended response is **B**. Loss of circulating fluid volume related to internal bleeding causes a decrease in blood pressure, a hallmark manifestation of hypovolemic shock. Although pulse rate increases in shock states, as part of the body's effort to compensate for decreased circulating fluid volume, the increase in Response **D** is still within normal pulse range, and thus is not significant. Neither pain nor weakness is specific enough to be of greatest significance in the development of hypovolemic shock.

4. The intended response is **B**. Shock states are characterized by two pathophysiologic features: a decrease in cardiac output, and a subsequent decrease in tissue oxygenation. The patient in shock will evidence increases in both pulse and respiratory rates as a result of the body's effort to compensate for decreased circulating fluid volume and decreased tissue oxygenation. The nurse should administer oxygen to the patient to increase tissue oxygenation and sustain organ function.

5. The intended response is **B**. Respiratory acidosis is associated with hypoventilation (decreased respiratory rate and depth) or hypoxygenation. The presence of fluids in the lungs indicated by crackles upon auscultation decreases the effectiveness of both venti-

lation and oxygenation, placing the patient at risk for respiratory acidosis. Repeated episodes of vomiting would cause a loss of stomach acids, with resultant risk for metabolic alkalosis. Acute pain in areas other than the chest increases the metabolic rate, thus increasing the respiratory rate. Rapid and deep "blowing" respirations are evidence of the body's efforts to "blow off" excess acid via loss of carbon dioxide.

6. The intended response is **C**. The patient's admission blood gas values indicate respiratory acidosis, with a decreased pH, increased CO_2, and decreased O_2. An increase in arterial blood pH toward normal parameters indicates a resolution of the acidotic state.

7. The intended response is **B**. The medication order is incomplete, because no frequency for PRN doses has been specified. The remaining responses are all incorrect.

8. The intended response is **D**. The presence of metal-based implants such as artificial joints or permanent pacemakers prohibits the use of MRI as a diagnostic test. Allergy to iodine (as contained in shellfish) is associated with the use of iodine-based dyes in radiologic studies. MRI does not require a patient to be NPO or to have any special diet prior to testing. History of hypertension is not significant to this diagnostic test.

9. The intended response is **B**. A decrease in hemoglobin value indicates a decrease in the number of oxygen transport cells in the blood, causing symptoms of tissue hypoxygenation (fatigue, shortness of breath, dizziness, mental lethargy, etc.) Bruising may be associated with a decrease in platelets (clotting cells). Recurrent infections may be related to a change in white blood cell count or function. Periodic cramping pain in the lower extremities suggests an impairment of arterial blood flow unrelated to hemoglobin value.

10. The intended response is **B**. As with any invasive procedure, bleeding from a bone marrow aspiration puncture site is a considerable risk. Prevention and control of postprocedure bleeding is of priority following bone marrow aspiration. Firm pressure should be applied to the puncture site until oozing of blood is no longer evident. The nurse should continue to monitor the puncture site pressure dressing at frequent intervals for evidence of bleeding. Both administration of analgesia and monitoring of vital signs are indicated for postprocedure care, but neither assumes the priority of the prevention and control of bleeding.

11. The intended response is **C**. Even with careful crossmatch and type procedures, there is always a risk that a patient receiving a transfusion of blood or blood products may develop a transfusion reaction, indicated by the development of classic immune response related signs such as urticaria, headache, fever and chills, and low back pain.

12. The intended response is **D**. Standards of sterile technique indicate that any object not within clear view on a sterile field is not considered sterile. An object that has fallen to

the floor is unsterile, and, placed on a sterile field, will also contaminate all remaining objects on the field.

13. The intended response is **B**. The specific gravity of urine represents the proportion of the urine sample that is solid matter. Specific gravity will increase (more solid matter, less fluid) in fluid volume deficit, and will contrastingly decrease in fluid volume excess. None of the remaining responses will fluctuate related to fluid status.

14. The intended response is **D**. Urgency, frequency, and dysuria are all classic symptoms of urinary tract infection (UTI). Culture testing of a urine sample would provide information regarding the infecting organism(s).

15. The intended response is **C**. Because the patient with renal insufficiency is prone to fluid volume excess related to decreased urinary production, strict monitoring (ideally, hourly) of intake and output is essential in preventing fluid imbalance. Fluid intake is usually restricted for this patient. Routine blood pressure monitoring (every 8 hours) is too infrequent to monitor fluid status and potential complications of fluid excess. Body weights should be measured daily, as changes in body weight provide essential information regarding fluid status.

16. The intended response is **C**. The head of the bed should not be elevated more than 30 degrees in order to avoid neck flexion, which would interfere with drainage of cerebrospinal fluid in the spinal canal. The remaining interventions are appropriate in the care of a patient with increased intracranial pressure.

17. The intended response is **A**. Parkinson's disease is an irreversible degenerative neuromuscular disease involving loss of purposeful behaviors such as gait stability and facial and vocal expression, coupled with an increase in nonpurposeful behaviors such as trembling of the extremities and repetitive "pill rolling" hand movements. Because of these neuromuscular changes, the patient is at high risk for injury. Although the remaining responses are appropriate to this neuromuscular disorder, none assumes priority in terms of the risk to patient safety.

18. The intended response is **C**. Ventricular tachycardia is a potentially lethal cardiac arrhythmia which significantly decreases cardiac output. The nurse should check the patient's pulse to determine whether immediate initiation of CPR is indicated. If the patient is pulseless, the nurse may then position the patient supine and place a cardiac board beneath the chest area for use during cardiac compressions. The appropriate antiarrhythmic medication in VT is lidocaine (Xylocaine). An Ambu bag may be needed in CPR, but only after the establishment of cardiac/respiratory arrest.

19. The intended response is **A**. The 6 second ECG monitor strip indicates normal sinus rhythm (NSR), with a rate between 60–100 bpm, a regular rhythm, and characterized by P wave preceding tall and peaked QRS and followed by T wave. No intervention is indicated for this cardiac pattern.

20. The intended response is **C**. Loop diuretics (e.g., Lasix) increase potassium loss in urine, and thus are a common cause of hypokalemia. A significant decrease in urinary output (less than 30 mL/hr) is associated with hyperkalemia, as potassium excretion through urine is markedly decreased. Lactose intolerance is associated with a decreased intake of dairy products, which could result in hypocalcemia. Because fruits are a primary source of potassium, a diet low in fat and cholesterol would not be associated with a risk for hypokalemia.

21. The intended response is **B**. Because potassium is normally excreted primarily in urine, the nurse preparing to administer this electrolyte per IV drip should first assure that urinary output is minimally 30 mL/hour. The remaining clinical parameters are not associated with effects of potassium on the body.

22. The intended response is **A**. Acute hypoglycemia may be readily reversed via the administration of a simple form of glucose, such as apple juice or orange juice. Administration of more complex forms of glucose, such as in saltines or toast, is not rapid enough to reverse this condition. Offering the patient cookies is contraindicated, as this may overcompensate for hypoglycemia and elevate blood glucose above desired range.

23. The intended response is **B**. Hyperkalemia and the potentially lethal cardiac arrhythmias associated with this electrolyte imbalance are complications of DKA. As rapid-acting insulin is administered to the patient to reverse the ketoacidosis, serum potassium levels may drop precipitously. For these reasons, the nurse should closely monitor serum K^+ levels for this patient. Serum BUN, Hct, and Na^+ may all be elevated related to the dehydration associated with DKA; but none is at the monitoring priority of potassium.

24. The intended response is **C**. Thrombocytopenia, a decrease in the number of platelets, places a patient at risk for bleeding. Use of sharps, such as venipuncture or injection needles, should be limited as much as possible to prevent oozing of blood from puncture sites.

25. The intended response is **B**. Use of deodorants or talcs interferes with mammographic screening. No restriction of oral intake is necessary prior to this diagnostic test. Although some women may experience minimal breast tenderness following mammography, there is no need to restrict wearing of undergarments or constrictive clothing posttest. IV fluids are neither indicated nor used for this diagnostic testing.

26. The intended response is **B**. Daily self-assessment of pulse is essential in monitoring pacemaker function. A pulse rate lower than the minimal pacing rate should be reported to the physician. Although persons with cardiac disease may have a need for restriction of fluid intake or sexual activity, these restrictions are not related to pacemaker function. There is no need for a patient with a pacemaker to perform daily measurements of urinary output.

27. The intended response is **B**. Pain experience in acute myocardial infarction increases the metabolic rate, which thus increases oxygen demand and consumption by the heart. As oxygen supply to the heart is already compromised, increases in oxygen demand may cause extended cardiac damage in infarction. Analgesia is administered not only to reduce the experience of pain, but also to reduce the potential extension of myocardial damage. Although the remaining responses would be appropriate in the nursing care of a patient experiencing acute myocardial infarction, none assumes the priority of analgesic administration.

28. The intended response is **C**. The appearance of increased congestion of lung fields and sinus tachycardia in a patient recovering from acute myocardial infarction would suggest the onset of left heart failure. Increasing congestion of venous circulation evidenced by neck vein distention and edema is associated with right heart failure. Because left heart failure causes decreased cardiac output, oliguria is a hallmark manifestation of this cardiac disorder.

29. The intended response is **D**. A patient with a deep vein thrombosis should be maintained on complete bed rest to decrease risk of embolus development. The remaining responses are all appropriate in the care of this patient.

30. The intended response is **C**. Because the overproduction of antidiuretic hormone (ADH) in SIADH causes significant fluid retention and oliguria, Fluid Volume Excess is a priority diagnosis. Body Image Disturbance would be more appropriately associated with acromegaly, as this endocrine disturbance leads to distressing alterations in physical appearance. Pain is not a clinical manifestation associated with SIADH. Altered Nutrition: Less Than Body Requirements would be a diagnosis associated with hyperthyroidism, because the metabolic rate, and thus nutritional needs, are accelerated by excessive production of thyroid hormone.

31. The intended response is **D**. Bending, stooping, or slumping postures may increase reflux and thus magnify gastric discomfort. No foods should be taken within a few hours prior to bedtime. Alcohol exacerbates GERD, and should thus be avoided entirely. Gaviscon is ineffective unless taken on a "full stomach" after meals.

32. The intended response is **C**. Loss of turgor of the skin is an indication of fluid volume deficit (dehydration). A weak, rapid pulse and hypotension are associated with fluid volume deficit. Central venous pressure decreases as dehydration causes less filling pressure in the right atrium of the heart.

33. The intended response is **A**. An elevation of temperature indicating a febrile state should be reported to the surgeon, as preexisting infection represents a significant surgical risk. The remaining responses are within acceptable parameters for a surgical candidate.

34. The intended response is **B**. Administration of antiemetic medication such as Compazine (prochlorperazine maleate) or Reglan (metoclopramide) at regularly scheduled intervals is the most effective management of the predictable chemotherapeutic side effects of nausea and vomiting. Although upright positioning and small, frequent feedings will reduce the risk of gastric reflux, neither intervention will reduce the nausea and vomiting triggered by chemotherapeutic medications. Because dehydration secondary to vomiting is a concern, oral fluids should be encouraged as much as tolerated by the patient.

35. The intended response is **B**. Dysfunctional uterine bleeding can lead to loss of RBCs and hemoglobin, causing an anemic state.

36. The intended response is **A**. The patient with gout may experience impaired physical mobility secondary to the pain and swelling of the inflamed joint. Gout as an inflammatory process is not related to risk for or presence of infection. Although gout is associated with accumulation of uric acid, etiology of this form of arthritis is most often related to abnormal purine metabolism, and not altered urinary elimination. Gout typically involves a solitary joint (such as the great toe), and no impairment of peripheral perfusion is associated.

37. The intended response is **A**. As the pulling force and counterforce of traction is exerted, muscle is extended, thus reducing the spastic pain of muscle contractions associated with fracture. Traction exerts no effect on arterial circulation or muscle strength and mass. Decreased sensation in the affected limb indicates paresthesia, and should be investigated.

38. The intended response is **C**. Classic presentation of thrombophlebitis includes inflammation with localized redness, swelling, warmth, and tenderness.

39. The intended response is **B**. The presence of renal calculus in the urinary tract causes irritation of urinary structures with resulting bleeding. A burning sensation with urination, foul odor, or fever would suggest urinary tract infection.

40. The intended response is **B**. Because osteomyelitis is an infectious process in bone marrow, elevation of temperature along with elevation of WBC over 10,000 are classic clinical presentations.

41. The intended response is **B**. An understanding of the patient's normal eating habits, cultural customs, and food likes and dislikes will allow the nurse and patient to tailor a diet and treatment plan as close to the patient's own lifestyle as possible. This increases the likelihood that the patient will be able to comply with her treatment plan for an extended period of time. **A, C,** and **D** are all appropriate assessment strategies that will provide important information to the nurse and patient in developing the plan of care. However, the question asked specifically about diet planning, and **B** is the only answer that addresses diet specifically.

42. The intended response is **C**. Research has shown that pregnancies complicated by gestational diabetes have no greater incidence of intrauterine fetal demise than other normal pregnancies, as long as the patient maintains tight glycemic control. **A** and **D** are incorrect because there is a greater risk of intrauterine fetal demise in both insulin-dependent and gestational diabetic women when they are under poor glycemic control. **B** is incorrect because diabetic women are not routinely induced early, secondary to the increased risk of respiratory distress syndrome in infants of diabetic mothers. Rather, these patients are monitored closely, and only delivered early if there is evidence of maternal and/or fetal compromise making preterm delivery desirable.

43. The intended response is **A**. Diet manipulation is the principal intervention for the management of gestational diabetes. Having the patient move various diet exchanges from one meal or snack to another frequently corrects the blood glucose elevation. **B** is incorrect because although exercise is helpful in normalizing blood glucose levels, it is not appropriate as the first intervention. Additionally, testing after vigorous exercise may result in falsely low and misleading blood glucose results. **C** is incorrect because insulin administration is not usually initiated during pregnancy until diet therapy has proven to be ineffective. With only mild glucose elevations and no adjustments in diet, it is too soon to assume that diet alone has failed. **D** is incorrect because although poor testing technique can alter results, it is unlikely that the errors would only occur in the evening.

44. The intended response is **B**. One of the goals of dietary management of gestational diabetes is to assist the patient to maintain reasonable maternal weight gain and minimize fetal macrosomia. Appropriate weight gain in the final weeks of pregnancy should not exceed approximately 1–2 lbs/week. **A** is incorrect because this is a normal finding in diabetic pregnancies. Infants of diabetic mothers frequently have immature respiratory systems until very close to term. **C** is incorrect because this normal finding indicates that the fetus is growing at an appropriate rate and is unlikely to be macrosomic. **D** is incorrect because this is a normal finding for all pregnancies.

45. The intended response is **D**. Uncorrected magnesium sulfate toxicity can result in respiratory depression/arrest, and death. Calcium gluconate is the appropriate antidote for magnesium toxicity. **A, B,** and **C** are all appropriate interventions in caring for the pregnant patient with preeclampsia receiving magnesium sulfate for seizure prophylaxis. These strategies are aimed at providing appropriate therapy while avoiding toxicity. However, this question asks which is the most important intervention once a patient is identified as having toxic magnesium levels. The only response that addresses care for the magnesium toxic patient is **D.**

46. The intended response is **C**. All the assessments require intervention on the part of the nurse, but only newborn respiratory depression is associated with narcotic administration within 3–4 hours after administration.

47. The intended response is **D**. With the administration of magnesium sulfate, respiratory depression is a risk. Routinely the client should be assessed for the following: respira-

tions, deep tendon reflexes, urinary output, level of consciousness, and shortness of breath. **A, B,** and **C** are within the normal limits.

48. The intended response is **B**. During epidural administration, maternal hypotension with subsequent decrease in placental circulation is a risk. **B** addresses this concept. Hypotension, not hypertension, is prevented with the previous interventions. **C** and **D** are not prevented with this treatment.

49. The intended response is **D**. This is an open ended statement which will let the client express her concerns regarding her daughter. **A, B,** and **C** disregard the patient's feelings and close communication.

50. The intended response is **C**. Methergine is contraindicated if the client is hypertensive, because of the vasoconstrictive properties of this medication.

51. The intended response is **C**. All of the other interventions are appropriate to alleviate nasal stuffiness. Increasing fluid intake should be encouraged.

52. The intended response is **A**. Newborns exposed to cocaine in utero usually display the characteristics described in **A**. Other characteristics include irritability, increased startle response, inability to console, and elevated respiratory and heart rates. Also of significance is the increased risk of SIDS death. **B, C,** and **D** do not address these characteristics.

53. The intended response is **B**. This illustrates the defense mechanism of rationalization. It shows justification of behavior by offering a socially acceptable, intellectual explanation for an impulsive act or decision. Reaction formation is seen when the client expresses attitudes and statements which are the opposite of those which may seem angry or unacceptable. Repression is seen when ideas and/or impulses are pushed into the unconscious where they cannot be recalled. Sublimation is seen when the client diverts unacceptable impulses into socially acceptable activities.

54. The intended response is **C**. Clients who are anxious respond best to a calm, directive approach. Because reality may be distorted, complex directions or responses which require focus on the part of the client are unrealistic at this time. Therefore, referring to unit policy in response **A**, or expecting an insightful response such as **B**, will probably not be successful. Response **D** would be inappropriate at this time, since the client is not a danger to himself or others. A less restrictive means of limiting behavior would be more appropriate.

55. The intended response is **D**. Response **D** indicates that rapport and trust have begun to develop between the client and nurse. The client is willing to look at new behaviors to effect more positive outcomes in the future. In response **A** the client has not recognized the need for change in relation to the problem. Response **B** indicates that the patient may be experiencing some symptomatic relief that could be related to medication, but

may be seen as manipulative and also may indicate a relationship that is more social than therapeutic.

56. The intended response is **B**. Lithium is excreted by the kidney. Clients who have a sodium deficiency, or who are receiving diuretics, such as Lasix, are predisposed to lithium retention and resultant toxicity. Response **A**, Prolixin, is a phenothiazine which may be used with lithium to control psychotic behavior. Response **C**, Tegretol, is often used alone or with lithium to control bipolar symptoms. Response **D**, Antabuse, used as an alcohol deterrent in alcoholism, can be used with lithium.

57. The intended response is **B**. A history of previous suicide attempts is a strong risk factor for an adolescent male, along with the other factors listed. Responses **A, C,** and **D** are all important risk factors to be considered with this client.

58. The intended response is **C**. Akathisia is an extrapyramidal side effect of antipsychotic medication and is not seen in clients who are taking lithium. All other answers are consistent with signs of lithium toxicity. Symptoms of lithium toxicity include ataxia, muscle twitching, vomiting and diarrhea, confusion, slurred speech, and lethargy.

59. The intended response is **D**. Depressed clients often feel a sense of powerlessness. Allowing the client involvement and choices in procedures, diet, schedules, and activities assists in increasing feelings of control, power, and worth. These interventions are demonstrated in responses **A, B,** and **C.**

60. The intended response is **C**. Clients who are experiencing moderate to severe anxiety are easily agitated and respond well to a calm environment. A firm, but calm, reassuring approach works better than distraction. Anxious clients respond well to relaxation techniques, teaching regarding the physical effects of anxiety, and identification of the causes of their anxiety so that it may be better managed.

61. The intended response is **A**. Compulsive rituals such as hand washing demonstrate undoing, a defense mechanism which attempts to decrease anxiety by decreasing the effect of the obsessional fear. Response **B** is when the client expresses attitudes and statements which are the opposite of those which may seem angry or unacceptable. Response **C** is when the client retreats from the current threatening or anxious situation to an earlier, more comfortable and dependent level. Response **D** is when the client redirects feelings from one person to another person.

62. The intended response is **C**. During a short-term, first-time admission it would be unrealistic to expect insight into anxiety or its causes. Psychotropic medication and staff interventions will assist the client in achievement of responses **A, B,** and **D** during a short-term stay.

63. The intended response is **D**. The child is in the preschool years. This is a time when fantasy rules. It is important to prepare these children close to the actual event so they do not have the time to have their fantasy distort the event. One to four hours is manageable for the preschooler, yet leaves enough time for the RN to creatively use the child's natural fantasy for medical play. **A** is too lengthy a time for the preschool age group. Their concept of time is minimal and this prolonged framework will increase their fears. **B** is too brief a time. It does not allow for any therapeutic play, which is the most effective means of teaching in this age group. Although the preschooler does have simple concrete understanding of events, it is important to prepare them **C**. Focus on their senses—what they will see, smell, hear, feel, and taste—during the procedure.

64. The intended response is **D**. During late infancy and throughout the toddler years, separation anxiety is an expected developmental fear. It is a demonstration of the strong bond between the child and the primary caregivers. The nursing focus should be in supporting the established bond. Toddlers are very ritualistic and seek comfort in the familiar. A child experiencing separation anxiety may progress through the stages of anger, protest, and then withdrawal. If a child readily attaches to strangers or does not demonstrate fear of the unknown, the child may be in withdrawal.

65. The intended response is **D**; affected hemoglobin sickles under situations of decreased oxygen or decreased hydration. During a vaso-occlusive crisis, these sickled RBCs clump and clog in the smaller vasculature. The vessel occlusion leads to ischemia and tissue/organ necrosis or death. The goal is to prevent situations that increase tissue oxygen needs or cause dehydration. A scheduled exercise routine would increase his BMR and therefore challenge his ability to balance his oxygen supply and demand. **A** and **C** help reduce his body's need for oxygen. **B** keeps the blood more fluid and less likely to clump and result in crisis.

66. The intended response is **C**. The school-age child uses drawings and diagrams every day at school as learning tools. This is a method that is developmentally appropriate and familiar. **A** would work best for preschool children, taking advantage of their tendency to fantasize and their limited cognitive abilities. **B** and **D** would be too complex for a school-age child.

67. The intended response is **A**. The support bar is to keep the cast in the abducted position. It is very tempting to use it to lift or turn the child. Using the bar in this manner will damage the cast and could injure the child. **B,** petaling the edges with tape, smooths the rough edges and provides some water protection. A child in a hip spica cast, **C**, will be unable to bend at the hip, and therefore will need a bed pan for toileting. The hip spica abducts the hips, and the legs are spread wide. Because of the spread to the legs and the extra weight of the cast, transporting the child is very difficult. Carts are often used, but they cannot go up and down staircases. It is advisable for safety and convenience to place the child on a ground level floor. Escape routes, **D,** should be planned, and the child, even if old enough, should never be left unattended in a home because he or she would be helpless.

68. The intended response is **A.** Celiac disease is an inborn error of metabolism. The individual is intolerant to the protein component gluten found in wheat, barley, oats, and rye. The breakdown component of gluten becomes toxic to the intestinal villi, leading to malabsorption. Demyelinization of the nervous system, **B,** is found in an inherited disease of protein metabolism—PKU. Celiac disease leads to malabsorption of fats first, and then proteins, carbohydrates, and vitamins. Fluids, **C,** are mainly regulated by the kidneys and large intestine, which are unaffected. Celiac will not lead to projectile vomiting, **D.**

69. The intended response is **B.** Nephrotic syndrome is characterized by increased permeability of the glomerular membrane to plasma proteins. The protein is lost in the urine, resulting in proteinuria. The loss of serum protein pulls water from the vascular system into the tissues, leading to edema. The body senses low filtration through the kidney and tries to save Na^+ and H_2O. The saved fluids are further shifted to the tissues in a vicious circle. The net result is severe generalized edema, massive proteinuria, and a normal to decreased BP from hypovolemia. **A** is incorrect because of the mild periorbital edema. **C** is characteristic of glomerulonephritis. Hematuria, **D,** is not characteristic of nephrotic syndrome.

70. The intended response is **C.** The mist tent provides a special environment in which oxygen or humidity can be manipulated. For it to be effective, the child must be in the tent, and the sides tucked under the mattress. Care must be taken to not open the environment too frequently. Layering linen is done to ease changing the bed. The blankets, sheets, and the child's pajamas will become moist frequently, and the patient may become chilled. **A,** wiping down the wall frequently, will involve opening up the environment, thus decreasing its effectiveness. **B,** open ends, will allow O_2 or humidity to leave the special environment and reduce its effectiveness. **D,** removing the child, defeats the purpose of the tent. To reduce anxiety, toys and familiar objects may be placed in the tent. Items in the tent should appeal to the child's senses and developmental level.

71. The intended response is **B.** Thick tenacious mucus inhibits the flow of pancreatic enzymes into the small intestine. Without the pancreatic enzymes, fats and fat-soluble enzymes cannot be digested and absorbed. The enzymes are taken with each meal and with snacks. **A:** it is important that the child expectorates the mucus. Cough suppressants inhibit the removal of mucus and contaminants, which increases the child's risk for respiratory infection. **C:** due to thick mucus and resulting impairment of respiratory function, a child with cystic fibrosis will demonstrate coarse breathing sounds. Chest physiotherapy is used as a means to help clear the lungs. **D:** proper use of pancreatic enzymes will allow digestion and uptake of fats. No fat restrictions are needed.

72. The intended response is **D.** Capillary refill time could be prolonged in states of dehydration. **A:** as a child becomes significantly dehydrated, you will find loss of tears. This is in response to the body conserving fluids. **B:** one of the body's compensating mecha-

nisms for a lowered vascular volume is tachycardia. The body tries to maintain pressure and blood circulation by increasing its heart rate.

73. The intended response is **A**. It is important that critical medications such as Digoxin are not mixed with food or drink. Mixing it increases the volume the child must consume, and there is no way to evaluate what quantity of the medication has been consumed if all of the mixture is not taken. **B:** once the surgical wound is healed, there is no need to restrict the child's play activities. **C:** vomiting, anorexia, and bradycardia may all be indicators of digoxin toxicity. **D:** it is commonly thought that bananas are the only fruit high in K$^+$. Citrus and strawberries are also high and offer another good food option.

74. The intended response is **B**. It is important to push fluids in order to help flush the chemotherapeutic agent out of the body, thereby limiting its toxic effects. Overall hydration of the body is needed during chemotherapy. The CBC is monitored as part of the assessment for infection and anemia. Pain medication should be offered and administered as directed in order to provide client comfort, which can help the client to continue to perform routine activities.

75. The intended response is **D**. **A** are nonsteroidal antiinflammatory drugs. **B** are sedative/hypnotics. **C** are actual chemotherapy drugs.

76. The intended response is **A**. Fibrosis may and does occur with some clients; however, it is not a *common* effect and is considered an unusual occurrence. **B, C,** and **D** are commonly expected side effects of radiation.

77. The intended response is **C**. This statement clearly indicates that the client has not yet accepted her change in body image (the alopecia) resulting from the chemotherapy. **A, B,** and **D** are all answers that indicate a healthy attitude and acceptance of this temporary condition.

78. The intended response is **C**. Three meals a day can be difficult for the client undergoing chemotherapy and/or radiation; therefore, supplements or healthy snacks are needed. Raw vegetables and fruits should be limited because of their risk of carrying and transmitting infectious agents. **B:** small, frequent meals that are high in calories and protein are best for the client during chemotherapy. **D:** soft, bland, cold foods are therapeutic and more easily tolerated for the client with nausea and loss of appetite.

79. The intended response is **A**. **B:** T-lymphocytes function as either helper cells that activate the beta cells (T-4 cells) or as suppressor cells (T-8 cells) that call off the attack on the invading substance. **C:** macrophages serve as the alarm that alerts the immune system of an invasion.

80. The intended response is **D**. Bright red drainage indicates active bleeding, and the physician should be notified of this occurrence immediately. **A:** warm, mobile extremities indicate circulation. **B:** wrist pain when arm is dependent is expected due to increased edema. **C:** fractured areas should be elevated to decrease edema, but mild edema of the fingers is expected in this type of injury.

81. The intended response is **D**. Placement of a damp cast on a hard surface may cause pressure and indentation of the soft tissue underneath. **A:** casts should be left open and uncovered until completely dry. **B:** if handling is necessary while cast is still damp, only the palms of the hands should be used to prevent indentation of the cast by fingers. **C:** elevation of the casted extremity is necessary to decrease edema.

82. The intended response is **B**. The client in Buck's traction for a hip fracture should not be removed from traction for activities in order to maintain proper bone alignment, immobilization, and to permit healing. **A, C,** and **D** are all activities appropriate for the client in Buck's traction.

83. The intended response is **A**. Compromising with the angry and/or depressed patient helps to give him or her the feeling of having control. Explain the rationale for your request in a non-threatening manner and offer assistance. If the patient is premedicated before moving or changing positions, it will be less painful, and the patient will be more apt to comply. **B** and **C** are rude and inappropriate responses that should not be used. **D** would provide therapy after the fact, and a little too late to prevent the initial stages of skin breakdown.

84. The intended response is **B**. Uric acid levels above normal indicate purine metabolism, which results in hyperuricemia, whereby the uric acid crystals are deposited in various joints, usually in that of the great toe, causing painful clinical manifestations. Treatment includes an acid ash diet to create a more alkaline urine to prevent uric acid precipitation. Elevation of the extremities or joint aids in decreasing edema; and colchicine is the antiinflammatory agent of choice for gout, as it inhibits lactic acid production by leukocytes. Lactic acid and ascorbic acid levels have no indication in the treatment or diagnosis of gout. An alkaline ash diet would cause urine acidity, which would cause uric acid deposits in the urine. NSAID therapy is helpful in pain management of gout, but is not therapeutic in preventing further attacks and/or halting the current attack of gout. Probenecid blocks the reabsorption and promotes excretion of urates, but again is not as effective in treating acute attacks as colchicine. All other interventions mentioned would cause the client more discomfort and pain.

85. The intended response is **C**. Clients on steroids are prone to high glucose levels, loss of potassium, and breakdown of proteins; therefore, their diets should be low in carbohydrates to keep glucose levels within normal range, high potassium to compensate for the loss of this substance, and high protein to replace the lost protein.

86. The intended response is **C**. Verify the rhythm in another lead and assure that all three electrodes are in place. **A:** this is not your first action; it will come later. **B:** there is no mention of pulselessness. CPR is only initiated after determining there is no pulse. **D:** verifying the rhythm is most essential, but even if asystole were confirmed, defibrillation is not a treatment for asystole.

87. The intended response is **C**. Early defibrillation is proven to be most beneficial for V-tach without a pulse a V-fib. **A:** IV access is not first priority. American Heart Association standards and research prove that early defibrillation is priority if V-fib is identified. IV access will come secondary to defib.

88. The intended response is **B**. Checking the stability of the patient is crucial. Determining pulse versus pulselessness is a critical element is deciding what future interventions or treatments are correct. **A:** defibrillating a patient prior to determining the patient's heart rhythm and prior to determining pulselessness could do more harm than good. **C:** there is no mention of a lost airway and patient is receiving 15 L/min of oxygen. Intubation is too drastic a measure without further data. **D:** CPR is never initiated without first determining that the patient has no pulse.

89. The intended response is **A**. pH below 7.35 would indicate acidosis. CO_2 levels within normal limits (35–45) show it is not respiratory. HCO_3 below normal limits (25) indicates a loss of bicarb, which is a metabolic condition. Disorientation, lethargy, and sweet, fruity breath are characteristic of diabetic ketoacidosis. **B:** an alkalosis pH would be greater than 7.45. **C:** if it were a respiratory-related imbalance, the CO_2 level would not be within normal limits (35–45). **D:** if it were a respiratory-related imbalance, the CO_2 level would not be within normal limits (35–45). An alkalosis pH would be greater than 7.45.

90. The intended response is **B**. A supine position with head elevated approximately 30° provides for maximum diaphragmatic functioning and facilitates cerebral venous flow. When the body is totally supine with feet raised, venous return is less affected. When the head is flat, cerebral congestion is enhanced. A head elevated to 90° is likely to impede diaphragmatic functioning.

91. The intended response is **A**. The pupillary response and elevated blood pressure indicate serious cerebral or brain stem involvement. The action required goes beyond the license of the nurse and requires either surgical intervention or medication. **B, C,** and **D** in this instance would delay effective and necessary intervention.

92. The intended response is **D**. An increase in intracranial pressure from a head injury will cause the systolic blood pressure to rise. Cerebral congestion due to brain swelling or abnormal distribution of fluids will cause the pulse to be slow and bounding. A is incorrect because the pulse rate will not be tachycardia. Respirations, however, could be

irregular. **B** is incorrect because the pulse pressure does not narrow; it widens. **C** is incorrect because the blood pressure is not low.

93. The intended response is **B**. Mannitol is an osmotic diuretic that reduces cerebrospinal pressure by drawing water from intracranial fluids back into plasma. Lasix is used with mannitol to treat cerebral edema and facilitate diuresis. Procardia is not effective in reducing cerebral edema. It acts on the myocardium of the heart. Phenobarbital is a central nervous system depressant. Reserpine is an antihypertensive, but will not effectively reduce cerebral edema as needed.

94. The intended response is **A**. Muscle paralysis seen in the acute phase of Guillain-Barré syndrome is a serious threat to respiratory function. The most serious complication is respiratory failure. Reducing anxieties, maintaining motor function, and promoting adequate nutrition are important goals, but the most critical goal is preventing life threats by maintaining respiratory function.

95. The intended response is **B**. The presence of the gag reflex indicates normal swallowing. Stating that she is hungry and touching the NG tube are not indicators that the patient might tolerate oral feedings, because they do not have an impact on the return of physiological functioning. The quality of respirations has no bearing on the return of swallowing and the gag reflex.

96. The intended response is **D**. Any loss, real or perceived, should be accompanied by an adequate grieving period. The other responses will be appropriate at a later time, when the patient is ready for recovery. These actions will not be effective until the patient has grieved the loss.

97. The intended response is **C**. The parathyroid gland secretes the hormone, parathormone, which regulates calcium levels in the blood. Accidental removal of a parathyroid gland could alter the serum calcium level. The parathyroid gland has no action on potassium, sodium chloride, or albumin levels.

98. The intended response is **B**. Early hearing deficits involve difficulty with high frequency sounds. Therefore, the nurse should use a low frequency voice and talk slowly and distinctly. Raising the voice will not help. Visual speech and writing can be used later, if needed.

99. The intended response is **C**. Cerebral edema often occurs after a stroke, which causes a decrease in the level of consciousness and creates a variety of symptoms. After a few days, when edema subsides, symptoms tend to disappear. This response provides factual information without giving false hope. Telling someone not to give up hope or to be patient does not demonstrate acceptance of the level of concern and does not offer an explanation of what is happening. Telling her that it is too soon to tell may be true, but it offers no support or explanation.

100. The intended response is **B.** Heparin injections should be administered in rotating sites to prevent hematoma formation. The thigh should not be the only site used. Sites should be rotated. The skin should not be squeezed or pinched to prevent traumatization. The Z-track technique is not necessary.

101. The intended response is **A.** In diabetes insipidus, a deficiency of ADH prevents the kidneys from reabsorbing water. **B:** Graves' disease causes an increase in the metabolic rate, which leads to increased sweating—related to increased temperature, not urine production. **C:** Addison's disease does cause loss of fluids, but not to the extreme of 5 liters a day. **D:** Cushing's syndrome results in an elevation in blood sodium, which causes polydipsia and water retention, not excretion.

102. The intended response is **C.** IV potassium should never be given IV push, because it may cause lethal cardiac arrhythmias. **A:** potassium must be diluted prior to IV administration because it may cause lethal cardiac arrhythmias. **B:** although the drug and dose are the same, the route must also be ordered by the doctor. Changing the route without a doctor's order is illegal.

103. The intended response is **A.** IV calcium counteracts the effect of hypermagnesemia on the nervous and cardiovascular systems. It is the reciprocal of magnesium. **B, C,** and **D** do not reverse or counteract magnesium.

104. The intended response is **D.** A normal lab value of total serum calcium is 8.5—10.0 mg/dL. **A:** 4.5–5.5 mg/dL is the normal level for free calcium. **B:** indicates hypercalcemia. **C:** bound calcium accounts for one-half of the total serum calcium; this level would indicate hypercalcemia.

105. The intended response is **D.** Drinking electrolyte-rich fluids not only replaces the fluid content lost due to sweating, it also replaces critical electrolytes lost. **A:** reducing the exercise level to avoid sweating may be counterproductive at the patient's physical fitness level and may inhibit the patient from reaching an aerobic exercise level. **B:** allowing the sweat to evaporate naturally will not correct the loss of electrolytes. **C:** increasing water intake will only replace fluids, not essential electrolytes.

106. The intended response is **D.** Citrus fruits, raisins, green leafy vegetables, and baked potatoes are all potassium-rich foods which will help increase the patient's potassium level. **A:** this indicates the patient is in need of nursing teaching. Certain foods contain potassium, which may increase potassium levels. **B:** supplemental potassium by pill ingestion is a possible treatment, but foods containing potassium naturally will be easier to ingest and less expensive. **C:** these foods are high in calcium, fat, and sodium, not potassium.

107. The intended response is **A**. Lasix as a diuretic is an essential element of the treatment of heart failure and would only be withheld if the potassium serum value was below normal limits.

108. The intended response is **B**. Crackles (rales) upon auscultation of the chest indicates pulmonary congestion associated with left heart failure. Chest pain is not a characteristic sign of either left or right heart failure. Abdominal ascites and extremity edema are associated with the circulatory congestion of right heart failure.

109. The intended response is **C**. Vomiting occurs in digitalis toxicity, as in most drug toxicities, evidencing the body's effort to rid itself of the toxin. **A:** weight gain and dyspnea would indicate increasing hypervolemia and respiratory congestion in heart failure. **B:** weakness and muscle cramps are indications of potassium disturbances associated with heart failure and its treatment. **D:** hypertension and headache are not associated with digitalis use or toxicity.

110. The intended response is **D**. Because pulmonary edema is characterized by severe circulatory congestion and hypervolemia, an intravenous infusion rate of 150 mL/hr (3600 mL/24 hr) is much too rapid, and would worsen the patient's circulatory and respiratory status. The remaining orders are appropriate for this diagnosis.

Index

Note: Page numbers in *italics* indicate illustrations; those followed by t indicate tables.

A

ABCs, as memory aid, 21, *21*
Abruptio placentae, 224
Accidental injuries, in children, 318
Acid-base balance, mechanisms of, 142
Acid-base imbalances. *See also* Acidosis; Alkalosis
  arterial blood CO_2 in, 143
  arterial blood HCO_3 in, 144
  arterial blood pH in, 141–142
  compensatory mechanisms in, 142
  identification of, 141–144
  inadequate elimination and, 159–161
Acidosis
  metabolic, 143, 149–150, 154, 155
    anorexia and, 159
    in diabetes, 149, 155, 197, 198, 204–205, 208
    inadequate elimination and, 159–161
    in renal disease, 159
  pH in, 142
  respiratory, 143, 144, 145–146, 152–154
Acquired immunodeficiency syndrome. *See* AIDS
Acronyms, 21
Acrostics, 21
Action plan
  creation of, 3–5
  sample, 4t
Active transport, 219
Activity, 233–244
  in diabetes, 202, 207
Activity intolerance, inadequate elimination and, 160
Adaptation
  nursing interventions for, 261
  physical, 261
  psychological, 260–261, *261*
Addison's disease, 196t
Adolescents

body image of, 294
development of, 293–295
  cognitive, 294
  social, 296
growth of, 293
nutrition for, 314
sex education for, 299–300
special concerns and problems of, 294–295
Adrenal cortex, 196t
Aerobic metabolism, 303
AIDS, 170, *171*
  universal precautions for, 174, 176–178, 179, 181–182
Airway management, in children, 304–305
Airway obstruction, 97–99
Alcohol, in pregnancy, 226
Aldosterone, 196t, 207
Alkalosis
  metabolic, 144
  pH in, 142
  respiratory, 146–148
Alveolar collapse, in immobilization, 237–238
Alzheimer's disease, 186, 187, 192–193
Aminophylline, for asthma, 98
Amniotic fluid, meconium staining of, 228
Amniotic membrane, 222
Amyotrophic lateral sclerosis (ALS), 187, 191
Anaerobic metabolism, 304
Analgesia. *See* Pain management
Analysis, 27–31, 37–38
  in cognitive process model, *65*, 68
  errors in, 29
  incomplete, 29
  reasoning exercises for, 30–31
  of test-taking strengths and weaknesses, 56, *57*
Anasarca, 132
Anemia, 116, 126
  renal insufficiency and, 163
  sickle cell, 116, 307, 321–322
Anesthesia, peristalsis and, 326–327
Angina, 125, 126